PEDIATRIC
CARE PLANS

PEDIATRIC CARE PLANS

Sharon Ennis Axton, RN, MS, PNP

Terry Fugate, RN, MSN

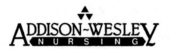

A Division of The Benjamin/Cummings Publishing Company, Inc.
Redwood City, California • Menlo Park, California
Reading, Massachusetts • New York • Don Mills, Ontario
Wokingham, U.K. • Amsterdam • Bonn • Sydney
Singapore • Tokyo • Madrid • San Juan

SPONSORING EDITOR: Mark McCormick
PRODUCTION COORDINATOR: Alyssa Wolf
BOOK DESIGNER: Paula Schlosser
COVER DESIGNER: John Martucci
COPY EDITOR: Barbara Fuller
PROOFREADER: Kate Kimmelman
INDEXER: William J. Richardson Associates
MANUFACTURING SUPERVISOR: Merry Free Osborn
COMPOSITON: The Clarinda Company

Care has been taken to confirm the accuracy of information presented in this book. The authors, editors, and publisher, however, cannot accept responsibility for errors or omissions or for consequences from application of the information in this book and make no warranty, express or implied, with respect to its contents.

The authors and publisher have exerted every effort to ensure that drug selections and dosages set forth in this text are in accord with current recommendations and practice at the time of publication. However, in view of ongoing research, changes in government regulations, and the constant flow of information relating to drug therapy and drug reactions, the reader is urged to check the package inserts of all drugs for any change in indications of dosage and for added warnings and precautions. This is particularly important when the recommended agent is a new and/or infrequently employed drug. Mention of a particular generic or brand name drug is not an endorsement, nor an implication that it is preferable to other named or unnamed agents.

Library of Congress Cataloging-in-Publication Data

Axton, Sharon Ennis.
    Pediatric care plans/Sharon Ennis Axton, Terry Fugate.
       p.   cm.
    Includes index.
    ISBN 0-8053-0905-5
    1. Pediatric nursing—Handbooks, manuals, etc. 2. Nursing care
plans—Handbooks, manuals, etc.   I. Fugate, Terry.   II. Title.
    [DNLM: 1. Patient Care Planning—handbooks. 2. Pediatric Nursing—
handbooks.   WY 39 A972p]
RJ245.A885 1993
610.73'62—dc20
DNLM/DLC
for Library of Congress   92-49364
                                                    CIP

ISBN 0-8053-0905-5
   5 6 7 8 9 10-CRS-99

Addison-Wesley Nursing
A Division of The Benjamin/Cummings Publishing Company, Inc.
390 Bridge Parkway
Redwood City, California 94065

Preface

The desire to write a book of nursing care plans for noncritical hospitalized children arose from our past experience as practicing nurses and educators. We realized that a source was needed to help identify nursing diagnoses for these patients and their families. Both nursing students and practicing nurses have verified this need.

Pediatric nurses are ever-present at the child's bedside, constantly assessing, planning, implementing, and evaluating the care needed by the child and the family. The increasing complexity and acuity of hospitalized children places many demands on the pediatric nurse. This book is designed to help bridge the gap between theoretical knowledge and clinical application in an inpatient pediatric setting. From our past experience and observation of other nurses in this setting, it has become evident that time management is often a major concern. We hope that this book will help nurses form quick and accurate nursing diagnoses and will provide the basis for the development of individualized nursing care plans. To facilitate this process, we correlate nursing diagnoses with some of the most common pediatric medical diagnoses.

Most of the nursing diagnoses are those accepted by the North American Nursing Diagnosis Association (NANDA). On a few occasions, it was necessary to use nursing diagnoses that are not on the NANDA list. These are identified by asterisks.

Nursing students, graduate nurses, practicing pediatric nurses, and nurse educators will find this book useful in planning care for hospitalized children. A special feature of this book is the discharge planning which is incorporated into each care plan, identified by the 🏠 logo. We hope that nurses who use this book will gain personal satisfaction in providing comprehensive pediatric nursing care.

We would like to express our appreciation to all of our colleagues (educators and practicing nurses) who, through their encouragement and support, have contributed to our personal and professional growth. We would also like to acknowledge our nursing students for their enthusiasm, which is a continual source of inspiration.

Sharon Ennis Axton

Terry Fugate

REVIEWERS

Peggy Battistini
Columbus College
Cougar Drive
Columbus, GA 31993
(404) 568-2053

Sandy Chacko
Des Moines Area Community
    College
1125 Hancock Drive
Boone, IA 50036
(515) 432-7203

Daniel Chaussee
University of Mary
7500 University Drive
Bismark, ND 58504
(701) 255-1724

Judith Davis
Samuel Merritt College
370 Hawthorne Ave
Oakland, CA 90609
(510) 420-6011

Florencetta Gibson
Northeast Louisiana University
700 University Avenue
Monroe, LA 71207
(318) 342-1640

Mary Ellen Howell
    (née Brown)
Women's Center of Carolina
    Hospital System
Box 5906 (home)
Florence, SC 29502
(803) 393-5350

Carole Kenner
University of Cincinnati
3110 Vine Street
Cincinnati, OH 45221
(513) 558-5228

Elizabeth Lambertz
St. Luke's Hospital
3555 Army St.
San Francisco, CA 94110
(415) 749-1846

Kathy Pittman
Florida State University
Tallahassee, FL 32306-3051
(904) 644-3296

Deborah Scott
University of Louisville
H.S.C. Carmichael Building
Louisville, KY 40292
(502) 588-5825

Susan Sorenson
Bellin College
929 Cass Street
Green Bay, WI 54301
(414) 433-3560

Contents

FIVE
Care of Children with Hemopoietic Dysfunction and Neoplasms

181

SIX
Care of Children with Hepatic Dysfunction

215

Introduction

The goal of *Pediatric Care Plans* is to assist practicing nurses, nurse educators, and students in implementing the nursing process for pediatric patients. This book provides a quick reference for correlating frequently encountered pediatric medical diagnoses with nursing diagnoses. Most of the nursing diagnoses are those accepted by the North American Nursing Diagnosis Association (NANDA). On a few occasions, it was necessary to use nursing diagnoses that are not on the NANDA list. These are identified by asterisks. A special feature of this book is the discharge planning which is incorporated into each care plan, identified by the 🏠 logo. Each diagnostic entry has a standard set of components:

Medical Diagnosis.

Pathophysiology. This is a basic and brief overview of the pathophysiology of the medical diagnosis.

Primary Nursing Diagnosis. This can be stated as either actual or at high risk for occurring. The nurse writing the care plan makes the determination.

Definition. This refers only to the nursing diagnosis and not to the medical diagnosis.

Possibly Related To. The rationale for the selection of each nursing diagnosis is inherent in this statement.

Characteristics. These are of the selected nursing diagnosis and of the identified medical diagnosis. The list presents possible signs and symptoms specific to the identified nursing and medical diagnoses.

Expected Outcomes. Listing expected outcomes is the next step in the nursing process after identification of the nursing diagnosis. Expected outcomes may be listed on a nursing care plan as patient goals or objectives. Outcomes are written as specifically as possible so that they can be measured and easily evaluated. Directions are sometimes included to help individualize the expected outcomes for each infant/child. For example, Expected Outcomes might read as follows:

> Child will have adequate cardiac output as evidenced by heart rate within acceptable range (state specific highest and lowest rates for each child).

To individualize this statement, the nurse needs to include the highest and lowest acceptable heart rates for each child. The range will vary depending upon the child's age and disease state. The expected outcome for a 1-month-old infant with normal cardiac function would read:

> Infant will have adequate cardiac output as evidenced by heart rate of 100 to 160 beats/minute.

Possible Nursing Interventions. These are ways in which the nurse can assist the infant/child and/or family to achieve the expected outcomes. Some of these interventions are *independent* nursing actions, whereas others are *collaborative* (the nurse implements the physician's orders). For example, a nursing intervention to "elevate head of bed at a "30° angle" could be instituted for an infant or child with increased intracranial pressure without a specific order from the physician. This would be an independent nursing intervention. A nursing intervention to "administer antibiotic on schedule" depends upon the physician's order.

Evaluation for Charting. This section, which deals with the final step in the nursing process, evaluates the expected outcomes and, to some extent, the identified nursing interventions. Statements made here direct the reader to describe or state results. For example, the reader may be directed to "describe breath sounds." This would be correlated with the expected outcome, "infant/child will have clear and equal breath sounds" and with a nursing intervention such as "assess and record breath sounds every 4 hours and PRN."

Evaluation is an ongoing process; the evaluation statement may need to be changed frequently. For this reason, the nurse may wish to include this part of the nursing process in the daily charting, noting on the nursing care plan under the evaluation column "see nurses' notes," stating the date and time, and initialing the note. This section includes documentation for all appropriate forms, such as flowsheets, graphic sheets, or nurses' notes.

Nursing Diagnoses. Following the primary nursing diagnosis are one to two associated nursing diagnoses that are prioritized and carried through the nursing process. The nurse writing the care plan decides if these are actual nursing diagnoses or if the patient is at high risk for the selected nursing diagnoses.

Related Nursing Diagnoses. These are nursing diagnoses that are most likely to be included in a nursing care plan for an infant or child with the stated medical diagnosis. Many of these nursing diagnoses are actual; the patient is at high risk for others. The nurse determines which. The related nursing diagnoses are in priority order for an infant/child with the stated medical diagnosis. However, the needs and condition of the infant or child will determine whether the nurse must reorder the priorities. All related nursing diagnoses are completely developed through the nursing process and can be found in the text; refer to the index for location.

To use this book most efficiently, scan the Table of Contents for the applicable medical diagnosis. After finding it in the text, review the accompanying nursing care plan and related nursing diagnoses and select the appropriate expected outcomes and nursing interventions. Write those on the nursing care plan and then implement them. Later, at intervals that you designate when writing the care plan, evaluate the infant's or child's response to your nursing interventions and record your findings.

ONE

CARE OF CHILDREN WITH CARDIOVASCULAR DYSFUNCTION

1

PROCEDURE

Cardiac Catheterization

DESCRIPTION Cardiac catheterization is an invasive procedure used to diagnose congenital heart defects that may require surgical correction. Certain cardiac defects may also be corrected without surgical intervention during cardiac catheterization. Objectives for cardiac catheterization include measurement of oxygen saturation and pressures within the chambers and great vessels, measurement of cardiac output and function, visualization of the structures of the heart, and evaluation of the blood flow through the heart. Other procedures that may be performed during catheterization include the creation or closure of atrial septal defects, the insertion of pacer wires, and the assessment of a child's hemodynamic response to certain medications.

During cardiac catheterization, the physician inserts a thin, flexible, radiopaque catheter through an artery and/or vein and into the chambers of the heart. One of the femoral vessels is most often used, but vessels in the jugular, axillary, and antecubital fossa areas are other possibilities. To gain access to the vessels, the physician uses percutaneous entry or a cutdown. This procedure is done under fluoroscopy, allowing for visualization of the catheter's movement and location. Both right-sided and left-sided catheterizations can be performed. To enter the right side of the heart, the physician usually inserts a catheter into the right femoral vein, then passes it into the superior or inferior vena cava and advances it into the right atrium, the right ventricle, and the pulmonary artery. The left side of the heart can be entered by passing the catheter through the former foramen ovale to the left atrium and ventricle, or by passing the catheter retrograde through the femoral artery, through the aorta, and across the aortic valve. At the end of the procedure, the catheter is removed. Pressure is applied to the insertion site or the cutdown sutures.

The injection of contrast material (angiography) into the great vessels or chambers of the heart during catheterization can facilitate their visualization. The contrast medium may cause nausea, a generalized burning sensation, allergic rashes, central nervous system symptoms, tachycardia, hypotension, and/or anaphylactic shock. Complications other than contrast medium reactions include arrhythmias, bleeding, perforation, tamponade, cardiac perforation, cerebrovascular accident, thrombosis, hematoma, and/or cardiopulmonary arrest.

The child undergoing a cardiac catheterization is not allowed to eat or drink for at least 4 to 6 hours prior to the procedure. Preoperative medications vary among institutions but usually include an analgesic (such as meperidine or morphine) to help the child relax. A combination of meperidine (Demerol), promethazine (Phenergan), and chlorpromazine (Thorazine), called Toronto Mix or Pediatric Cocktail, is often used to sedate the child. In many institutions, cardiac catheterizations are performed on an outpatient basis if the child is in stable condition. The child is admitted the day of catheterization and is usually discharged 5 to 6 hours after the procedure.

PRE-CARDIAC CATHETERIZATION NURSING CARE PLAN

PRIMARY NURSING DIAGNOSIS

Anxiety: Parental

DEFINITION   Feeling of apprehension resulting from an unknown cause

POSSIBLY RELATED TO
Cardiac catheterization
Unknown heart defect of child
Unknown prognosis for child
Fear of undesirable outcome for child

CHARACTERISTICS
Verbalization of apprehension or nervousness
Inability to relax
Anticipation of misfortune for child during the cardiac catheterization
Inappropriate or hostile behavior toward health care team
Inability to concentrate
Reports of somatic discomfort

EXPECTED OUTCOMES Parents will demonstrate decreased anxiety as evidenced by

verbalization of decreased anxiety.

ability to relax.

lack of statements indicating anticipated misfortune for the child.

lack of inappropriate or hostile behavior.

ability to concentrate.

decreased reports of somatic discomfort.

POSSIBLE NURSING INTERVENTIONS

Listen to the parents' concerns and complaints. Encourage expression of feelings to health care team, family, or friends regarding the procedure and its implications.

Explain the cardiac catheterization procedure and instruct the parents in home care. Keep explanations simple and concise; use illustrations. Repeat explanations as necessary.

Answer any questions parents may have regarding the procedure, child's care, or child's condition.

Dispel any misinformation.

Remove excess stimulation from the environment.

Record interactions with parents.

EVALUATION FOR CHARTING

Describe parents' behavior and level of anxiety.

State whether parents were able to verbalize an understanding of explanations regarding the procedure, child's care, and child's condition.

Describe any measures used to decrease the parents' anxiety. State effectiveness of measures.

NURSING DIAGNOSIS

Knowledge Deficit: Parental

DEFINITION Lack of information concerning the child's disease and care

POSSIBLY RELATED TO

Misconceptions or inaccurate information concerning cardiac catheterization, possibly caused by

fear of cardiac catheterization procedure
fear of cardiac catheterization outcome
sensory overload

Cognitive or cultural-language limitations

CHARACTERISTICS
Verbalization by parents indicating lack of knowledge
Relation of incorrect information to members of the health
    care team
Requests for information

EXPECTED OUTCOMES   Parents will have an adequate
knowledge base concerning the child's cardiac catheterization
and care as evidenced by

ability to correctly state information previously taught
    regarding the cardiac catheterization procedure and
    home care.
ability to relate appropriate information to the health
    care team.

POSSIBLE NURSING INTERVENTIONS
Listen to parents' concerns and fears.

Assess and record parents' knowledge concerning the cardiac
catheterization. Encourage questions.

Provide parents with information about the cardiac
catheterization, including

preoperative medication.
preparation of the catheter insertion site.
equipment.
monitoring of child during the procedure.
x-ray films.
any diversional activities available for the child (e.g.,
    cassette tapes) should the child be awake during the
    procedure.
time frame for the procedure.
condition of child (sleepiness) after the procedure.
care of child after the procedure (assessment of vital signs,
    cardiovascular assessment, site assessment, initial diet
    of clear liquids).

Use pictures as necessary to facilitate teaching.

Provide parents with any available literature or booklets concerning cardiac catheterization.

Arrange a preliminary visit to the catheterization laboratory.

Assign a primary nurse as usual spokesperson to parents.

When indicated, obtain an interpreter.

Dispel any incorrect information.

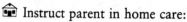 Instruct parent in home care:

> observation of the catheterization site for bleeding, swelling, redness, drainage.
> observation of the extremity for paleness, pain.
> site care.
> monitoring of child's temperature.
> monitoring of child's extremity for any numbness.
> diet.
> hygiene.
> activity.

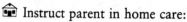 Identify sources of support or information that the parents may contact for assistance after the child's discharge.

EVALUATION FOR CHARTING

State whether parents verbalized a knowledge deficit.

 State whether parents were able to repeat information correctly.

Describe any measures used to facilitate parent teaching.

RELATED NURSING DIAGNOSES

Knowledge Deficit: Child *related to*

a. invasive procedure
b. home care after procedure

Decreased Cardiac Output *related to*
congenital heart defect

Fear: Child/Family *related to*

a. invasive procedure
b. outcome of cardiac catheterization

Compromised Family Coping *related to*

a. child's hospitalization
b. invasive procedure
c. potential for child to have a fatal or chronic disease

POST-CARDIAC CATHETERIZATION NURSING CARE PLAN

PRIMARY NURSING DIAGNOSIS

Decreased Cardiac Output

DEFINITION   Decrease in the amount of blood that leaves the left ventricle

POSSIBLY RELATED TO
Dysrhythmias secondary to catheter irritation
Septal perforation
Hemorrhage
Shock
Reaction to contrast medium
Reaction to sedation
Cardiopulmonary arrest

CHARACTERISTICS
Tachycardia
Hypotension
Unequal, decreased, or absent peripheral pulses
Excessive bleeding from catheter insertion site
Cool, clammy extremities
Prolonged capillary refill, longer than 2 to 3 seconds
Decreased urine output
Hematoma
Cardiopulmonary arrest

EXPECTED OUTCOMES   Child will have an adequate cardiac output as evidenced by

heart rate within acceptable range (state specific highest and lowest rates for each child).
blood pressure within acceptable range (state specific highest and lowest pressures for each child).

strong and equal peripheral pulses.

minimal bleeding from catheterization site.

brisk capillary refill, within 2 to 3 seconds.

skin warm to touch.

regular heart rate and rhythm.

adequate urine output (state specific highest and lowest outputs for each child, minimum 1 to 2 ml/kg/hr).

Possible Nursing Interventions

Assess and record child's vital signs every 15 minutes until stable, then every 30 minutes for two times, then every hour for 4 hours, or as otherwise indicated.

Assess and record the following with vital signs or per postcatheterization protocol:

condition of catheter site or dressing. Notify physician of excessive drainage.

peripheral pulses. If indicated, use a Doppler device to locate pulses.

capillary refill.

skin temperature and color.

signs/symptoms of decreased cardiac output (such as those listed under **Characteristics**).

When indicated, initiate use of cardiac monitor. Evaluate and record results of EKG strips.

Keep accurate record of intake and output.

Have emergency medications and equipment ready.

Evaluation for Charting

State highest and lowest vital signs.

Describe quality of peripheral pulses, capillary refill, and skin temperature and color.

Describe condition of catheterization site or dressing.

Describe any signs/symptoms of decreased cardiac output noted (such as those listed under **Characteristics**).

State intake and output.

Describe any measures used (such as cardiac monitor or Doppler) to further assess cardiac status.

Describe any therapeutic measures used to improve cardiac output. State their effectiveness.

NURSING DIAGNOSIS

Altered Tissue Perfusion: Peripheral

DEFINITION   Inadequate amount of blood and oxygen being delivered to the tissues in the body

POSSIBLY RELATED TO
Hemorrhage from catheterization site
Arterial or venous clots obstructing blood flow
Decreased cardiac output

CHARACTERISTICS   Catheterized extremity may have the following characteristics:

cool, clammy
pale or mottled
decreased intensity of pulses
spasms of artery
thrombus
prolonged capillary refill, longer than 2 to 3 seconds
excessive bleeding at catheterization site
hematoma
edema
decreased movement or sensation

EXPECTED OUTCOMES   Child's catheterized extremity will have adequate supply of blood and oxygen as evidenced by

skin warm to touch.
pink color.
strong, equal peripheral pulses.
brisk capillary refill, within 2 to 3 seconds.
adequate movement and sensation as compared to other
    extremities.
lack of signs/symptoms of altered peripheral perfusion (such
    as those listed under **Characteristics**).

POSSIBLE NURSING INTERVENTIONS
Assess and record the following with vital signs or per postcatheterization protocol:

condition of catheterization site or dressing. Notify
    physician of excessive drainage.

peripheral pulses. If indicated, use a Doppler device to locate pulses.

capillary refill.

skin temperature and color.

signs/symptoms of altered peripheral tissue perfusion (such as those listed under **Characteristics**). Notify physician of any abnormalities.

Minimize movement and attempt to prevent flexion of catheterized extremity.

Maintain bedrest for child as indicated.

When indicated,

elevate extremity to facilitate venous return (especially if extremity is edematous).

apply additional direct pressure or reinforce dressing at the catheterization site.

apply heat to contralateral extremity to maintain circulation to catheterized extremity by reflex vasodilation. (Do not apply heat directly to the catheterized extremity as this will increase the oxygen requirements of already-compromised tissue.)

EVALUATION FOR CHARTING

Describe any signs/symptoms of altered peripheral tissue perfusion noted (such as those listed under **Characteristics**).

Describe quality of peripheral pulses, capillary refill, and skin temperature and color.

Describe condition of catheterization site or dressing.

Describe any therapeutic measures used to improve peripheral perfusion. State their effectiveness.

RELATED NURSING DIAGNOSES

Altered Comfort* _related to_
catheter insertion site

---

*Non–NANDA diagnosis.

Infection: High Risk *related to*
   invasive procedure

Fluid Volume Deficit *related to*
   a. vomiting secondary to medications
   b. diuresis caused by contrast medium

Compromised Family Coping *related to*
   outcome of procedure

MEDICAL DIAGNOSIS

Congenital Heart Disease

PATHOPHYSIOLOGY Congenital heart disease (CHD) occurs in approximately eight of one thousand live births. In most cases the specific cause is unknown. Inheritance, genetic predisposition, and environmental influences (such as viruses, alcohol, and drugs) have been associated with CHD. Certain chromosomal aberrations, such as trisomies 13, 18, and 21, also increase the risk of CHD.

Congenital heart defects can be categorized as either acyanotic or cyanotic lesions. Cardiovascular surgery can be performed for palliation and/or correction of many cardiac defects.

The pathophysiologies of twelve congenital heart defects are presented here. Preoperative and intermediate postoperative nursing care plans follow. The postoperative nursing care plan applies to children who have been moved out of the intensive care unit setting. For immediate postoperative care, consult a pediatric critical care nursing care plan book.

Acyanotic Heart Defects

Atrial Septal Defect An atrial septal defect (ASD), an opening between the right and left atrium, occurs in approximately 15% of all congenital cardiac defects. An ASD can vary in size and location in the septum and can be associated with other cardiac defects. Some of the oxygenated blood going to the left atrium is shunted through the ASD to the right atrium; thus, an ASD is a left-to-right shunt. From the right atrium, the blood passes through the tricuspid valve to the right ventricle; it then recirculates through the lungs, increasing the blood flow to the lungs. Pulmonary vascular changes occur very slowly, and increased pulmonary vascular resistance usually does not occur until early adulthood. Small ASDs may close spontaneously. Surgical intervention to close the ASD is usually done on children between 2 and 4 years of age. Earlier closure is recommended if the child is experiencing problems. Most children with an ASD are asymptomatic, and the diagnosis is based on a crescendo-decrescendo systolic ejection murmur heard during a routine physical examination.

Aortic Stenosis   Aortic stenosis (AS) is an obstruction of the aortic outflow tract that causes resistance to ejection of blood from the left ventricle. It can be supravalvular, valvular, or subvalvular, with valvular being the most common. Pressure builds on the left side of the heart and causes increased pressure in the pulmonary veins. The increased pulmonary vascular pressure causes fluid to leak into the interstitial spaces, resulting in pulmonary edema. Surgical intervention is necessary to correct the defect. Infants with AS can manifest symptoms of left ventricular failure and low cardiac output such as respiratory distress, faint peripheral pulses, decreased urine output, and poor feeding. If AS is not severe, it may go undiagnosed until preadolescence, when the child may manifest symptoms such as fainting, dizziness, epigastric pain, or exercise intolerance. Acute dysrhythmias may develop and result in sudden death following exertion in some individuals.

Atrioventricular Canal Defect   Atrioventricular canal defect, also called endocardial cushion defect, is a large central hole in the heart with free communication between all four chambers. A left-to-right, right-to-left, and/or bidirectional shunt may exist. Oxygenated blood is recirculated to the lungs. Increased blood flow going under increased pressure to the lungs can lead to increased pulmonary vascular resistance and pulmonary hypertension, which can ultimately result in congestive heart failure. Complete surgical repair is usually performed before a child is 2 years of age. Prior to surgical repair, medical management of congestive heart failure may be necessary. Cyanosis is the main clinical manifestation.

Coarctation of the Aorta   Coarctation of the aorta (COA) is a narrowing of the aorta that can vary from mild constriction to total occlusion. The most common location is juxtaductal (at the junction of the ductus arteriosus on the aortic arch). The degree of narrowing determines the severity of the symptoms. In juxtaductal coarctation, blood flow to the lower part of the body is decreased, manifested by diminished pulses in the lower extremities. Pressure builds proximal to the obstruction and results in upper extremity hypertension. Surgical correction is recommended when the defect is identified and the patient is symptomatic. Clinical manifestations of congestive heart failure may be present in symptomatic infants with COA. Children with COA may be asymptomatic, and the defect is first detected during a routine physical examination when upper extremity systemic hypertension, weak or absent femoral pulses, and a heart murmur are present.

Patent Ductus Arteriosus   The ductus arteriosus, a connection between the pulmonary artery and the descending aorta, is a normal pathway in fetal circulation that usually closes permanently during the first few weeks of life. Failure of the ductus arteriosus to close results in a left-to-right shunt. Oxygenated blood flows from the aorta into the pulmonary artery and is recirculated through the lungs. The lungs then receive increased blood flow under increased pressure. If the patent ductus arteriosus (PDA) is not corrected, irreversible pulmonary vascular disease can result. Some PDAs may close spontaneously. Surgical ligation or the use of prostaglandin inhibitor (indomethacin) is recommended for closure of PDAs in preterm infants who are symptomatic. Older infants and children who have not had spontaneous closure will also require closure by surgical intervention. Clinical manifestations may include a machinery-like murmur associated with a thrill, a widened pulse pressure, frequent respiratory infections, failure to thrive, and signs/symptoms of congestive heart failure.

Pulmonary Stenosis   Pulmonary stenosis results when an obstruction interferes with blood flow out of the right ventricle. The obstruction can vary in degree from mild to severe and can be supravalvular, valvular, or subvalvular. Pressure builds in the right ventricle and can result in right ventricular hypertrophy. In young infants, this increase in pressure may cause the foramen ovale to reopen, resulting in right-to-left shunting of unoxygenated blood. If pulmonary stenosis is severe, systemic venous engorgement results and can lead to congestive heart failure. Balloon angioplasty or surgical intervention may be required to correct the defect. Clinical manifestations may include a systolic ejection murmur, dyspnea, cyanosis, fatigue, and signs/symptoms of congestive heart failure.

Ventricular Septal Defect   A ventricular septal defect (VSD), an abnormal opening between the left and right ventricles, is the most common heart lesion. It can vary in size, location in the septum, and number (there can be multiple VSDs). A VSD is often associated with other, more complex defects. It causes a left-to-right shunt that results in increased blood flow going to the lungs under increased pressure. This increased flow is of blood that has already been oxygenated and is recirculating through the lungs.

Irreversible pulmonary vascular changes can result (usually when the child is around 2 years of age) if the condition is not corrected. Approximately 75% of all VSDs close spontaneously sometime during the first 2 years of life. Surgical intervention for closure of the VSD is required when the child is symptomatic and the defect does not close spontaneously. Clinical manifestations may include a loud, harsh, pansystolic murmur; frequent respiratory infections; failure to thrive; and signs/symptoms of congestive heart failure.

Cyanotic Heart Defects

Tetralogy of Fallot   Tetralogy of Fallot (TOF) has four components: pulmonary stenosis, ventricular septal defect, an overriding aorta, and right ventricular hypertrophy (creating a boot-shaped heart as seen on x-ray). The pattern of blood flow in this defect is determined by the degree of pulmonary stenosis. If pulmonary stenosis is severe, pressure builds in the right ventricle and unoxygenated blood passes through the VSD into the overriding aorta (right-to-left shunt) producing cyanosis. If the pulmonary stenosis is mild and the pressure in the right ventricle is not increased, the blood shunts left to right through the VSD and the child is acyanotic. In time, the pulmonary stenosis becomes more severe and the child becomes more cyanotic as less blood flows to the lungs. Hypoxic, or "tet," spells occur in some children with TOF. These spells are thought to occur as a result of a transient increase in obstruction of the right ventricle outflow tract causing cyanosis and a decreased level of consciousness. Tet spells can be treated by placing the child in the knee-chest position, which is thought to increase venous return to the heart and dilate the right ventricle and should decrease the pulmonary outflow obstruction. Surgical correction involves closing the VSD and resectioning the infundibular stenosis or enlarging the right ventricular outflow tract. Clinical manifestations may include cyanosis, hypoxemia, increased hemoglobin and hematocrit, and a pansystolic murmur. Since surgical repair is usually done early (before the child is 2 years of age), squatting, once common, is rarely seen now.

Total Anomalous Pulmonary Venous Connection

Total anomalous pulmonary venous connection (TAPVC), also called total anomalous pulmonary venous return (TAPVR), occurs when the pulmonary veins do not connect to the left atrium; instead, they connect to the right atrium or to one of the systemic veins draining toward the right atrium (such as the superior vena cava or the inferior vena cava). The blood flow pattern in the heart depends on where the pulmonary veins connect (above or below the diaphragm) and on the presence or absence of pulmonary venous obstruction. In all types of TAPVC, the right atrium ultimately receives systemic blood as well as the blood returning from the lungs. This increased blood flow to the right atrium results in hypertrophy of the right side of the heart. The only way for blood flow to reach the left atrium is through an associated atrial septal defect or a patent foramen ovale. When there is no pulmonary venous obstruction, excessive blood flow to the lungs occurs, which can result in congestive heart failure. If pulmonary venous congestion is present, blood flow to the lungs is decreased and cyanosis can be marked. Pulmonary venous pressure rises proximal to the obstruction, resulting in pulmonary edema.

Surgical correction is required to repair TAPVC. Clinical manifestations include cyanosis, a blowing systolic murmur, a venous hum, tachypnea, feeding difficulties, repeated upper respiratory infections, and signs/symptoms of congestive heart failure.

Transposition of the Great Arteries   In transposition of the great arteries (TGA), the aorta arises from the right ventricle and the pulmonary artery arises from the left ventricle. This results in two separate circulatory systems. Blood from the systemic circulation enters the right atrium and passes to the right ventricle and out the aorta back to the rest of the body without going to the lungs for oxygenation. The pulmonary veins empty into the left atrium. The oxygenated blood goes to the left ventricle, out the pulmonary artery, and back to the lungs. Associated lesions (atrial septal defect, ventricular septal defect, and patent ductus arteriosus) are usually present and account for any mixing of oxygenated and unoxygenated blood. Balloon septostomy can be performed as a palliative procedure during cardiac catheterization in order to enlarge the interatrial communication and mixing of blood, resulting in a dramatic increase in arterial oxygenation. Surgeries for total correction involve intraatrial redirection of blood flow or arterial switch procedures. Clinical manifestations may include cyanosis and signs/symptoms of congestive heart failure.

Tricuspid Atresia   Tricuspid atresia is total occlusion of the tricuspid valve. There is no communication between the right atrium and the right ventricle. Other anomalies, such as atrial septal defect (ASD), ventricular septal defect (VSD), or patent ductus arteriosus (PDA), are commonly present. The right ventricle is usually small, and the pulmonary arteries may also be small. Blood returning from the body empties into the right atrium and cannot pass into the right ventricle; therefore, the blood goes through the ASD to the left atrium. From the left atrium, blood flows to the left ventricle, and a portion of this blood goes to the lungs via a VSD. If no VSD is present, the blood can flow to the lungs via a PDA. In infants with a PDA, prostaglandin E1 can be given to maintain the patency of the ductus arteriosus. Palliative surgery designed to increase blood flow to the lungs may also be done prior to total correction. Total repair involves creating communication between the right atrium (or right ventricle) and the pulmonary artery. The most consistent clinical manifestation is cyanosis in conjunction with tachypnea and dyspnea.

Truncus Arteriosus   Truncus arteriosus is characterized by a single vessel that arises from the left and right ventricles and overrides a ventricular septal defect (VSD). Blood from both ventricles enters the single vessel and flows to the lung and to the rest of the body. Blood flow to the lungs is usually under systemic pressure, depending on the type of truncus present. Infants with truncus arteriosus are usually at high risk for early pulmonary vascular disease because the blood flows under increased pressure to the lungs. Corrective surgery is usually performed in the first 2 years of life. Palliative surgery may be done prior to corrective surgery and is aimed at decreasing pulmonary blood flow. Corrective surgery involves closing the VSD in such a way that the truncus arteriosus only receives outflow from the left ventricle. The pulmonary arteries are then excised from the truncus and attached to the right ventricle. Clinical manifestations include cyanosis and signs/symptoms of congestive heart failure.

PREOPERATIVE NURSING CARE PLAN

PRIMARY NURSING DIAGNOSIS
Knowledge Deficit: Child/Family

DEFINITION   Lack of information concerning the child's disease and care

POSSIBLY RELATED TO
>   Sensory overload (too much to learn all at once)
>   Cognitive or cultural-language limitations

Misconceptions, lack of information, or inaccurate information

Lack of exposure

CHARACTERISTICS

Verbalization by child/family indicating lack of knowledge

Relation of incorrect information to members of the health care team

Inability to repeat correctly and comprehend information taught

Inability to correctly demonstrate previously taught skills

Inappropriate or hostile behavior

EXPECTED OUTCOMES   Child/family will have an adequate knowledge base concerning disease state and upcoming surgical procedure and care as evidenced by

ability to state information correctly.

ability to demonstrate skills correctly.

willingness to participate in learning process.

appropriate questions.

lack of inappropriate or hostile behavior.

POSSIBLE NURSING INTERVENTIONS

Assess and record current level of knowledge.

Listen to concerns and fears of child/family.

Give correct information and literature to child/family.

Teach at appropriate level.

Correct any misinformation.

Demonstrate skills.

Assist and observe child/family in performing skills that have been taught. Record their ability to perform skills.

Encourage questions and provide nonjudgmental learning environment.

🏠 Assign primary nurse as usual spokesperson to provide consistency.

Assess and record child's/family's knowledge of and participation in care regarding

equipment and procedures.

chest physiotherapy.

medication administration.

Assess and record child's/family's participation in
  visit to pediatric ICU setting and introduction to nurses in
    that area.
  visit to recovery room.

Instruct child/family in any areas needing improvement.
Record results.

Identify sources of support/information that parents may
contact for assistance after discharge.

EVALUATION FOR CHARTING
State current level of knowledge.

State whether child/family verbalized a knowledge deficit.

Note whether child/family were able to restate taught
information correctly.

State whether child/family were able to perform skills
previously taught. Describe abilities.

Describe any inappropriate or hostile behavior.

Describe child's/family's knowledge of and participation in
care. State any areas needing improvement and information
provided. Describe child's/family's responses.

NURSING DIAGNOSIS

Fear: Child/Family

DEFINITION   Feeling of apprehension resulting from a
known cause

POSSIBLY RELATED TO
Outcome of surgical procedure
Pain and discomfort following surgery
Unfamiliar surroundings
Forced contact with strangers
Treatments and procedures

CHARACTERISTICS
Uncooperativeness
Regressed behavior
Hostile behavior
Restlessness
Inability to recall previously taught information
Decreased communication
Decreased attention span

EXPECTED OUTCOMES   Child/family will exhibit only a minimal amount of fear as evidenced by

> ability to relate appropriately to family members and members of the health care team.
> lack of regressed or hostile behavior.
> ability to rest and sleep when indicated.
> ability to restate information previously taught.
> ability to participate in care.
> ability to separate for short periods when indicated.
> ability to express fears to members of the health care team.

NURSING INTERVENTIONS

Assess and record level of child's/family's fears and their sources.

Decrease child's/family's fears when possible by

> encouraging family members to stay with child.
> encouraging child/family members to participate in care.
> assigning same staff members to provide care for child.
> spending extra time with child when family members are unable to be present.
> encouraging family members to bring in familiar articles and toys from home.

Initiate age-appropriate therapeutic play, when indicated.

Encourage child/family to express fears to members of the health care team.

Encourage child/family to meet basic needs, such as eating and resting appropriately. Assist them as needed.

EVALUATION FOR CHARTING

State any identified sources of child's/family's fears.

Describe any signs/symptoms of fear manifested by the child/parents (such as those listed under **Characteristics**).

Describe any measures used to help alleviate fear. State effectiveness of measures.

State whether child's fear decreases if family members stay and participate in child's care.

State whether child/family were able to separate for short periods so that family members could meet their own basic needs.

State whether child/family were able to understand information given to them about the child's illness.

RELATED NURSING DIAGNOSES

Decreased Cardiac Output *related to*

a. fluid volume excess
b. increased blood flow to the lungs
c. pulmonary hypertension
d. congenital heart defect

Activity Intolerance *related to*
fatigue, weakness secondary to

a. disease process
b. circulatory compromise

Infection: High Risk *related to*
debilitated physical status

Altered Growth and Development *related to*
decreased oxygenation

POSTOPERATIVE, POST–PEDIATRIC ICU NURSING CARE PLAN

PRIMARY NURSING DIAGNOSIS

Decreased Cardiac Output

DEFINITION   Decrease in the amount of blood that leaves the left ventricle

POSSIBLY RELATED TO
Surgical complications:

thrombus
ineffective circulation
interference with electrical conduction
dysrhythmias
tachycardia or bradycardia

CHARACTERISTICS

Tachycardia/bradycardia
Dysrhythmias
Hypotension/hypertension
Unequal, decreased, or absent peripheral pulses
Cyanosis
Prolonged capillary refill, longer than 2 or 3 seconds
Murmur, gallop, rub, click
Cool, pale skin
Fever
Activity intolerance
Fatigue
Decreased urine output

EXPECTED OUTCOMES   Child will maintain an adequate
cardiac output as evidenced by

vital signs within acceptable ranges (state specific highest and
lowest parameters).
strong and equal peripheral pulses.
brisk capillary refill, within 2 to 3 seconds.
skin warm to touch.
lack of murmur, gallop, rub, click, cyanosis, fatigue,
activity intolerance.
adequate urine output (state specific highest and lowest
outputs for each child, minimum 1 to 2 ml/kg/hr).

POSSIBLE NURSING INTERVENTIONS

Assess and record the following every 4 hours and PRN:

vital signs
peripheral pulses
capillary refill
any signs/symptoms of decreased cardiac output (such as
those listed under **Characteristics**)

Assess and record condition of dressing and/or incision site
every shift and PRN. Notify physician of excessive drainage.

Administer cardiac drugs (such as digoxin) on schedule.
Assess and record effectiveness and any signs/symptoms of
toxicity (e.g., bradycardia, vomiting). Monitor and record
digoxin levels. Notify physician if results are out of the

acceptable range. Assess and record apical rate for 1 full minute before giving digoxin. Do not give medication if apical rate is below 100 beats/minute in infants, below 70 beats/minute for older children, or below specific parameters indicated. Two nurses should check dosage prior to each administration.

Ensure that chest physiotherapy is done effectively and on schedule. Protect suture line during treatment. Record effectiveness of treatments.

Keep accurate record of intake and output.

☖ Assess and record child's/family's knowledge of and participation in care regarding

    medication administration.
    chest physiotherapy, if indicated.
    monitoring of child's intake and output.
    identification of any signs/symptoms of decreased cardiac
       output (such as those listed under **Characteristics**).

EVALUATION FOR CHARTING

State highest and lowest vital signs.

Describe quality of peripheral pulses and capillary refill.

Describe any signs/symptoms of decreased cardiac output (such as those listed under **Characteristics**).

Describe condition of dressing and/or incision site.

Indicate whether medications were administered on schedule. Describe effectiveness and any side effects noted.

State digoxin levels. If levels were out of the acceptable range, describe any corrective measures implemented.

Indicate whether chest physiotherapy was performed on schedule. Describe how child tolerated procedure. State effectiveness of procedure.

State intake and output.

☖ Describe child's/family's knowledge of and participation in care related to maintaining an adequate cardiac output. State any areas needing improvement and information provided. Describe child's/family's responses.

NURSING DIAGNOSIS
Altered Comfort*

DEFINITION   Condition in which an individual experiences discomfort

POSSIBLY RELATED TO
Incision site
Treatments and procedures

CHARACTERISTICS
Verbal communication of discomfort or tenderness
Crying unrelieved by usual comfort measures
Facial grimacing
Restlessness
Physical signs/symptoms:

tachycardia
tachypnea/bradypnea
increased blood pressure
diaphoresis

EXPECTED OUTCOMES   Child will be free of severe and/or constant discomfort as evidenced by

verbal communication of comfort.
lack of constant crying.
lack of restlessness.
heart rate within acceptable range (state specific highest and lowest rates for each child).
respiratory rate within acceptable range (state specific highest and lowest rates for each child).
blood pressure within acceptable range (state specific highest and lowest pressures for each child).
lack of diaphoresis.

POSSIBLE NURSING INTERVENTIONS
Assess and record any signs/symptoms of discomfort (such as those listed under **Characteristics**) at least once/shift.

Handle child gently.

---

*Non-NANDA diagnosis.

When indicated, administer analgesics on schedule. Assess and record effectiveness.

Encourage family members to stay and comfort child when possible.

EVALUATION FOR CHARTING
State range of vital signs.

Describe any signs/symptoms of discomfort.

Describe any therapeutic measures used to increase child's comfort. State their effectiveness.

RELATED NURSING DIAGNOSES

Infection: High Risk *related to*
surgical procedure

Compromised Family Coping *related to*
a. child's surgery
b. child's hospitalization
c. lack of support systems
d. financial considerations

Activity Intolerance *related to*
postoperative status

Altered Growth and Development *related to*
underlying disease process

Congestive Heart Failure

PATHOPHYSIOLOGY   Congestive heart failure (CHF) is a group of signs and symptoms that reflect the heart's inability to effectively pump blood to meet the metabolic requirements of the body. The name congestive heart failure is misleading; the heart does not actually have to fail. Congestive heart failure can result from increased blood volume, obstruction to outflow from the ventricles, decreased contractility, and/or high cardiac output demands. The most common cause of CHF in children is altered hemodynamics secondary to congenital heart defects.

By the time CHF is present, the body has already made some acute adjustments in an attempt to maintain and improve cardiac output. The sympathetic nervous system responds to decreased blood pressure detected by vascular stretch receptors and baroreceptors. Catecholamines increase venous tone in order to improve blood return to the heart. Another compensatory mechanism maximizes blood supply to the heart, lungs, and brain by decreasing circulation to the skin, extremities, stomach, intestines, and kidneys. Decreased blood flow to the kidneys stimulates the release of renin, angiotensin, and aldosterone. As a result, the kidneys retain fluid and sodium, which initially aids in cardiac output. However, hypervolemia ultimately occurs and increases the work load on the already stressed cardiac musculature.

It is difficult to clinically separate right-sided and left-sided heart failure in children; the two usually occur together. If one chamber fails, failure in the opposite chamber is only a matter of time. Right-sided heart failure causes increased central venous pressure, resulting in systemic congestion and edema. Elevated pressure in the inferior vena cava causes hepatomegaly. With left-sided heart failure, the pressure in the left atrium rises, and blood returning from the lungs via the pulmonary veins is unable to enter the left atrium. Pressure then begins to rise in the pulmonary vasculature. Fluid leaks out of the pulmonary capillaries into the interstitial spaces, resulting in pulmonary edema.

PRIMARY NURSING DIAGNOSIS
Decreased Cardiac Output

DEFINITION   Decrease in the amount of blood that leaves the left ventricle

POSSIBLY RELATED TO
Increased volume
Obstruction to outflow
Decreased contractility
High cardiac output demands
These four conditions can result from

hypervolemia
fluid volume overload
increased volume of blood circulating through the heart
increased flow of blood to the lungs
congenital heart defect
acquired heart defect
dysrhythmias
myocarditis
myopathies
anemia
endocrine and/or metabolic disorders

Noncardiovascular diseases (e.g., respiratory disease, anemia, metabolic disorders, renal disorders, endocrine disorders)

CHARACTERISTICS
Tachycardia
Tachypnea
Dyspnea at rest
Costal retractions
Nasal flaring
Crackles
Cough
Poor peripheral circulation, cold extremities
Pallor and mottling of skin
Transient duskiness of skin
Cyanosis
Diaphoresis (especially over head and neck)
Hypotension
Rapid, weak peripheral pulses
Prolonged capillary refill, longer than 2 to 3 seconds

Narrow pulse pressure
Distended neck veins in older children
Gallop rhythm
Cardiomegaly revealed on chest x-ray
Edema (periorbital, sacral, scrotal, peripheral)
Rapid weight gain
Hepatosplenomegaly
Feeding difficulty
Decreased urine output (less than 0.5 to 1 ml/kg/hr)
Weakness
Exercise intolerance
Fatigue
Growth rate slower than normal

EXPECTED OUTCOMES Child will maintain an adequate
cardiac output as evidenced by

heart rate within acceptable range (state specific highest and
lowest rates for each child).
respiratory rate within acceptable range (state specific highest
and lowest rates for each child).
clear and equal breath sounds bilaterally.
blood pressure within acceptable range (state specific highest
and lowest pressures for each child).
pulse pressure within acceptable limits of 20 to 50 mm/Hg.
normal sinus rhythm.
skin warm to touch.
brisk capillary refill, within 2 to 3 seconds.
appropriate heart size as seen on chest x-ray.
adequate urine output (state specific highest and lowest
output for each child, minimum 1 to 2 ml/kg/hr).
steady progress on growth curve.
lack of signs/symptoms of decreased cardiac output (such as
those listed under **Characteristics**).

POSSIBLE NURSING INTERVENTIONS
Assess and record the following every 2 to 4 hours and PRN:

apical heart rate
blood pressure
respiratory rate
signs/symptoms of decreased cardiac output (such as those
listed under **Characteristics**)

Evaluate and record results of EKG strips.

Keep accurate record of intake and output.

Administer cardiac drugs (e.g., digoxin) on schedule. Assess and record effectiveness and any signs/symptoms of toxicity (e.g., bradycardia, vomiting). Assess and record apical rate for 1 full minute before giving digoxin. Do not give medication if apical rate is below 100 beats/minute in infants, below 70 beats/minute in older children, or below specific parameters indicated. Two nurses should check the dosage prior to each administration.

Monitor and record digoxin levels. Notify physician if levels are out of the acceptable range.

Administer diuretics (e.g., furosemide) on schedule. Assess and record effectiveness and any side effects (e.g., hypokalemia, dehydration).

Elevate head of bed at 30° angle (can use infant seat).

Organize nursing care to allow child uninterrupted rest periods.

Check and record results of chest x-ray, when indicated.

🏠 Assess and record child's/family's knowledge of and participation in care regarding

> medication administration.
> positioning with head elevated.
> maintainance of sufficient rest periods.
> monitoring of intake and output.
> identification of any signs/symptoms of decreased cardiac output (such as those listed under **Characteristics**).

🏠 Instruct child/family in any areas needing improvement. Record results.

EVALUATION FOR CHARTING

State highest and lowest heart rates, respiratory rates, and blood pressures.

Describe cardiac rhythm and breath sounds.

Describe activity tolerance.

Describe any signs/symptoms of decreased cardiac output noted (such as those listed under **Characteristics**).

Document EKG interpretation.

State intake and output.

Indicate whether medications were administered on schedule. Describe effectiveness and any side effects noted.

State digoxin levels. If levels were out of the acceptable range, describe any corrective measures implemented.

Indicate whether head of bed was elevated.

Indicate whether child had uninterrupted rest periods.

State result of chest x-ray, when indicated.

🏠 Describe child's/family's knowledge of and participation in care related to maintaining an adequate cardiac output. State any areas needing improvement and information provided. Describe child's/family's responses.

NURSING DIAGNOSIS
Ineffective Breathing Pattern

DEFINITION   Breathing pattern that results in inadequate oxygen consumption (failure to meet the cellular requirements of the body)

POSSIBLY RELATED TO
Decreased cardiac output
Pulmonary hypertension
Increased flow of blood to the lungs
Pulmonary edema
Congenital heart defect
Fatigue

CHARACTERISTICS
Tachypnea
Dyspnea
Costal retractions
Nasal flaring
Grunting
Fatigue
Pallor, mottling

Cyanosis
Crackles
Use of accessory muscles
Head bobbing (for an infant)
Dry, hacking cough
Orthopnea
Shortness of breath
Activity intolerance

EXPECTED OUTCOMES   Child will have an effective breathing pattern as evidenced by

respiratory rate within acceptable range (state highest and lowest rates for each child).
clear and equal breath sounds.
lack of any signs/symptoms of ineffective breathing pattern (such as those listed under **Characteristics**).

POSSIBLE NURSING INTERVENTIONS
Assess and record the following every 2 to 4 hours and PRN:

breath sounds
vital signs
signs/symptoms of ineffective breathing pattern (such as those listed under **Characteristics**)

Administer humidified oxygen in correct amount and route of delivery. Record percent of oxygen and route of delivery. Assess and record effectiveness of therapy.

Elevate head of bed at 30° angle (may use infant seat).

Ensure that chest physiotherapy is done effectively and on schedule. Record effectiveness and child's response to treatment. Modification of the procedure may be necessary if child becomes stressed.

Suction if child is unable to cough up secretions. Record amount and characteristics of secretions.

Assess and record child's/family's knowledge of and participation in care regarding

chest physiotherapy
positioning with head elevated
identification of any signs/symptoms of ineffective breathing pattern (such as those listed under **Characteristics**)

Instruct family in any areas needing improvement. Record results.

EVALUATION FOR CHARTING

Describe breath sounds.

State highest and lowest respiratory rates.

Describe any signs/symptoms of ineffective breathing pattern noted (such as those listed under **Characteristics**).

State amount and route of oxygen delivery. Describe effectiveness.

Indicate whether head of bed was elevated.

Indicate whether chest physiotherapy was performed on schedule. Describe how child tolerated procedure. State effectiveness of procedure.

State frequency of suctioning and describe amount and characteristics of secretions.

Describe any therapeutic measures used to maintain an effective breathing pattern. State their effectiveness.

 Describe child's/family's knowledge of and participation in care related to maintaining an effective breathing pattern. State any areas needing improvement and information provided. Describe child's/family's responses.

RELATED NURSING DIAGNOSES

Fluid Volume Excess _related to_

    a. edema secondary to decreased cardiac output
    b. decreased urine output

Altered Nutrition: Less than Body Requirements
related to

    a. respiratory distress
    b. fatigue
    c. feeding difficulty
    d. increased metabolic demands

Activity Intolerance _related to_

    a. decreased cardiac output
    b. respiratory distress

c. fatigue
d. decreased oxygen supply and increased oxygen needs

Compromised Family Coping *related to*

a. hospitalization of child
b. illness involving major body organ
c. added stress of chronic illness on family system
d. knowledge deficit

MEDICAL DIAGNOSIS

Hypertension

PATHOPHYSIOLOGY   Systemic arterial hypertension is becoming an increasingly common health problem in children and adolescents, although it is still more prevalent in adults. Hypertension is usually defined as an elevation of the systolic and/or diastolic blood pressures above the acceptable range for a given age and sex. Blood pressure readings above the ninetieth percentile for age and sex on three separate occasions over a 6- to 12-month period is one criterion for diagnosing hypertension in children.

Hypertension can be either primary or secondary. Primary hypertension, also called essential hypertension, has no known cause, although genetic and environmental factors may play a role in its development. This is the most common form of hypertension in the adult population and may at times have its origin in childhood. Identified environmental factors that may contribute to the condition include stress, increased sodium intake, and obesity. Secondary hypertension results from an existing pathological process such as renal disease, endocrine disorders, and cardiovascular disease. It can also occur as a side effect of steroid therapy for chronic illness.

Research has led to speculation that primary hypertension may originate in the kidneys. Renal ischemia results in the release of renin. Renin in turn causes the eventual formation of angiotensin II, a pressor agent that constricts the arterioles, thus elevating blood pressure. Angiotensin II decreases the glomerular filtration rate by its vasoconstrictive action and causes the release of aldosterone from the adrenal cortex. Aldosterone promotes sodium and water retention, resulting in increased blood volume and increased blood pressure.

Children with primary hypertension may be asymptomatic. Blood pressure should be checked routinely for all children 3 years of age and older.

PRIMARY NURSING DIAGNOSIS
Decreased Cardiac Output

DEFINITION   Decrease in the amount of blood that leaves the left ventricle

POSSIBLY RELATED TO
> Increased systemic vascular resistance
> Fluid volume overload
> Underlying disease process (specify)
> Impaired elasticity of the vessels

CHARACTERISTICS
> Tachycardia
> Palpitations
> Bounding carotid and radial pulses
> Delayed femoral pulse compared to radial pulse
> Absent or diminished lower extremity pulses
> Flushing of skin
> Headache
> Visual disturbance
> Epistaxis
> Chest pain
> Fatigue

EXPECTED OUTCOMES   Child will maintain an adequate cardiac output as evidenced by

> heart rate within acceptable range (state specific highest and lowest rates for each child).
> blood pressure within acceptable range (state specific highest and lowest pressures for each child).
> strong and equal peripheral pulses.
> absence of
>> flushing.
>> headache.
>> epistaxis.
>> visual disturbance.
>> chest pain.
>> fatigue.

POSSIBLE NURSING INTERVENTIONS
> Assess and record the following every 2 to 4 hours and PRN:
>> heart rate and blood pressure

signs/symptoms of decreased cardiac output (such as those listed under **Characteristics**)

Administer diuretics and antihypertensives on schedule. Assess and record effectiveness and any side effects (e.g., dizziness, headache, GI disturbance, hypokalemia).

Weigh child on same scale at same time each day.

Keep accurate record of intake and output.

🖬 Assess and record child's/family's knowledge of and participation in care regarding

accurate procedure for obtaining blood pressure.
dietary considerations (sodium reduction).
weight reduction.
exercise.
identification of any signs/symptoms of decreased cardiac output (such as those listed under **Characteristics**).

🖬 Instruct child/family in any areas needing improvement. Record results.

EVALUATION FOR CHARTING

State highest and lowest heart rates and blood pressures.

Describe any signs/symptoms of decreased cardiac output noted (such as those listed under **Characteristics**).

Indicate whether medications were administered on schedule. Describe effectiveness and any side effects noted.

State child's weight and determine whether it has increased or decreased since previous weighing.

State intake and output.

🖬 Describe child's/family's knowledge of and participation in care related to maintaining an adequate cardiac output. State any areas needing improvement and information provided. Describe child's/family's responses.

NURSING DIAGNOSIS
Noncompliance

DEFINITION   Inability or unwillingness of an individual to adhere to therapeutic recommendations

POSSIBLY RELATED TO
Asymptomatic condition
Side effects of medication
Dietary restrictions
Forgetfulness in taking medications
Lack of family support
Developmental stage of life

CHARACTERISTICS
Evidence of increase in or return of symptoms
Weight gain
Edema
Inability to attain set goals
Verbalization of difficulty in maintaining set goals
Failure to keep appointments

EXPECTED OUTCOMES Child will comply with therapeutic recommendations as evidenced by

blood pressure within acceptable range (state highest and
lowest pressures for each child).
lack of sudden weight gain and edema.
evidence of weight loss, if appropriate.
attainment of set goals.
ability to follow altered diet (reduced sodium).
keeping of clinic appointments after discharge.

POSSIBLE NURSING INTERVENTIONS
Assess and record the following every 2 to 4 hours and PRN:

blood pressure
signs/symptoms of noncompliance (such as those listed
under **Characteristics**)

Weigh child on same scale at same time each day.

⌂ Assess and record child's/family's knowledge of and
participation in care regarding

dietary restrictions and ways to help child adhere to diet.
importance of continuing to take medications even if the
child is asymptomatic.
accurate procedure for taking blood pressure.
importance of keeping regular appointments after
discharge.

🏠 Instruct child/family in any areas needing improvement. Record results.

EVALUATION FOR CHARTING

State highest and lowest blood pressures.

State child's weight and determine whether it has increased or decreased since previous weighing.

Describe any successful measures used to help child/family comply with therapeutic recommendations.

🏠 Describe child's/family's knowledge of and participation in care related to identification of potential noncompliant behavior. State any areas needing improvement and information provided. Describe child's/family's responses.

RELATED NURSING DIAGNOSES

Knowledge Deficit: Child/Family *related to*

a. disease process
b. continuing home management (including diet, exercise, medications)

Activity Intolerance *related to*

a. fatigue
b. side effects of medication

Altered Comfort* *related to*

a. headache
b. chest pain
c. side effects of medication

Compromised Family Coping *related to*
needed changes in lifestyle

---

*Non–NANDA diagnosis.

MEDICAL DIAGNOSIS
Infective Endocarditis

PATHOPHYSIOLOGY   Infective endocarditis includes both bacterial and nonbacterial endocarditis. Bacterial endocarditis is most often caused by *Streptococcus viridans,* although staphylococcal endocarditis has become more common over the past 2 decades. Fungal organisms (e.g., *Candida albicans*) may cause nonbacterial endocarditis.

Although children who do not have a cardiac malformation can develop infective endocarditis, congenital heart disease is the overwhelming predisposing factor for this condition. Children with cardiac lesions associated with a high velocity of blood being injected into a chamber or vessel are most susceptible to infective endocarditis; at highest risk are children with ventricular septal defects, left-sided valvular disease, and systemic-pulmonary arterial communications. The turbulent blood flow created by these lesions results in areas of cardiac tissue damage. Circulating infectious organisms can become entrapped in these eroded sites and form vegetations, which then grow, damage valves, interfere with cardiac function, or break off and become emboli that can cause infarcts.

Infectious agents may be introduced into the child's circulation during a variety of procedures. Surgical or dental procedures can be implicated in most cases of infective endocarditis. Children who have undergone cardiac surgery for a systemic-to-pulmonary artery shunt, valve replacement, or valve conduit repair are at high risk. Children with cyanotic heart disease who have poor dental hygiene are also at risk.

The early signs and symptoms of infective endocarditis can be vague. The child may experience unexplained fevers, malaise, chills, nausea, joint pain, and/or myalgia. Depending on the virulence of the infectious organism, a variety of cardiovascular changes can follow.

Prior to antibiotics, infective endocarditis was fatal. Complications continue to occur in approximately 50% of children with this disease. The most common complication is cardiac failure due to vegetations involving the aortic or mitral valves. Other complications include congestive heart failure, sequelae of pulmonary or neurologic emboli, mycotic aneurysms, acquired ventricular septal defect, and heart block. Fungal endocarditis, which often occurs in immunosuppressed or debilitated children, is difficult to manage and still has a poor prognosis.

The incidence of infective endocarditis can be reduced in susceptible children by using antimicrobial prophylaxis prior to and after dental work and surgery. However, proper oral hygiene and routine dental care are also important.

Treatment of infective endocarditis involves intravenous antibiotics for approximately 6 weeks, instituted immediately upon diagnosis. Bedrest, digitalis, sodium restriction, and diuretic therapy may also be indicated. Surgical removal of vegetations or replacement of an infected valve may also be necessary.

PRIMARY NURSING DIAGNOSIS
Decreased Cardiac Output

DEFINITION   Decrease in the amount of blood that leaves the left ventricle

POSSIBLY RELATED TO
Invasion of the endocardium by bacterial or nonbacterial agents secondary to

congenital heart defect
dental procedures
surgical procedures
immunosuppression

CHARACTERISTICS
Fatigue
Activity intolerance
Tachycardia
Tachypnea
Hypotension
Decreased urine output
Abdominal pain
Cough
Dyspnea
Orthopnea
Crackles

Edema
Cardiomegaly revealed on chest x-ray
Gallop rhythm
Hepatomegaly
Anorexia

EXPECTED OUTCOMES   Child will maintain an adequate
cardiac output as evidenced by

> heart rate within acceptable range (state specific highest and
> lowest rates for each child).
> respiratory rate within acceptable range (state specific highest
> and lowest rates for each child).
> blood pressure within acceptable range (state specific highest
> and lowest pressures for each child).
> clear and equal breath sounds bilaterally.
> appropriate heart size on chest x-ray.
> adequate urine output (state specific highest and lowest
> outputs for each child, minimum 1 to 2 ml/kg/hr).
> lack of signs/symptoms of decreased cardiac output (such as
> those listed under **Characteristics**).

POSSIBLE NURSING INTERVENTIONS
Assess and record the following every 2 to 4 hours and PRN:

> heart rate, respiratory rate, and blood pressure.
> signs/symptoms of decreased cardiac output (such as those
> listed under **Characteristics**).

Organize nursing care to allow child uninterrupted rest
periods.

Keep accurate record of intake and output.

Check and record results of chest x-ray, when indicated.

Elevate head of bed at 30° angle.

Administer cardiac drugs (e.g., digoxin) on schedule. Assess
and record effectiveness and any signs/symptoms of toxicity
(e.g., bradycardia, vomiting). Assess and record apical rate
for 1 full minute before giving digoxin. Do not give
medication if apical rate is below 100 beats/minute in infants
below 70 beats/minute in older children, or below specific
parameters indicated. Two nurses should check the dosage
prior to each administration.

Monitor and record digoxin levels. Notify physician if levels are out of the acceptable range.

Administer diuretics (e.g., furosemide) on schedule. Assess and record effectiveness and any side effects (e.g., hypokalemia, dehydration).

🏠 Assess and record child's/family's knowledge of and participation in care regarding

> medication administration.
> positioning with head elevated.
> maintainance of sufficient rest periods.
> monitoring of intake and output.
> identification of any signs/symptoms of decreased cardiac output (such as those listed under **Characteristics**).

🏠 Instruct child/family in any areas needing improvement. Record results.

EVALUATION FOR CHARTING

State highest and lowest heart rates, respiratory rates, and blood pressures.

Describe breath sounds and respiratory effort.

Describe any signs/symptoms of decreased cardiac output noted (such as those listed under **Characteristics**).

State intake and output.

Indicate whether medications were administered on schedule. Describe effectiveness and any side effects noted.

State digoxin levels. If levels were out of the acceptable range, describe any corrective measures implemented.

State result of chest x-ray, when indicated.

Indicate whether child had uninterrupted rest periods.

Indicate whether head of bed was elevated.

Describe any therapeutic measures used to improve cardiac output. State their effectiveness.

🏠 Describe child's/family's knowledge of and participation in care related to maintaining an adequate cardiac output. State any areas needing improvement and information provided. Describe child's/family's responses.

NURSING DIAGNOSIS
Activity Intolerance

DEFINITION   Insufficient psychosocial, emotional, or physiological ability to perform required or desired activities

POSSIBLY RELATED TO
Hypermetabolic state secondary to persistent fever
Insufficient oxygenation secondary to decreased cardiac output
Myalgia
Arthralgia

CHARACTERISTICS
Fatigue
Weakness
Dyspnea
Tachypnea
Tachycardia
Headache
Verbalization of weakness or fatigue
Inability to perform age-appropriate activities of daily living
Inability to play
Impaired ability to ambulate

EXPECTED OUTCOMES   Child will have appropriate activity for age as evidenced by

heart rate within acceptable range (state specific highest and lowest rates for each child).
respiratory rate within acceptable range (state specific highest and lowest rates for each child).
blood pressure within acceptable range (state specific highest and lowest pressures for each child).
ability to ambulate.
ability to perform activities of daily living (age-appropriate).
ability to play (age-appropriate).
lack of signs of activity intolerance (such as those listed under **Characteristics**).

POSSIBLE NURSING INTERVENTIONS
Assess and record child's baseline activity tolerance.

Assess and record child's baseline and activity vital signs every 4 hours and PRN.

Organize nursing care to allow child uninterrupted rest periods.

Assist with activities of daily living, ambulation, and repositioning, as needed.

Assist in choosing play activities appropriate for child's energy level.

Assist child with slowly increasing activity level, as indicated.

Encourage parents to assist their child with certain activities.

If indicated, administer antipyretics or analgesics on schedule. Record effectiveness.

🏠 Assess and record child's/family's knowledge of and participation in care regarding

identification of any signs of activity intolerance (such as those listed under **Characteristics**).
alterations in activities of daily living, ambulation, repositioning, and play to correspond to child's activity level.

🏠 Instruct child/family in any areas needing improvement. Record results.

EVALUATION FOR CHARTING

Describe any signs of activity intolerance noted (such as those listed under **Characteristics**).

State range of baseline and activity vital signs.

State whether child was able to have uninterrupted rest periods during the shift.

🏠 Describe child's ability to participate in activities of daily living, repositioning, ambulation, and play.

🏠 Describe parents' involvement in child's care. Describe child's response.

Describe any therapeutic measures used to gradually increase the child's activity tolerance. State their effectiveness.

🏠 Describe child's/family's knowledge of and participation in care related to the child's activity intolerance. State any areas needing improvement and information provided. Describe child's/family's responses.

RELATED NURSING DIAGNOSES

Actual Infection* *related to*

invasion of the endocardium by bacterial or non-bacterial agents

Ineffective Breathing Pattern *related to*

a. decreased cardiac output
b. congenital heart defect

Altered Level of Consciousness* *related to*

a. cerebral abscesses
b. emboli

Anxiety: Parental *related to*

a. lengthy hospitalization of child
b. activity intolerance of child
c. uncertain prognosis for child
d. potential serious complications

*Non-NANDA diagnosis.

MEDICAL DIAGNOSIS

Rheumatic Fever

PATHOPHYSIOLOGY Acute rheumatic fever (ARF) is a systemic inflammatory disease that occurs following an upper respiratory infection by group A beta-hemolytic streptococcus. It is unclear as to how the antecedent streptococcal infection leads to ARF. Some theorize that it is a type of autoimmune process. *Streptococci* and normal connective tissues, such as those found in the myocardium, have similar antigen-determinant sites. The body's immune system produces antibodies that begin to destroy the invading *Streptococci* but also destroy the normal cells found in connective tissue. This results in inflammation at the site of tissue destruction. The inflammatory process causes lymphocytes and plasma cells to infiltrate cardiac tissue and joints. Inflamed joints—large joints, such as the knees, elbows, hips, shoulders, and wrists—become red, warm, and extremely painful. This joint inflammation (arthritis) is reversible and migratory in nature. Inflammatory lesions, called Aschoff's bodies, form in the heart and produce swelling and alteration in the connective tissue. Most commonly affected are the mitral and aortic valves. Children who develop carditis during the initial attack may sustain sequelae, depending on the severity of the carditis.

Diagnosis is usually based on the modified Jones criteria. Acute rheumatic fever is suspected if a child manifests two major or one major and two minor criteria and if there is evidence of a recent group A beta-hemolytic streptococcal infection. Major manifestations include carditis, polyarthritis, subcutaneous nodules, erythema marginatum, and chorea. Minor manifestations are fever, arthralgia, previous history of ARF, prolonged P–R interval on EKG, leukocytosis, elevated erythrocyte sedimentation rate, and positive C-reactive protein.

Acute rheumatic fever can occur in children of all ages, but it primarily affects those between 5 and 15 years of age. Adequate treatment of group A beta-hemolytic streptococcal upper respiratory infections with antibiotics will prevent ARF.

PRIMARY NURSING DIAGNOSIS
Decreased Cardiac Output

DEFINITION   Decrease in the amount of blood that leaves the left ventricle

POSSIBLY RELATED TO

Inflammation and destruction of the connective tissue in the myocardium

Scarring and stenosis of heart valves (usually mitral and/or aortic)

Backflow or regurgitation of blood through heart valves (mitral or aortic insufficiency)

CHARACTERISTICS

Tachycardia

Murmurs

Fever

EKG changes, prolonged P–R interval

Signs of right heart failure (e.g., hepatomegaly, edema, distended neck veins)

Cardiomegaly revealed on chest x-ray

Chest pain

Pericardial friction rub

EXPECTED OUTCOMES   Child will maintain an adequate cardiac output as evidenced by

heart rate within acceptable range (state specific highest and lowest rates for each child).

normal sinus rhythm.

temperature within acceptable range of 36.5° C to 37.2° C.

appropriate heart size on chest x-ray.

absence of

chest pain.
pericardial friction rub.
edema.
hepatomegaly.
distended neck veins.

POSSIBLE NURSING INTERVENTIONS

Assess and record the following every 2 to 4 hours and PRN:

heart rate and temperature.

signs/symptoms of decreased cardiac output (such as those listed under **Characteristics**).

Evaluate and record results of EKG strips.

Check and record results of chest x-ray, when indicated.

Ensure maintenance of bedrest or periods of rest alternating with passive activities.

Organize nursing care to allow child uninterrupted rest periods.

Administer salicylates (aspirin) on schedule. Assess and record effectiveness and any signs/symptoms of toxicity (e.g., tinnitus, GI disturbance, headache, irritability, ketosis).

Administer steroids (prednisone) on schedule. Assess and record effectiveness and any side effects (e.g., sodium retention, fluid retention, potassium loss).

If indicated, administer antibiotics on schedule. Assess and record effectiveness and any side effects (e.g., rash, diarrhea).

Assess and record child's/family's knowledge of and participation in care regarding

medication administration; need for prophylactic antibiotic therapy.
maintenance of sufficient rest periods.
identification of any signs/symptoms of decreased cardiac output (such as those listed under **Characteristics**).

Instruct child/family in any areas needing improvement. Record results.

EVALUATION FOR CHARTING

State highest and lowest heart rates and temperatures.

Describe cardiac rhythm.

Describe any signs/symptoms of decreased cardiac output noted (such as those listed under **Characteristics**).

Document EKG interpretation.

State results of chest x-ray, when indicated.

Indicate whether bedrest (or rest periods) were sufficiently maintained.

Indicate whether medications were administered on schedule. Describe effectiveness and any side effects noted.

State salicylate levels. If levels were out of the acceptable range, describe any corrective measures implemented.

Describe child's/family's knowledge of and participation in care related to maintaining an adequate cardiac output. State any areas needing improvement and information provided. Describe child's/family's responses.

NURSING DIAGNOSIS
Altered Comfort*

DEFINITION Condition in which an individual experiences discomfort

POSSIBLY RELATED TO
Joint tenderness
Chest pain
Dyspnea

CHARACTERISTICS
Swollen, red, warm joints
Verbal communication of pain or tenderness
Crying unrelieved by usual comfort measures
Moaning
Facial grimacing
Physical signs/symptoms:

tachycardia
tachypnea/bradypnea
increased blood pressure
diaphoresis
restlessness

EXPECTED OUTCOMES Child will be free of severe and/or constant discomfort as evidenced by

decrease in swelling, redness, and warmness of joints.
verbal communication of comfort.
lack of constant crying or moaning.
lack of facial expression of discomfort.

---

*Non–NANDA diagnosis.

heart rate within acceptable range (state specific highest and lowest rates for each child).

respiratory rate within acceptable range (state specific highest and lowest rates for each child).

blood pressure within acceptable range (state specific highest and lowest pressures for each child).

lack of diaphoresis and extreme restlessness. ·

POSSIBLE NURSING INTERVENTIONS

Assess and record any signs/symptoms of discomfort (such as those listed under **Characteristics**) at least once/shift.

Handle child gently.

Administer salicylates (aspirin) on schedule. Assess and record effectiveness and any signs/symptoms of toxicity (e.g., tinnitus, GI disturbance, headache, irritability, ketosis).

Encourage family members to stay and comfort child when possible.

If indicated, perform limited passive range-of-motion exercises to help increase comfort.

Use diversional activities (e.g., music, television), when appropriate.

If indicated, use a bed cradle and heat to increase comfort.

Assess and record child's/family's knowledge of and participation in care regarding

medication administration.
passive range-of-motion exercises.
appropriate diversional activities.

Instruct child/family in any areas needing improvement. Record results.

EVALUATION FOR CHARTING

State range of vital signs.

Describe any signs/symptoms of discomfort.

Indicate whether medications were administered on schedule. Describe effectiveness and any side effects noted.

State salicylate levels. If levels were out of the acceptable range, describe any corrective measures implemented.

Describe any successful measures used to reduce discomfort.

Describe child's/family's knowledge of and participation in care related to alleviating discomfort. State any areas needing improvement and information provided. Describe child's/family's responses.

RELATED NURSING DIAGNOSES

Activity Intolerance *related to*

a. joint inflammation
b. cardiac inflammation

Injury: High Risk *related to*
involuntary movements of the muscles in the extremities

Knowledge Deficit: Child/Family *related to*

a. disease process
b. continuing home management (including medications and limited activity)

Body Image Disturbance *related to*
side effects of steroids

Two

CARE OF CHILDREN WITH ENDOCRINE DYSFUNCTION

Diabetes Insipidus

PATHOPHYSIOLOGY   Children with diabetes insipidus either lack antidiuretic hormone (ADH) or have decreased renal responsiveness to ADH. Central or neurogenic diabetes insipidus results from decreased production of ADH. Incomplete formation of the pituitary gland may cause central diabetes insipidus. Central nervous system insults, including head trauma, infections, intracranial lesions, and brain surgery, may also cause central diabetes insipidus, which can be transient. In nephrogenic diabetes insipidus, an X-linked, recessive genetic defect, the kidneys are unresponsive to ADH.

Antidiuretic hormone, which is produced in the hypothalamus, is stored and released from the posterior pituitary gland. Normally the body is able to conserve water when the distal renal tubules respond to ADH stimulation. When circulating ADH levels are low or when the kidneys are not responsive to normal levels of ADH, collecting tubules do not reabsorb free water; instead the water is lost in the urine. Interstitial and intracellular water is pulled into the intravascular space and lost in the urine as well. This water loss occurs even in the presence of increased serum osmolality and hypovolemia, resulting in hypernatremia.

Children with diabetes insipidus experience polyuria and polydipsia, usually preferring water to quench their excessive thirst. Significant dehydration can occur if the child is unable to maintain adequate fluid intake.

PRIMARY NURSING DIAGNOSIS
Fluid Volume Deficit

DEFINITION   Decrease in the amount of circulating fluid volume

POSSIBLY RELATED TO
Polyuria secondary to

lack of ADH
kidneys unresponsive to ADH

CHARACTERISTICS
Polyuria
Polydipsia
Nocturia
Enuresis
Intense thirst and preference for water
Dilute urine, specific gravity less than 1.008
Weight loss
Poor skin turgor
Dry mucous membranes
Sunken fontanel
Decreased urine osmolality (less than 280 mOsm/L)
Increased serum sodium (greater than 145 mEq/L, usually
     160 to 200 mEq/L)
Increased serum osmolality (greater than 300 mOsm/L)
Decreased urine sodium (less than 130 mEq/24 hr)
Tachycardia, hypotension
Cool extremities
Weak peripheral pulses
Prolonged capillary refill, longer than 2 to 3 seconds
Irritability

EXPECTED OUTCOMES   Child will have adequate fluid
volume as evidenced by

adequate fluid intake, IV and/or oral (state specific amount
     of intake needed for each child).
adequate urine output (state specific highest and lowest
     outputs for each child, minimum 1 to 2 ml/kg/hr).
urine specific gravity from 1.008 to 1.020.
urine osmolality from 500 to 800 mOsm/L.
serum osmolality from 280 to 295 mOsm/L.
serum sodium from 138 to 145 mEq/L.
urine sodium from 130 to 200 mEq/24 hr.
moist mucous membranes.
rapid skin recoil.
heart rate and blood pressure within acceptable ranges (state
     specific highest and lowest parameters for each child).

lack of signs/symptoms of fluid volume deficit (such as those listed under **Characteristics**).

POSSIBLE NURSING INTERVENTIONS

Keep accurate record of intake and output.

Administer oral and IV fluids as ordered, including urine output replacement. Intravenous fluids with low sodium (1/16 to 1/8 normal saline) and low glucose (2.5%) concentrations may be used.

Assess and record

heart rate and blood pressure every 4 hours.
IV fluids and condition of IV site every hour.
signs/symptoms of fluid volume deficit (such as those listed under **Characteristics**) every 4 hours and PRN.
laboratory values, as indicated. Report any abnormalities to the physician.

Check and record urine specific gravity every 4 hours or as indicated.

Weigh child on same scale at same time each day.

Assist with water deprivation testing.

Administer vasopressin on schedule by the prescribed route. Assess and record effectiveness and side effects (e.g., abdominal cramping and tachycardia/bradycardia or other signs of hypersensitivity).

🏠 Assess and record child's/family's knowledge of and participation in care regarding

monitoring of child's intake and output.
identification of any signs/symptoms of fluid volume deficit (such as those listed under **Characteristics**).
medication administration.

🏠 Instruct child/family in any areas needing improvement. Record results.

EVALUATION FOR CHARTING

State intake and output.

Describe any signs/symptoms of fluid volume deficit noted (such as those listed under **Characteristics**).

State highest and lowest urine specific gravity values.

State condition of IV site.

State child's current weight and indicate whether it has increased or decreased since previous weighing.

Describe status of mucous membranes and skin turgor.

Describe any therapeutic measures used to maintain adequate fluid volume. State their effectiveness.

State whether vasopressin was given on schedule. Describe effectiveness and side effects.

⌂ Describe child's/family's knowledge of and participation in care related to maintaining adequate fluid volume. State any areas needing improvement and information provided. Describe child's/family's responses.

NURSING DIAGNOSIS
Electrolyte Imbalance: Sodium Excess*

DEFINITION   Disturbance in the level of the body's sodium

POSSIBLY RELATED TO
Polyuria secondary to

lack of ADH
unresponsiveness of kidneys to ADH

CHARACTERISTICS
Increased serum sodium (greater than 145 mEq/L, usually
160 to 200 mEq/L)
Lethargy
Dry mucous membranes
Flushed skin
Intense thirst
Seizures
Coma

EXPECTED OUTCOMES   Child will have adequate sodium balance as evidenced by

serum sodium from 138 to 145 mEq/L.

_____
*Non−NANDA diagnosis.

appropriate level of consciousness for age.

moist mucous membranes.

lack of signs/symptoms of sodium excess (such as those listed under **Characteristics**).

POSSIBLE NURSING INTERVENTIONS

Assess and record

signs/symptoms of sodium excess (such as those listed under **Characteristics**) every 4 hours and PRN.

neurological vital signs every 4 hours and PRN.

laboratory values, as indicated. Report abnormalities to the physician.

Administer oral and IV fluids as ordered, including urine output replacement. Intravenous fluids with low sodium (1/16 to 1/8 normal saline) and low glucose (2.5%) concentrations may be used.

Administer vasopressin on schedule by the prescribed route. Assess and record effectiveness and side effects (e.g., abdominal cramping and tachycardia/bradycardia or other signs of hypersensitivity).

Keep accurate record of intake and output.

Provide mouth care every 4 hours and PRN.

🏠 Assess and record child's/family's knowledge of and participation in care regarding

monitoring of child's intake and output.

identification of any signs/symptoms of sodium excess (such as those listed under **Characteristics**).

medication administration.

🏠 Instruct child/family in areas needing improvement. Record results.

EVALUATION FOR CHARTING

Describe child's neurological status.

State current laboratory values.

Describe any signs/symptoms of sodium excess noted (such as those listed under **Characteristics**).

State intake and output.

Describe any therapeutic measures used to correct sodium excess. State their effectiveness.

State whether vasopressin was given on schedule. Describe effectiveness and side effects.

⌂ Describe child's/family's knowledge of and participation in care related to maintaining adequate fluid volume. State any areas needing improvement and information provided. Describe child's/family's responses.

RELATED NURSING DIAGNOSES

Altered Level of Consciousness* *related to* hypernatremia

Decreased Cardiac Output *related to* circulatory compromise secondary to severe fluid volume deficit

Altered Parenting *related to*
a. child's hospitalization
b. child's need for chronic medication administration
c. knowledge deficit

Compromised Family Coping *related to*
a. underlying disease state
b. knowledge deficit

---

*Non–NANDA diagnosis.

Diabetes Mellitus

PATHOPHYSIOLOGY The most common endocrine disease of childhood is diabetes mellitus. In the child with this chronic disease, insulin-producing beta cells in the pancreatic islets of Langerhans have been destroyed or reduced in number, creating a deficiency in insulin. This adversely affects carbohydrate, protein, and fat metabolism.

Glucose is the primary energy source for most cells. Insulin facilitates the uptake of intravascular glucose by muscle and fat cells, facilitates the storage of glucose (as glycogen) in the liver and muscle cells, and indirectly prevents fat metabolism. Insufficient insulin leads to hyperglycemia because intravascular glucose is unable to enter the cells. The liver responds to lack of intracellular glucose by initiating gluconeogenesis and glycogenolysis, further contributing to the hyperglycemia. This hyperglycemia causes an osmotic diuresis, leading to excessive water loss, electrolyte imbalance, and, eventually, dehydration.

The inability of glucose to enter the cells triggers catabolism. In this process, the body uses fat and protein for energy, and despite increased food intake, weight loss occurs. When fat is used for energy, the liver converts the increased free fatty acids in the blood to ketone bodies. The circulating ketone bodies accumulate in substantial numbers, altering the serum pH, resulting in ketoacidosis. During acidosis, total body potassium can be significantly decreased. Signs of the rise in acetone and ketoacid levels are a fruity breath, Kussmaul breathing, abdominal pains, and vomiting. Once vomiting begins, the excessive fluid losses can no longer be balanced by increased intake, and the child's condition can quickly deteriorate.

The classic presentation of diabetes in children includes a history of polyuria, polydipsia, polyphagia, and weight loss. Many children present initially with ketoacidosis. The child with diabetic ketoacidosis (DKA) presents with the classic signs and symptoms and also with hyperglycemia (glucose greater than 300 mg/dL), ketonemia, acidosis (pH less than 7.30, bicarbonate less than 15 mEq/L), glucosuria, and ketonuria.

Acute treatment of diabetes focuses on returning the child to a balanced metabolic state. Long-term treatment attempts to promote normal growth and development and emphasizes independence and self-management in order to reduce adverse psychosocial effects. Treatment includes child/family education on self blood glucose monitoring, insulin administration, diet, exercise, and hyperglycemia/hypoglycemia management.

PRIMARY NURSING DIAGNOSIS
Altered Metabolic Function*

DEFINITION Imbalance or altered utilization of specific body biochemicals

POSSIBLY RELATED TO
> Insufficient insulin secondary to ineffective beta cells in pancreatic islets
> Increased insulin requirements secondary to infection, stress, and/or illness
> Unstable serum glucose levels

CHARACTERISTICS
> Hyperglycemia, hypoglycemia, or fluctuating blood glucose levels
> Signs/symptoms of hyperglycemia (slow onset):
>> polyuria
>> polydipsia
>> polyphagia
>> weight loss
>> enuresis in a previously toilet-trained child
>> lethargy or stupor
>> warm, flushed, dry skin
>> weakness
>> nausea/vomiting
>> acetone (fruity) breath
>> abdominal pain
>> Kussmaul breathing
>> dehydration

---

*Non−NANDA diagnosis.

glucosuria
ketonuria
metabolic acidosis

Signs/symptoms of hypoglycemia (rapid onset):
excessive sweating
faintness
dizziness
poor coordination
pallor
cool skin
pounding of heart
trembling
impaired vision
personality changes
irritability
headache
hunger
inability to awaken

EXPECTED OUTCOMES   Child will maintain adequate metabolic function as evidenced by

stable blood glucose level from 70 to 180 mg/dL.
lack of signs/symptoms of hyperglycemia (such as those listed under **Characteristics**).
lack of signs/symptoms of hypoglycemia (such as those listed under **Characteristics**).

POSSIBLE NURSING INTERVENTIONS
Assess and record

vital signs and neurological status every 1 to 4 hours and PRN.
blood glucose levels as ordered and PRN. Fasting, preprandial, peak postprandial, and 3 A.M. blood glucose levels may be needed. Assist child/family with self-blood glucose monitoring PRN.
signs/symptoms of hyperglycemia or hypoglycemia (such as those listed under **Characteristics**) every 2 to 4 hours and PRN.
IV fluids and condition of IV site every hour.

Maintain diabetic flow sheet. Include blood glucose levels, insulin dose, injection site, clinical observations, urine test results, and intake and output.

Keep accurate record of intake and output.

Weigh child on same scale at same time each day.

Administer IV maintenance and replacement fluids and supplements (potassium, bicarbonate) as indicated. (If child is in DKA, bolus with normal saline or Ringer's lactate, followed by an isotonic solution over 24 hours. Add dextrose to the IV fluids when the plasma glucose approaches 300 mg/dL. Attempt to maintain plasma glucose concentrations from 200 to 300 mg/dL). Assess and record child's response.

When indicated, administer insulin drip following institutional policies for solution and tubing changes and use of a pump. (If child is in DKA, start with regular insulin 0.1 U/kg IV push, followed by regular insulin 50 units in 500 ml half-normal saline to run at 1 ml/kg/hr, which equals 0.1 U/kg/hr). Adjust insulin drip as indicated. Assess and record child's response.

When indicated, administer subcutaneous insulin on schedule. Assess and record effectiveness.

If child is hypoglycemic, administer orange juice (4 oz), regular soda (4 oz), or glucose tablets to provide approximately 10 grams of carbohydrate or 40 calories. Repeat if child does not feel better in 10 to 15 minutes. If severe hypoglycemia occurs and the child is unable to swallow, administer glucagon, as indicated. Assess and record child's response.

🏠 Assess and record child's/family's knowledge of and participation in care regarding

> glucose monitoring.
> insulin dosage adjustment.
> insulin administration and site rotation.
> diet and exercise.
> identification of any signs/symptoms of hyperglycemia or hypoglycemia and the correct action for each.

🏠 Instruct child/family in any areas needing improvement. Record results.

EVALUATION FOR CHARTING
State highest and lowest blood glucose levels and urine test results.

Describe any signs/symptoms of hyperglycemia or hypoglycemia noted (such as those listed under **Characteristics**).

Describe any therapeutic measures used to correct hyperglycemia or hypoglycemia. State effectiveness of measures.

State intake and output.

State child's current weight and indicate whether it has increased or decreased since previous weighing.

State condition of IV site.

🏠 Describe child's/family's knowledge of and participation in care related to maintaining adequate metabolic function. State any areas needing improvement and information provided. Describe child's/family's responses.

NURSING DIAGNOSIS
Fluid Volume Deficit

DEFINITION   Decrease in the amount of circulating fluid volume

POSSIBLY RELATED TO
Osmotic diuresis secondary to hyperglycemia
Vomiting
Decreased oral intake

CHARACTERISTICS
Polyuria
Flushed, dry skin
Dry mucous membranes
Poor skin turgor
Weight loss
Tachycardia
Hypotension
Lack of tears

EXPECTED OUTCOMES   Child will have an adequate fluid volume as evidenced by

adequate fluid intake, IV or oral (state specific amount for each child).

adequate urine output (state specific highest and lowest
outputs for each child, minimum 1 to 2 ml/kg/hr).
moist mucous membranes.
rapid skin recoil.
lack of weight loss.
heart rate and blood pressure within acceptable ranges (state
specific highest and lowest parameters for each child).

POSSIBLE NURSING INTERVENTIONS
Keep accurate record of intake and output.

Administer IV maintenance and replacement fluids and
supplements (potassium, bicarbonate), as indicated. (If child
is in DKA, bolus with normal saline or Ringer's lactate,
followed by an isotonic solution over 24 hours. Add dextrose
to the IV fluids when the plasma glucose approaches 300
mg/dL. Attempt to maintain plasma glucose concentrations
from 200 to 300 mg/dL). Assess and record child's response.

Assess and record

condition of IV site every hour.
signs/symptoms of fluid volume deficit (such as those listed
under **Characteristics**).
heart rate and blood pressure every 2 to 4 hours and
PRN.

Provide mouth care every 4 hours and PRN.

Weigh child on same scale at same time each day.

EVALUATION FOR CHARTING
State intake and output.

State type of IV fluids used and describe condition of IV site.

Describe status of mucous membranes and skin turgor.

State highest and lowest heart rates and blood pressures.

State child's current weight and indicate whether it has
increased or decreased since previous weighing.

Describe any therapeutic measures used to maintain adequate
fluid volume. State their effectiveness.

NURSING DIAGNOSIS

Electrolyte Imbalance: Sodium Losses and Potassium Losses*

DEFINITION   Disturbance in the level of the body's sodium and potassium

POSSIBLY RELATED TO

Sodium losses secondary to vomiting and osmotic diuresis
Temporarily increased extracellular potassium (false high) secondary to

acidosis
insulin deficiency
dehydration

Potassium losses secondary to

polyuria
insulin administration
dilution resulting from rehydration
correction of acidosis (potassium reenters the cell)

CHARACTERISTICS

Hyponatremia, with the following signs/symptoms:

weakness
delirium

Hyperkalemia, with the following signs/symptoms:

EKG changes: spiked T waves, widened QRS complexes, flattened P waves, ectopic beats
weakness
flushed skin

Hypokalemia, with the following signs/symptoms:

EKG changes: flattened T waves, peaked P waves, ectopic beats
hypotension and rapid pulse
coma

EXPECTED OUTCOMES   Child will maintain adequate electrolyte balance as evidenced by

---

*Non–NANDA diagnosis.

serum sodium from 138 to 145 mEq/L.
serum potassium from 3.5 to 5.0 mEq/L.
normal sinus rhythm and EKG configuration.
lack of signs/symptoms of electrolyte imbalance (such as
    those listed under **Characteristics**).

POSSIBLE NURSING INTERVENTIONS
Assess and record

heart rate and blood pressure every 2 to 4 hours and
    PRN.
signs/symptoms of electrolyte imbalance (such as those
    listed under **Characteristics**) every 4 hours and PRN.
IV fluids and condition of IV site every hour.
laboratory values as indicated. Report abnormalities to the
    physician.

When indicated, initiate use of a cardiac monitor. Evaluate
and record results of EKG strips at least once/shift.

Ensure that proper supplements are added to IV fluids.

EVALUATION FOR CHARTING
State highest and lowest heart rates and blood pressures.

Document EKG interpretation.

Describe any signs/symptoms of electrolyte imbalance noted
(such as those listed under **Characteristics**).

State current laboratory values.

Describe condition of IV site.

Describe any therapeutic measures used to restore electrolyte
balance. State their effectiveness.

RELATED NURSING DIAGNOSES

Knowledge Deficit: Child/Parental *related to*
a. newly diagnosed illness
b. child/family request for information
c. child/family statements of misinformation
d. noncompliance with child's treatment
e. mismanagement of child's illness
f. anxiety regarding care regimen

Altered Nutrition: Less than Body Requirements
related to
    weight loss despite polyphagia secondary to catabolic state

Compromised Family Coping *related to*
a. newly diagnosed chronic illness
b. need for continual monitoring of blood glucose, urine acetone, diet, and exercise on a daily basis
c. fluctuating blood glucose despite compliance with treatment
d. frequent hospitalizations
e. lack of support or financial resources
f. stress of child's chronic illness on family

Syndrome of Inappropriate Secretion of Antidiuretic Hormone

PATHOPHYSIOLOGY The syndrome of inappropriate secretion of antidiuretic hormone (SIADH) occurs with an excessive or increased secretion of antidiuretic hormone (ADH). Normally ADH is released from the posterior pituitary gland in response to the physiological stimuli of hypovolemia or increased serum osmotic pressure (hyperosmolality), but in SIADH this is not the case. The increased ADH levels in SIADH often involve an abnormal response of the intracranial osmoreceptors of the hypothalamus. Decreased venous return may also stimulate thoracic volume receptors, resulting in water retention and hyponatremia.

The inappropriate or excessive secretion of ADH results in increased reabsorption of water from the renal tubules. This causes intravascular fluid overload, and the fluid then shifts into the intracellular space. Characteristics of SIADH are serum hypoosmolality and hyponatremia associated with urine hyperosmolality and high urine sodium levels. Clinical manifestations, consistent with water intoxication, improve with water restriction.

Syndrome of inappropriate secretion of antidiuretic hormone is associated with a number of clinical conditions, especially those involving the nervous system, such as meningitis, encephalitis, brain tumors and abscesses, Guillain-Barré syndrome, and seizures; it can also occur after neurosurgery. Syndrome of inappropriate secretion of antidiuretic hormone may also be a complication of pneumonia, tuberculosis, cystic fibrosis, perinatal asphyxia, repair of mitral valve insufficiency, use of positive pressure ventilators, and use of certain drugs, such as vincristine or vinblastine. Malignant tumors that ectopically produce ADH may cause SIADH as well. In many of these instances, SIADH can be a temporary condition.

PRIMARY NURSING DIAGNOSIS

Electrolyte Imbalance: Sodium Losses*

DEFINITION   Disturbance in the level of the body's sodium.

POSSIBLY RELATED TO
Excessive secretion of ADH resulting in

increased losses of sodium
increased intake of water

CHARACTERISTICS
Decreased serum sodium (usually less than 130 mEq/L)
Dilutional hypokalemia or normal potassium
Loss of appetite
Nausea
Vomiting
Headache
Irritability
Lethargy
Muscle twitching

If serum sodium falls below 110 mEq/L: possible personality
changes, including hostility and confusion; possible
neurological abnormalities, such as stupor, seizures, and
coma.

EXPECTED OUTCOMES   Child will have adequate sodium
balance as evidenced by

serum sodium from 138 to 145 mEq/L.
serum potassium from 3.5 to 5.0 mEq/L.
adequate urine output (state specific highest and lowest
outputs for each child, minimum 1 to 2 ml/kg/hr).
appropriate level of consciousness for age.
lack of nausea/vomiting.
lack of signs/symptoms of decreased serum sodium (such as
those listed under **Characteristics**).

POSSIBLE NURSING INTERVENTIONS
Assess and record

signs/symptoms of decreased serum sodium (such as those
listed under **Characteristics**) every 4 hours and PRN.

*Non-NANDA diagnosis.

neurological vital signs every 4 hours and PRN.

IV fluids and condition of IV site every hour.

laboratory values, as indicated. Record abnormalities and
notify the physician.

Keep accurate record of intake and output.

Restrict fluids, as indicated, and maintain negative water
balance. (Output should exceed intake.)

If serum sodium is very low, 3% saline with potassium
supplements, followed by a loop diuretic (such as Lasix),
may be indicated. Assess and record child's response.

EVALUATION FOR CHARTING

Describe child's neurological status.

Describe any signs/symptoms of decreased serum sodium
(such as those listed under **Characteristics.**)

State intake and output.

Describe condition of IV site.

State current laboratory values.

Describe any therapeutic measures used to restore serum
sodium balance. State their effectiveness.

NURSING DIAGNOSIS
Fluid Volume Excess

DEFINITION   Increase in the amount of circulating fluid volume
(which can eventually lead to interstitial or intracellular fluid overload)

POSSIBLY RELATED TO

Increased water reabsorption from renal tubules secondary to
excessive ADH secretion

CHARACTERISTICS

Decreased urine output
Decreased serum osmolality (less than 275 mOsm/L)
Decreased serum sodium (less than 130 mEq/L)
Increased urine osmolality (greater than 900 mOsm/L)
Urine osmolality inappropriately increased compared to
serum osmolality
Increased specific gravity (greater than 1.025)

Increased urine sodium
Positive water balance, with intake exceeding output
Edema
Sudden weight gain

EXPECTED OUTCOMES   Child will resume fluid balance as evidenced by

adequate urine output (state specific highest and lowest outputs for each child, minimum 1 to 2 ml/kg/hr).
serum sodium from 138 to 145 mEq/L.
serum osmolality from 280 to 295 mOsm/L.
urine osmolality from 500 to 800 mOsm/L (usually 1.5 to 3 times greater than serum osmolality).
urine specific gravity from 1.008 to 1.020.
lack of

sudden weight gain.
edema.

POSSIBLE NURSING INTERVENTIONS

Keep accurate record of intake and output.

Restrict fluid intake, as indicated, and maintain negative water balance, with output exceeding intake.

If serum sodium is very low, 3% saline with potassium supplements, followed by a loop diuretic (such as Lasix), may be indicated. Assess and record child's response.

Assess and record

signs/symptoms of fluid volume excess (such as those listed under **Characteristics**) every 4 hours and PRN.
laboratory values, as indicated. Report abnormalities to the physician.
IV fluid and condition of IV site every hour.

Check and record urine specific gravity every void or as ordered.

Weigh child on same scale at same time each day.

EVALUATION FOR CHARTING

State intake and output.

Describe any signs/symptoms of fluid volume excess noted (such as those listed under **Characteristics**).

State child's weight and indicate whether it has increased or decreased since previous weighing.

State current laboratory values.

State highest and lowest urine specific gravity values.

Describe condition of IV site.

RELATED NURSING DIAGNOSES

Altered Level of Consciousness* *related to*
cerebral edema secondary to hyponatremia resulting from increased intracellular fluid

Compromised Family Coping *related to*
child's underlying disease process

Knowledge Deficit: Child/Parental *related to*
a. child's underlying disease process
b. treatments and procedures

Body Image Disturbance *related to*
edema and sudden weight gain

---

*Non-NANDA diagnosis.

Three

CARE OF CHILDREN WITH FLUID AND ELECTROLYTE IMBALANCE

MEDICAL DIAGNOSIS

Burns

PATHOPHYSIOLOGY   Fire- and burn-related injuries are the second leading cause of accidental death in children under the age of 14. Thermal sources, electricity, chemical agents, and radioactive agents can all cause burn injuries.

Five interrelated factors are used to determine the severity of a burn: extent of the burn, depth of the burn, age of the child, medical history of the child, and part of the body burned. The extent of the burn injury is determined by estimating the percent of skin area covered by burns, accounting for the changing body proportions and body surface area of the growing child. The degree of involvement of the epidermis, dermis, and underlying structures determines the depth of the burn. In partial-thickness burns, only part of the skin has been damaged; in full-thickness burns, all skin layers are destroyed, including hair follicles, sweat glands, sebaceous glands, and nerves. Subcutaneous tissue, muscle, and bone may also be destroyed.

First- and second-degree burns are partial-thickness burns. In first-degree burns, the epidermis is damaged, resulting in redness, pain, and possibly edema. The wound blanches with pressure, and there is no blistering. In a second-degree burn, the injury involves the epidermis and extends into the dermis, resulting in a cherry red to glassy white appearance, edema, blister formation, exudate, severe pain, and possible damage to cutaneous nerve endings. With first- and second-degree burns, capillaries, hair follicles, sebaceous glands, and some protective functions usually remain intact. Most partial-thickness burns are able to heal by reepithelialization, especially if protected from further injury and infection.

Third- and fourth-degree burns are full-thickness burns. Third-degree burns vary in appearance from pearly white, tan, or brown to mahogany or black. Blisters are not present, and these burns are rarely painful because nerve endings have been damaged or destroyed. (Often, second-degree burns are also present with full-thickness burns; therefore, the child is not pain free). The tissue of a full-thickness burn is called *eschar*. Skin grafting is necessary as regeneration is not possible once the dermis and dermal structures are destroyed. Fourth-degree burns have the same characteristics as third-degree, but they extend into structures underlying the dermis, such as muscles, tendons, and bone.

Along with local pathological alterations, many systemic changes can occur as the body responds to a burn injury. Pulmonary, cardiovascular, metabolic, fluid and electrolyte, renal, gastrointestinal, and neurological problems can arise, as well as sepsis. Burned children under 4 years of age have a higher mortality rate than older children because they have a higher proportion of body surface area, a higher proportion of body fluid to mass, less effective cardiovascular responses to intravascular volume changes, and poor antibody response.

PRIMARY NURSING DIAGNOSIS
Fluid Volume Deficit

DEFINITION   Decrease in the amount of circulating fluid volume

POSSIBLY RELATED TO
Fluid loss from burn wound
Shift of plasma to interstitium

CHARACTERISTICS
Edema
Decreased urine output
Tachycardia
Hypotension
Increased urine specific gravity
Dry mucous membranes
Poor skin turgor

EXPECTED OUTCOMES   Child will have an adequate fluid volume as evidenced by

lack of edema.

adequate urine output (state specific highest and lowest outputs for each child, minimum 1 to 2 ml/kg/hr).

adequate fluid intake (state specific amount of PO and IV intake needed for each child).

heart rate and blood pressure within acceptable ranges (state specific highest and lowest parameters for each child).

urine specific gravity from 1.008 to 1.020.
moist mucous membranes.
rapid skin recoil.

POSSIBLE NURSING INTERVENTIONS

Keep accurate record of intake and output.

Assess and record

IV fluids and condition of IV site every hour.
heart rate and blood pressure every 4 hours and PRN.
signs/symptoms of fluid volume deficit (such as those listed
under **Characteristics**) every 4 hours and PRN.

Check and record urine specific gravity every void or as
indicated.

Weigh child on same scale at same time each day.

Provide mouth care every 4 hours and PRN.

⌂ Assess and record child's/family's knowledge of and
participation in care regarding

fluid intake.
monitoring of intake and output.
identification of any signs/symptoms of fluid volume
deficit (such as those listed under **Characteristics**).

⌂ Instruct child/family in any areas needing improvement.
Record results.

EVALUATION FOR CHARTING

State intake and output.

State type of IV fluids used and describe condition of IV site.

Describe status of mucous membranes and skin turgor.

State highest and lowest heart rates and blood pressures.

State child's current weight and indicate whether it has
increased or decreased since previous weighing.

Describe any therapeutic measures used to maintain adequate
fluid volume. State their effectiveness.

⌂ Describe child's/family's knowledge of and participation in
care related to improving fluid volume. State any areas

needing improvement and information provided. Describe child's/family's responses.

NURSING DIAGNOSIS
Pain

DEFINITION   Condition in which an individual experiences severe discomfort

POSSIBLY RELATED TO
>Thermal, electrical, chemical, or radioactive damage to or destruction of the skin and, sometimes, the underlying structures
>Burn dressing changes
>Exposed nerves

CHARACTERISTICS
>Crying or moaning
>Facial grimacing
>Verbal expression of pain
>Restlessness
>Guarding or protective behavior of burn site
>Physical signs/symptoms:

>>tachycardia
>>tachypnea
>>increased blood pressure

>Altered muscle tone (tenseness or listlessness)
>Rating of pain on pain-assessment tool

EXPECTED OUTCOMES   Child will have decreased pain or be free of pain as evidenced by

>lack of

>>crying or moaning.
>>facial grimacing.
>>restlessness.
>>guarding or protective behavior of burn site.
>>signs/symptoms of pain (such as those listed under **Characteristics**).

>heart rate, respiratory rate, and blood pressure within acceptable ranges (state specific highest and lowest parameters for each child).

verbal communication of comfort.

rating of decreased pain or no pain on pain-assessment tool.

POSSIBLE NURSING INTERVENTIONS

Assess and record any signs/symptoms of pain (such as those listed under **Characteristics**) every 2 to 4 hours. Use age-appropriate pain-assessment tool.

Handle child gently.

Administer analgesics and/or narcotics on schedule. Assess and record effectiveness.

Premedicate child as indicated before dressing changes, wound care, and treatments.

If age-appropriate, explain all procedures beforehand.

If age-appropriate, allow the child to participate in planning his or her care. Encourage the child to practice self-care (e.g. bathing, removing dressings).

Encourage family members to stay and comfort child when possible.

Allow family members to participate in care of child when possible.

When indicated, institute additional pain relief measures, such as relaxation, hypnosis, guided imagery, and music. Assess and record effectiveness.

Use diversional activities and distraction measures (e.g., toys, play activities, watching television, radio) when appropriate.

Assess and record child's/family's knowledge of and participation in care regarding

pain assessment.
use of additional pain relief measures.
administration of analgesics.

Instruct child/family in any areas needing improvement. Record results.

EVALUATION FOR CHARTING

Describe any signs/symptoms of pain noted (such as those listed under **Characteristics**).

State range of vital signs.

Describe any successful measures used to reduce or eliminate pain.

Describe effectiveness of analgesics and/or narcotics.

⌂ Describe child's/family's knowledge of and participation in care related to child's pain. State any areas needing improvement and information provided. Describe child's/family's responses.

RELATED NURSING DIAGNOSES

Infection: High Risk *related to*
   a. impaired skin integrity
   b. decreased resistance

Impaired Skin Integrity *related to*
   thermal, electrical, chemical, or radioactive injury

Impaired Physical Mobility *related to*
   a. pain
   b. dressings and splints

Compromised Family Coping *related to*
   a. guilt
   b. hospitalization of child
   c. scar formation

MEDICAL DIAGNOSIS

Diarrhea and Dehydration

PATHOPHYSIOLOGY   Diarrhea, an increase in the number, frequency, and fluidity of stools, can be either acute or chronic. Chronic diarrhea is defined as lasting longer than 2 weeks. Bowel habits vary considerably among individuals and must be considered when diagnosing diarrhea. Diarrhea has many different causes. Infection is a common one in children and can be either bacterial, viral, or parasitical. Others include food intolerance, such as an allergy to milk, ingestion of toxic substances, such as lead; drug intolerance, such as intolerance of antibiotics; bowel disease, such as Hirschsprung's disease; disaccharide deficiencies, such as deficiency of lactase; psychogenic factors, such as emotional stress; malabsorption, such as cystic fibrosis; and localized infections, such as otitis media.

Diarrhea results when contents are propelled through the intestines very rapidly, with little time for absorption of digested food, water, and electrolytes. The resultant stool is watery, is usually green, and contains undigested fats, undigested carbohydrates, and some undigested protein. Water loss can be up to ten times the normal rate. Electrolyte imbalance results, with losses of sodium, chloride, bicarbonate, and potassium.

When a viral infection is present, epithelial cells that line the intestinal tract are damaged and destroyed. The major cause of viral diarrhea is rotavirus. Bacterial infections can damage the intestinal mucosa in one of three ways: (1) organisms multiply and adhere to the mucosa, releasing an enterotoxin that interacts with the bowel mucosa and causes active water and electrolyte secretion; (2) in an inflammatory process, organisms invade the cells in the epithelium; or (3) organisms penetrate the gut wall and multiply intracellularly. Many organisms are responsible for bacterial diarrhea, including *Campylocbacter, Yersinia, Shigella, Salmonella, Staphylococcus aureus,* and *Escherichia coli.* One of the most common parasitic agents to cause diarrhea in children is *Giardia lamblia.*

Age, general health, climate, and environment are factors that can affect an individual's predisposition to diarrhea. Young children and children who are malnourished are more susceptible than others. Warm weather tends to make dehydration worse, and some organisms that cause diarrhea are more prevalent in warmer weather. Diarrhea also occurs more frequently where sanitation and refrigeration are problems and under crowded, substandard living conditions. Severe diarrhea is most common in infants and usually requires hospitalization.

The categorization of diarrhea can be related to the location in which it occurs along the alimentary tract. Inflammation of the stomach and intestines is called gastroenteritis; inflammation of the small intestines is enteritis; inflammation of the small intestines and colon is enterocolitis; and inflammation of the colon is colitis.

PRIMARY NURSING DIAGNOSIS
Fluid Volume Deficit

DEFINITION   Decrease in the amount of circulating fluid volume

POSSIBLY RELATED TO
An infection:

> systemic (from a virus, bacteria, or a parasite)
> local (e.g., otitis media or a urinary tract infection)

Food intolerance (e.g., mild allergy)
Drug intolerance (e.g., intolerance of antibiotics)
Inflammatory bowel disease (e.g., ulcerative colitis)
Malabsorption (e.g., cystic fibrosis)
Psychogenic factors (e.g., stress)

CHARACTERISTICS
Loose, watery stools (can be yellow or green and may
    contain mucus, pus, blood, and/or sugar)
Vomiting
Abdominal cramping
Abdominal distention
Hyperactive bowel sounds
Weight loss
Sunken fontanel
Sunken eyeballs
Dry mucous membranes
Poor skin turgor

Decreased urine output
Increased urine specific gravity
Fever

EXPECTED OUTCOMES   Infant will have an adequate fluid volume as evidenced by

adequate fluid intake, IV and/or oral (state specific amount of intake needed for each infant).
absence of

diarrhea.
mucus, pus, blood, and sugar in stool.
vomiting.
abdominal cramping and distention.
sunken eyeballs.

normal activity of bowel sounds (one every 10 to 30 seconds).
regaining of weight lost during illness.
flat fontanel.
rapid skin recoil.
adequate urine output (state specific highest and lowest outputs for each infant, minimum 1 to 2 ml/kg/hr).
urine specific gravity from 1.008 to 1.020.
temperature within acceptable range of 36.5°C to 37.2°C.

POSSIBLE NURSING INTERVENTIONS
Keep accurate record of intake and output. Weigh diapers for urine and stool output. Record frequency, color, odor, and consistency of stool. Measure and record amount and characteristics of any vomitus.

Assess and record

IV fluids and condition of IV site every hour.
bowel sounds every shift and PRN.
temperature every 4 hours and PRN.
signs/symptoms of fluid volume deficit (such as those listed under **Characteristics**) every 4 hours and PRN.

Weigh infant on same scale at same time each day without clothes.

Give mouth care every 4 hours and PRN.

Check and record urine specific gravity every 4 hours or as directed.

Report any of the following to the physician:

frequent stooling (more than three times/shift)
large amounts of vomitus
IV fluids infiltrated and unable to restart

🏠 Assess and record family's knowledge of and participation in care regarding

infant's need for appropriate fluids, when indicated.
need to offer infant a pacifier for comfort, when appropriate (especially if infant is NPO).
follow-up diet at home; when to reintroduce milk and solid foods.
monitoring of intake and output.
identification of any signs/symptoms of fluid volume deficit (such as those listed under **Characteristics**).

🏠 Instruct family in any areas needing improvement. Record results.

EVALUATION FOR CHARTING

State intake and output.

Describe condition of IV site.

State highest and lowest temperatures.

Describe any signs/symptoms of fluid volume deficit noted (such as those listed under **Characteristics**).

State highest and lowest urine specific gravity values.

Describe any therapeutic measures used to improve fluid volume deficit. State their effectiveness.

🏠 Describe family's knowledge of and participation in care related to improving fluid volume. State any areas needing improvement and information provided. Describe family's response.

NURSING DIAGNOSIS
Electrolyte Imbalance: Sodium Losses and Potassium Losses*

DEFINITION   Disturbance in the level of the body's sodium and potassium

---

*Non-NANDA diagnosis.

POSSIBLY RELATED TO
Frequent, loose, watery stools
Vomiting

CHARACTERISTICS
Hyponatremia

weakness
delirium
seizures

Hypokalemia

decreased muscle activity
EKG changes: flattened T waves, peaked P waves,
   ectopic beats
hypotension, rapid pulse
coma

EXPECTED OUTCOMES   Infant will maintain adequate
electrolyte balance as evidenced by

serum sodium from 138 to 145 mEq/L.
serum potassium from 3.5 to 5.0 mEq/L.
normal sinus rhythm and EKG configuration.
blood pressure within acceptable range (state highest and
   lowest pressures for each infant).
heart rate within acceptable range (state highest and
   lowest rates for each infant).
lack of signs/symptoms of electrolyte imbalance (such as
   those listed under **Characteristics**).

POSSIBLE NURSING INTERVENTIONS
Assess and record

heart rate and blood pressure every 4 hours and PRN.
laboratory values, as indicated. Report abnormalities to
   the physician.
signs/symptoms of electrolyte imbalance (such as those
   listed under **Characteristics**) every 4 hours and PRN.

Evaluate and record results of an EKG strip at least
once/shift.

EVALUATION FOR CHARTING
State highest and lowest heart rates and blood pressures.

Describe any signs/symptoms of electrolyte imbalance noted (such as those listed under **Characteristics**).

State current laboratory values.

Describe any therapeutic measures used to restore electrolyte balance. State their effectiveness.

NURSING DIAGNOSIS
Impaired Skin Integrity

DEFINITION   Interruption in integrity of the skin

POSSIBLY RELATED TO
Frequent perineal contact with acid stool
Superinfection of skin secondary to antibiotic therapy

CHARACTERISTICS
Discoloration of skin (reddened or shiny area)
Open or draining areas on skin

EXPECTED OUTCOMES   Infant will be free of signs/symptoms of impaired skin integrity as evidenced by

natural skin color of perineal area.
clean, intact skin.

POSSIBLE NURSING INTERVENTIONS
Bathe infant daily (or as indicated) with water. Use mild soap, when indicated.

Use lotion to moisturize infant's skin, when indicated. Lotion is contraindicated if a heat lamp is being used.

When indicated, apply a barrier ointment to perineal area after each diaper change. Change diapers and linens as soon as possible after elimination or soiling.

Treat any existing or potential breakdown area as soon as discovered by keeping area clean and dry and, if indicated, by exposing it to air.

🏠 Assess and record family's knowledge of and participation in care regarding

importance of keeping infant's perineal area clean and dry.
application of barrier medication.

identification of any signs/symptoms of impaired skin integrity (such as those listed under **Characteristics**).

🏠 Instruct family in any areas needing improvement.
Record results.

EVALUATION FOR CHARTING

Describe any potential or actual areas of skin breakdown.

Describe any therapeutic measures used to prevent or correct impaired skin integrity.

🏠 Describe family's knowledge of and participation in care related to improving infant's skin integrity. State any areas needing improvement and information provided. Describe family's response.

RELATED NURSING DIAGNOSES

Altered Nutrition: Less than Body Requirements
related to
   a. frequent, loose, watery stools
   b. vomiting

Decreased Cardiac Output *related to*
poor perfusion secondary to dehydration

Compromised Family Coping *related to*
hospitalization of infant

Four

CARE OF CHILDREN WITH GASTROINTESTINAL DYSFUNCTION

MEDICAL DIAGNOSIS
Appendicitis

PATHOPHYSIOLOGY The vermiform appendix is a blind sac located at the end of the cecum and serving no apparent function. Appendicitis, an inflammation of the vermiform appendix, is the most common surgical emergency of childhood, occurring most frequently in older children and adolescents. The walls of the appendix become inflamed when there is a physical obstruction of the lumen. This obstruction can be due to a hard, impacted mass of feces (fecalith) or to anatomic defects in the cecum. Obstruction leads to increased intraluminal pressure and distention, which causes compression and ischemia of the mucosal vessels. This compromised blood supply can lead to ulceration and bacterial invasion. Necrosis follows and can result in perforation, which allows feces and bacteria to escape and contaminate the peritoneal cavity and cause peritonitis. The signs and symptoms of appendicitis are diverse. They include periumbilical pain, later localized to the right upper quadrant; fever; vomiting; and reduced activity. The incidence of rupture is high—approximately 40% overall and more likely in the younger child. Treatment consists of laparotomy for removal of the appendix.

PREOPERATIVE NURSING CARE PLAN

PRIMARY NURSING DIAGNOSIS
Pain

DEFINITION Condition in which an individual experiences severe discomfort

POSSIBLY RELATED TO
  Inflammation
  Infection
  Pressure

CHARACTERISTICS

Verbal communication of pain

Crying unrelieved by usual comfort measures

Initially, generalized periumbilical pain

Later (a few hours), pain localized in the right lower
quadrant (McBurney's point)

Guarding of the abdomen

Tendency to lie quietly with the hips flexed (for infants)

Rebound tenderness

Decreased activity, self-imposed

Tenderness on rectal examination

Physical signs/symptoms:

tachycardia

tachypnea/bradypnea

increased blood pressure

diaphoresis

EXPECTED OUTCOMES   Child will be free of extreme pain
as evidenced by

verbal communication of decreased pain.

lack of constant crying.

heart rate within acceptable range (state specific highest and
lowest rates for each child).

respiratory rate within acceptable range (state specific highest
and lowest rates for each child).

blood pressure within acceptable range (state specific highest
and lowest pressures for each child).

decreased diaphoresis.

POSSIBLE NURSING INTERVENTIONS

Assess and record any signs/symptoms of pain (such as those
listed under **Characteristics**) every 2 hours and PRN.

Handle child gently. (Movement usually aggravates pain.)

Encourage family members to stay and comfort child when
possible.

Assess and record child's/family's knowledge of and
participation in care regarding preparation for impending
surgery.

Instruct child/family in any areas needing improvement.
Record results.

EVALUATION FOR CHARTING

State range of vital signs.

Describe characteristics of pain.

Describe any therapeutic measures used to decrease pain. State their effectiveness.

Describe child's/family's knowledge of and participation in care. State any areas needing improvement and information provided. Describe child's/family's responses.

NURSING DIAGNOSIS

Actual Infection*

DEFINITION   Condition in which microorganisms have invaded the body

POSSIBLY RELATED TO

Obstruction of the lumen leading to the appendix
Anatomic defect of the cecum

CHARACTERISTICS

Fever
Leukocytosis (usually not greater than 20,000 mm³)
Decreased activity, self-imposed
Listlessness
Decreased or absent bowel sounds
Vomiting
Diarrhea or constipation

EXPECTED OUTCOMES   Child will have decreased or stabilized signs/symptoms of infection as evidenced by

body temperature between 36.5°C and 38.4°C.

white blood cell count from 5,000 to 15,000 mm³.

stabilization of bowel sound activity.

decreased vomiting.

decreased diarrhea.

POSSIBLE NURSING INTERVENTIONS

Assess and record the following every 2 to 4 hours and PRN:

temperature

---

*Non-NANDA diagnosis.

signs/symptoms of infection (such as those listed under
Characteristics)

Maintain good hand-washing technique.

If indicated, ensure that child remains NPO.

Keep accurate record of intake and output. Record amount
and characteristics of any vomitus or diarrhea stools.

Check and record results of a complete blood count (CBC).
Notify physician if CBC results increase over previous
results.

If indicated, administer antibiotics on schedule and
antipyretics PRN. Assess and record effectiveness and any
side effects (e.g., rash, diarrhea.)

Position child in high Fowler's position if perforation is
possible.

EVALUATION FOR CHARTING
State highest and lowest temperatures.

Describe any signs/symptoms of infection (such as those
listed under **Characteristics**).

State intake and output. Describe characteristics of any
vomitus or diarrhea stools.

State results of CBC, if available.

State whether medications were administered on schedule.
Describe effectiveness and any side effects noted.

Describe any therapeutic measures used to treat the infection
and increase the child's level of comfort.

RELATED NURSING DIAGNOSES

Fear: Child *related to*
a. pain
b. hospitalization
c. unfamiliar surroundings
d. forced contact with strangers
e. treatments and procedures
f. impending surgery

Anxiety: Parental *related to*
a. pain experienced by child
b. outcome of surgery

Knowledge Deficit: Child/Family *related to*
a. care of child following surgery
b. misconception or inaccurate information concerning surgical procedure

Fluid Volume Deficit *related to*
a. vomiting
b. diarrhea

POSTOPERATIVE NURSING CARE PLAN

PRIMARY NURSING DIAGNOSIS

High Risk for Further Infection:*

DEFINITION   Condition in which the body is at risk for being invaded by additional microorganisms

POSSIBLY RELATED TO
Presence of invading organisms
Surgical wound
Compromised postoperative condition
Spread of organisms to peritoneum

CHARACTERISTICS
Fever
Redness
Swelling
Purulent wound drainage
Foul odor
Lethargy
Irritability
Altered white blood cell count (WBC)
Tachycardia

---

*Non-NANDA diagnosis.

EXPECTED OUTCOMES   Child will be free of infection as evidenced by

body temperature within the acceptable range of 36.5°C to 37.2°C.

clean wound site with minimal clear to serosanguineous drainage.

WBC within acceptable range (state specific highest and lowest counts for each child).

heart rate within acceptable range (state specific highest and lowest rates for each child).

lack of signs/symptoms of infection (such as those listed under **Characteristics**).

POSSIBLE NURSING INTERVENTIONS

Assess and record the following every 4 hours and PRN:

temperature and heart rate

any signs/symptoms of infection (such as those listed under **Characteristics**)

Maintain good hand-washing technique.

Ensure that wound care is done using aseptic technique. Assess and record amount and characteristics of drainage every 4 to 8 hours and PRN.

Obtain culture specimens (wound, blood) if indicated. Check results and notify physician of any abnormalities.

Check and record results of CBC. Notify physician if CBC results are out of the acceptable range.

Reposition child, as indicated. A low Fowler's position will help to localize infection and keep it from spreading upward.

Assist child with ambulation, as indicated.

Administer antibiotics on schedule and antipyretics PRN. Assess and record effectiveness and any side effects (e.g., rash, diarrhea).

Assess and record child's/family's knowledge of and participation in care regarding

medication administration.

incision site.

positioning in bed and gradual activity.

identification of any signs/symptoms of infection (such as those listed under **Characteristics**).

⌂ Instruct child/family in any areas needing improvement. Record results.

EVALUATION FOR CHARTING

State ranges of temperature and heart rate.

Describe wound site and amount and characteristics of any drainage.

State results of any cultures and/or CBCs, if available.

Describe any signs/symptoms of infection noted (such as those listed under **Characteristics**).

State whether antibiotics and antipyretics were administered on schedule. Describe effectiveness and any side effects noted.

State how often child was repositioned. Describe child's response to ambulation.

⌂ Describe child's/family's knowledge of and participation in care related to decreasing potential for further infection. State any areas needing improvement and information provided. Describe child's/family's response.

NURSING DIAGNOSIS
Fluid Volume Deficit

DEFINITION   Decrease in the amount of circulating fluid volume

POSSIBLY RELATED TO
Nausea/vomiting
Inability to tolerate PO fluids
Nasogastric suctioning
Third spacing of body fluid

CHARACTERISTICS
Tachycardia
Hypotension
Abdominal distention

Prolonged absence of bowel sounds
Nausea/vomiting
Dry mucous membranes
Poor skin turgor
Decreased urine output
Increased urine specific gravity

EXPECTED OUTCOMES   Child will have an adequate fluid volume as evidenced by

adequate IV fluid intake (state specific amount of intake needed for each child).
heart rate and blood pressure within acceptable range (state specific highest and lowest parameters for each child).
nondistended abdomen.
presence of bowel sounds.
absence of nausea/vomiting.
moist mucous membranes.
rapid skin recoil.
adequate urine output (state specific highest and lowest outputs for each child, minimum 1 to 2 ml/kg/hr).
urine specific gravity from 1.008 to 1.020.

POSSIBLE NURSING INTERVENTIONS

Keep accurate record of intake and output.

If indicated, keep NPO. When ordered, offer oral fluids when bowel sounds are present.

Assess and record

IV fluids and condition of IV site every hour.
heart rate and blood pressure every 4 hours and PRN.
bowel sounds every 2 to 4 hours and PRN.
any signs/symptoms of fluid volume deficit (such as those listed under **Characteristics**) every 4 hours and PRN.

If indicated, measure and record abdominal girth every shift.

Ensure that nasogastric tube is patent and connected to low intermittent suction. Irrigate, as indicated.

Check and record urine specific gravity every void or as indicated.

Assess and record child's/family's knowledge of and participation in care regarding

importance of offering child fluids, when indicated.
follow-up diet at home and reintroduction of solid foods.
monitoring of intake and output.
identification of any signs/symptoms of fluid volume
deficit (such as those listed under **Characteristics**).

🏠 Instruct child/family in any areas needing improvement.
Record results.

EVALUATION FOR CHARTING

State intake and output.

Describe condition of IV site.

State highest and lowest heart rates and blood pressures.

Describe bowel sounds.

Describe any signs/symptoms of fluid volume deficit noted
(such as those listed under **Characteristics**).

When indicated, state current abdominal girth and determine
whether it has increased since the previous measurement.

Describe amount and characteristics of nasogastric drainage.

Describe any therapeutic measures used to maintain adequate
fluid volume. State their effectiveness.

State highest and lowest urine specific gravity values.

🏠 Describe child's/family's knowledge of and participation in
care related to improving fluid balance. State any areas
needing improvement and information provided. Describe
child's/family's responses.

RELATED NURSING DIAGNOSES

Pain *related to*
   a. surgical incision
   b. invasive procedures

Compromised Family Coping *related to*
   a. surgical procedure
   b. child's hospitalization
   c. emergency nature of the illness

Electrolyte Imbalance (Specify)* *related to*
fluid volume deficit

Altered Nutrition: Less than Body Requirements
related to
a. nausea/vomiting
b. inability to tolerate food or fluids by mouth

---

*Non-NANDA diagnosis.

MEDICAL DIAGNOSIS

Bowel Obstruction

PATHOPHYSIOLOGY   Obstruction of the bowel occurs when either a disturbance in the muscular contractility of the bowel or a decrease/occlusion in the patency of the lumen of the bowel mechanically hinders the passage of intestinal contents. Surgical intervention is often necessary to correct the obstruction. The child's postoperative recovery is directly related to the preoperative state of the bowel, the presence of intraperitoneal infection, and whether or not an anastomosis was performed.

Intussusception

Intussusception is a telescoping of a portion of the intestine into a distal portion of the intestine. It is the most common intestinal obstruction in children ages 3 months to 6 years. In most cases of intussusception, the cause is unknown; possibilities include Meckel's diverticulum, an ileal polyp, lymphosarcoma, and adenovirus infections. The lumen of the bowel involved in the intussusception is partially obstructed and the vascular flow compromised, resulting in inflammation, edema, and bleeding. When complete bowel obstruction occurs, strangulation of the bowel can result. If untreated, intussusception can cause intestinal gangrene, peritonitis, and/or death. Prognosis is directly related to the duration of the intussusception prior to treatment.

The onset of intussusception is often sudden. The infant or child has paroxysmal attacks of severe abdominal pain accompanied by crying or screaming. The knees are drawn up to the chest and the infant/child can be restless, diaphoretic, and/or pale. Between the attacks of abdominal pain, the child may at first show no abnormal signs. As the condition worsens, the child becomes lethargic and weak. The abdomen becomes distended, vomitus may be bile stained, and the presence of blood and mucus give the stool a currant-jelly-like appearance. Eventually, the child may present in a shocklike state, with a weak, thready pulse, shallow respirations, grunting, and a fever as high as 41°C.

Intussusception reduction is usually an emergency procedure. If the child is not exhibiting signs of shock, the intussusception may be reduced by the hydrostatic pressure of air or a barium enema. If surgical intervention is necessary, manual reduction is first attempted. If the intussusception is not reducible by surgical manipulation, the involved bowel must be resected.

Malrotation

Malrotation occurs when the fetal bowel fails to rotate into its normal position. In most cases of malrotation, the cecum fails to move to the right lower quadrant and can eventually cause obstruction. Obstruction can occur if the duodenum becomes trapped behind peritoneal bands anchoring the abnormally placed cecum or if the mesentery of the small intestine is not attached properly and allows twisting of the intestine upon itself. This twisting is called *volvulus*. It can cause the bowel's blood supply to be compromised, resulting in bowel necrosis.

Children with malrotation of the gut and with volvulus usually present in the first few months of life with a history of bile-stained emesis after feedings. Abdominal distention may not be present early on, but radiographic films of the abdomen will show multiple distended bowel loops and a large bowel devoid of gas. Older children may present with a history of recurring attacks of abdominal pain or cyclic vomiting preceding the acute episode. In some cases of volvulus, vascular collapse occurs so rapidly that the child presents in shock preceded by vomiting, but with few other abdominal findings.

After correction of fluid and electrolyte disturbances and/or shock, a laporotomy is performed. During surgery the volvulus is untwisted, the bands between the cecum and the abdominal wall are divided, and the large intestine is straightened. Bowel resection and a jejunostomy or ileostomy may be necessary if a large portion of bowel has been compromised.

PREOPERATIVE NURSING CARE PLAN

PRIMARY NURSING DIAGNOSIS
Fluid Volume Deficit

DEFINITION   Decrease in the amount of circulating fluid volume

POSSIBLY RELATED TO

Vomiting

Third spacing of fluid secondary to infection

CHARACTERISTICS

Vomiting

Dry mucous membranes

Poor skin turgor

Decreased urine output

Increased urine specific gravity

Tachycardia

Hypotension

Abdominal distention

Sunken fontanel

Diminished or absent bowel sounds

Absence of tears when crying

EXPECTED OUTCOMES   Child will have an adequate fluid volume as evidenced by

adequate IV fluid intake (state specific amount of fluid intake needed for each child).

heart rate and blood pressure within acceptable ranges (state specific highest and lowest parameters for each child).

moist mucous membranes.

rapid skin recoil.

adequate urine output (state specific highest and lowest outputs for each child, minimum 1 to 2 ml/kg/hr).

urine specific gravity from 1.008 to 1.020.

absence of vomiting.

nondistended abdomen.

flat fontanel.

presence of bowel sounds.

presence of tears when crying.

POSSIBLE NURSING INTERVENTIONS

Keep accurate record of intake and output.

Keep child NPO. Ensure that nasogastric tube is patent and connected to low intermittent suction. Irrigate to maintain patency, as indicated.

Assess and record

IV fluids and condition of IV site every hour.

heart rate and blood pressure every 4 hours and PRN.
bowel sounds every 4 hours and PRN.
any signs/symptoms of fluid volume deficit (such as those
  listed under **Characteristics**) every 4 hours and PRN.

Check and record urine specific gravity every void or as
indicated.

If indicated, administer colloids. Assess and record
effectiveness.

If indicated, measure and record abdominal girth every 4
hours and PRN.

EVALUATION FOR CHARTING
State intake and output.

Describe amount and characteristics of nasogastric drainage.

Describe condition of IV site.

State highest and lowest heart rates and blood pressures.

Describe any signs/symptoms of fluid volume deficit noted
(such as those listed under **Characteristics**).

State highest and lowest urine specific gravity values.

When indicated, state current abdominal girth and determine
whether it has increased since the previous measurement.

Describe bowel sounds.

Describe any therapeutic measures taken to promote
adequate fluid volume. State their effectiveness.

NURSING DIAGNOSIS
Infection: High Risk

DEFINITION   Condition in which the body is at risk for being
invaded by microorganisms

POSSIBLY RELATED TO
Necrotic bowel and/or the release of intestinal contents into
  the peritoneal cavity, which may cause peritonitis

CHARACTERISTICS
Fever
Abdominal pain and/or tenderness

Abdominal distention
Lethargy
Diminished or absent bowel sounds
Vomiting
Diaphoresis
Increased white blood cell count (WBC)
Tachycardia
Pallor
Tachypnea
Hypotension

EXPECTED OUTCOMES   Child will have decreased symptoms or be free of infection as evidenced by

body temperature within acceptable range of 36.5°C to 37.2°C.
lack of abdominal pain/tenderness.
nondistended abdomen.
WBC within normal limits (state specific highest and lowest counts for each child).
heart rate, respiratory rate, and blood pressure within acceptable ranges (state specific parameters for each child).
presence of bowel sounds.
lack of

lethargy.
diaphoresis.
vomiting.
pallor.

POSSIBLE NURSING INTERVENTIONS

Assess and record the following every 2 to 4 hours and PRN:

vital signs
signs/symptoms of infection (such as those listed under **Characteristics**)

Maintain good hand-washing technique.

Check and record results of complete blood count (CBC).

Notify physician if CBC results are out of the acceptable range.

Administer antibiotics on schedule and antipyretics PRN.

Assess and record effectiveness and any side effects (e.g., rash, diarrhea).

Keep child NPO. Ensure that nasogastric tube is patent and connected to low intermittent suction. Irrigate to maintain patency, as indicated.

EVALUATION FOR CHARTING

State ranges of vital signs.

Describe any signs/symptoms of infection (such as those listed under **Characteristics**).

Describe amount and characteristics of emesis.

State results of current CBC.

State whether medications were administered on schedule. Describe effectiveness and any side effects noted.

Describe any therapeutic measures used to treat the infection. State their effectiveness.

RELATED NURSING DIAGNOSES

Electrolyte Imbalance: (Specify)* *related to*
  a. vomiting
  b. intestinal obstruction
  c. necrotic bowel

Pain *related to*
  a. intestinal vascular compromise
  b. intestinal obstruction

Anxiety: Child/Parental *related to*
  a. pain of the child
  b. emergency surgery
  c. outcome of the surgery

Knowledge Deficit: Parental *related to*
  a. diagnostic procedures such as administration of barium enema
  b. inaccurate information concerning child's illness or surgery
  c. postoperative care of child

---

*Non-NANDA diagnosis.

POSTOPERATIVE NURSING CARE PLAN

PRIMARY NURSING DIAGNOSIS
Fluid Volume Deficit

DEFINITION   Decrease in the amount of circulating fluid volume

POSSIBLY RELATED TO
Nasogastric drainage
Third spacing of fluid secondary to infection
Inability to tolerate oral fluids

CHARACTERISTICS
Vomiting
Dry mucous membranes
Poor skin turgor
Decreased urine output
Increased urine specific gravity
Tachycardia
Hypotension
Abdominal distention
Sunken fontanel
Prolonged absence of bowel sounds
Absence of tears when crying

EXPECTED OUTCOMES   Child will have an adequate fluid volume as evidenced by

adequate IV and PO fluid intake (state specific amount of fluid intake needed for each child).
heart rate and blood pressure within acceptable ranges (state specific highest and lowest parameters for each child).
moist mucous membranes.
rapid skin recoil.
adequate urine output (state specific highest and lowest outputs for each child, minimum 1 to 2 ml/kg/hr).
urine specific gravity from 1.008 to 1.020.
absence of vomiting.
nondistended abdomen.
flat fontanel.
presence of bowel sounds.
presence of tears when crying.

POSSIBLE NURSING INTERVENTIONS

Keep accurate record of intake and output.

When indicated,

keep NPO.

ensure that nasogastric tube is patent and connected to low intermittent suction or to gravity drainage. Irrigate to maintain patency.

replace nasogastric tube output with indicated type and amount of IV fluids.

start child on clear liquids (after the return of bowel function) and advance as tolerated.

Assess and record

IV fluids and condition of IV site every hour.

heart rate and blood pressure every 4 hours and PRN.

bowel sounds every 4 hours and PRN.

any signs/symptoms of fluid volume deficit (such as those listed under **Characteristics**) every 4 hours and PRN.

Check and record urine specific gravity every void or as indicated.

If third spacing of fluid has occurred, administer colloids followed by diuretics on schedule. Assess and record effectiveness.

If indicated, measure and record abdominal girth every 4 hours and PRN.

EVALUATION FOR CHARTING

State intake and output.

Describe amount and characteristics of nasogastric drainage.

Describe condition of IV site.

State highest and lowest heart rates and blood pressures.

Describe any signs/symptoms of fluid volume deficit noted (such as those listed under **Characteristics**).

State highest and lowest urine specific gravity values.

When indicated, state current abdominal girth and determine whether it has increased since the previous measurement.

Describe bowel sounds.

Describe any therapeutic measures to promote adequate fluid volume. State their effectiveness.

NURSING DIAGNOSIS
Pain

DEFINITION   Condition in which an individual experiences severe discomfort

POSSIBLY RELATED TO
Abdominal surgical incision

CHARACTERISTICS
Verbal communication of pain
Crying unrelieved by usual comfort measures
Guarding of the abdomen
Decreased activity, self-imposed
Physical signs/symptoms:

tachycardia
tachypnea/bradypnea
increased blood pressure
diaphoresis

Rating of pain on pain-assessment tool

EXPECTED OUTCOMES   Child will be free of extreme pain as evidenced by

verbal communication of decreased pain.
lack of constant crying.
heart rate, respiratory rate, and blood pressure within
    acceptable ranges (state specific parameters for each child).
decrease in or lack of diaphoresis.
increase in activity.
lack of abdominal guarding.
rating of decreased or no pain on pain-assessment tool.

POSSIBLE NURSING INTERVENTIONS
Assess and record any signs/symptoms of pain (such as those listed under **Characteristics**) every 2 hours and PRN. Use age-appropriate pain-assessment tool.

Handle child gently.

Encourage family members to stay and comfort child when possible.

Allow family members to participate in care of the child when possible.

Administer analgesics and/or narcotics on schedule. Assess and record effectiveness. Premedicate child before dressing changes or activities (e.g. bathing, ambulation), as indicated.

Monitor patient-controlled analgesia (PCA).

If age-appropriate, explain all procedures beforehand.

When indicated, institute additional pain relief measures, such as relaxation and music. Assess and record effectiveness.

Use diversional activities and distraction measures (e.g., toys, play activities, television) when appropriate.

🏠 Assess and record child's/family's knowledge of and participation in care regarding

> pain assessment.
> use of additional pain relief measures.
> use of diversional activities or distraction measures.
> administration of pain medication.

🏠 Instruct child/family in any areas needing improvement. Record results.

EVALUATION FOR CHARTING

Describe any signs/symptoms of pain noted (such as those listed under **Characteristics**).

State range of vital signs.

Describe any successful measures used to reduce or eliminate pain.

Describe effectiveness of analgesics and/or narcotics.

🏠 Describe child's/family's knowledge of and participation in care related to child's pain. State any areas needing improvement and information provided. Describe child's/ family's responses.

RELATED NURSING DIAGNOSES

High Risk for Further Infection* *related to*
    a. presence of invading microorganisms
    b. surgical wound
    c. compromised preoperative and postoperative condition

Electrolyte Imbalance: (Specify)* *related to*
fluid volume deficit

Fear: Child *related to*
    a. pain
    b. hospitalization
    c. treatments and procedures
    d. surgery
    e. forced contact with strangers
    f. unfamiliar surroundings

Compromised Family Coping *related to*
    a. situational health crisis of child
    b. surgery
    c. hospitalization

---

*Non-NANDA diagnosis.

MEDICAL DIAGNOSIS

Cleft Lip and Cleft Palate

PATHOPHYSIOLOGY   Cleft lip and cleft palate, the most common of all facial anomalies, may occur together or separately. Cleft lip, with or without cleft palate, is more common in boys than in girls. Isolated cleft palate occurs more often in girls.

Cleft lip results when the nasal and maxillary processes do not fuse due to hypoplasia of the mesenchymal layer of the lip. Cleft lip can vary from a slight indentation in the vermilion border to a widely opened cleft extending into the floor of the nose. Along with varying degrees of nasal distortions, supernumerary, deformed, or absent teeth may accompany cleft lip. Cleft lip may be unilateral or bilateral and usually involves the alveolar ridge. Unilateral cleft lip is usually on the left side. Bilateral cleft lip is often associated with cleft palate.

Cleft palate results when the two palatal shelves fail to fuse. The deformity varies in degree from involving only the uvula to extending into the soft and hard palates. Cleft palate can be unilateral, bilateral, or midline.

Several variations of cleft palate are associated with cleft lip. The midline of the soft palate may be affected, with the defect extending into one or both sides of the hard palate and exposing either one or both of the nasal cavities.

Feeding an infant with cleft lip and/or cleft palate can be challenging. The severity of the deformity will determine the difficulty of sucking for the infant and the types of adjustments necessary to maintain adequate caloric intake.

Cleft lip repair is usually performed at 1 to 2 months of age if the infant has shown adequate weight gain. The infant should also be free of any infections. In Z-plasty, the surgical technique most often used, a staggered suture line minimizes possible notching of the lip from retraction of the scar tissue. Immediately after the operation, a Logan clamp (a wire bow attached by adhesive tape to the cheeks) may be applied to take tension off the suture line.

Depending on the severity of the original deformity, revisions or nasal and cosmetic surgery may be needed as the child grows.

The timing of the surgical correction for cleft palate is individualized, depending on the size, shape, and degree of deformity. The goals for corrective surgery include joining the cleft segments, promoting intelligible and pleasant speech, reducing nasal regurgitation, and avoiding injury to the growing maxilla. The correction is generally performed before the child is 2 years of age to prevent the formation of faulty speech habits.

Postoperatively, the goals are to maintain a clean incision and to avoid strain on the suture line. Prevention of atelectasis and pneumonia is also important.

Complications associated with cleft lip and cleft palate include recurrent otitis media, hearing loss, dental decay, displacement of the maxillary arches, malposition of the teeth, and speech defects.

PREOPERATIVE NURSING CARE PLAN

PRIMARY NURSING DIAGNOSIS

Altered Nutrition: Less than Body Requirements

DEFINITION   Insufficient nutrients to meet body requirements

POSSIBLY RELATED TO
Sucking difficulties secondary to congenital orofacial defect prohibiting the infant from making an adequate seal around the nipple
Parental anxiety and frustration secondary to infant's tendency to choke on feedings

CHARACTERISTICS
Inadequate weight gain
Episodes of gagging and choking
Formula returned through the infant's nose

EXPECTED OUTCOMES   Infant will be adequately nourished as evidenced by

steady weight gain.
lack of or decreased episodes of gagging, choking, or formula returned through the nose.

sufficient caloric consumption (state range of calories needed for each infant).

POSSIBLE NURSING INTERVENTIONS

Keep accurate record of intake and output.

Assess and record any signs/symptoms of altered nutrition (such as those listed under **Characteristics**) every 4 hours and PRN.

Weigh infant on same scale at same time each day without clothes. Record results and compare to previous weight.

If indicated, maintain and record daily calorie counts.

Place infant in an upright or semisitting position during feedings. After feedings, place in an infant seat or on the side with head of bed elevated at a 30° angle.

Use an appropriate nipple for each infant (long and soft, cross-cut, preemie, Breck feeder, or lamb's). Place the nipple firmly in the infant's mouth on the side opposite the cleft.

Burp the infant frequently, every ½ to 1 oz (15 to 30 ml). (These infants have a tendency to swallow large amounts of air.)

To avoid distressing the infant, remove the nipple from the infant's mouth only for burping or when coughing warrants removal.

When indicated, limit feeding times to 30 to 45 minutes. Ensure that the infant consumes the appropriate amount of calories.

When indicated, feed the infant with a rubber-tipped medicine dropper, an Asepto syringe with a rubber tip, or a spoon.

When indicated, assist the mother with techniques to facilitate breast-feeding. Refer the mother to a local La Leche League chapter.

Assess and record family's knowledge of and participation in care regarding

> feeding techniques.
> positioning of infant.

monitoring of infant's weight gain and caloric consumption.

identification of signs/symptoms of altered nutrition (such as those listed under **Characteristics**).

🏠 Instruct family in any areas needing improvement.
Record results.

EVALUATION FOR CHARTING

State intake and output.

Describe any signs/symptoms of altered nutrition noted (such as those listed under **Characteristics**).

Describe how infant tolerated feedings. State effectiveness of positioning and feeding technique used.

State infant's current weight and determine whether it has increased or decreased since previous weighing.

🏠 Describe family's knowledge of and participation in care related to improving nutritional status. State any areas needing improvement and information provided. Describe family's response.

NURSING DIAGNOSIS
Altered Parenting

DEFINITION   Inability of the child's primary caregiver to provide a nurturing environment

POSSIBLY RELATED TO
Visible orofacial defect of infant
Difficulties in feeding infant
Infant's loud noises while eating
Frequent hospitalization of infant
Impaired parent-infant attachment

CHARACTERISTICS
Inappropriate parenting behaviors (such as inability to read infant's cues, to meet infant's basic needs, and/or to provide age-appropriate stimulation)
Lack of attachment behavior
Frequent verbalization of dissatisfaction with infant or infant's appearance
Verbalization of frustration in feeding infant

Verbalization of frustration with parental role
Evidence of infant abuse or neglect
Infant's failure to thrive or developmental delay

EXPECTED OUTCOMES   Parent will demonstrate appropriate parenting behaviors as evidenced by

increased attachment behaviors such as holding infant in en face position during feedings, seeking eye contact with infant, smiling at, and talking to infant, and holding infant close.
participation in infant's care.
provision of age-appropriate stimulation for infant.
verbalization of positive feelings regarding infant and infant's appearance.
happy, healthy infant with lack of

evidence of abuse or neglect.
failure to thrive.
developmental delay.

POSSIBLE NURSING INTERVENTIONS

Assess and record parent's interactions with the infant each shift and PRN.

Provide opportunities for the parent to observe and participate in the infant's care. Demonstrate appropriate stimulation for the infant, as well as holding, cuddling, feeding, and bathing. Record results.

Encourage family members to incorporate infant's care into their daily routine.

Allow parent to express feelings regarding infant's defect and any feeding difficulties.

Initiate consultation with social services to help the parent identify available supports and resources.

Encourage parent to seek the participation of other family members and friends in the feeding and care of the child.

Introduce the parent to other families with infants who have cleft lip and/or cleft palate and to families whose children have had lip and/or palate repairs.

Refer the parent to a support group.

EVALUATION FOR CHARTING

Describe any signs/symptoms of altered parenting noted (such as those listed under **Characteristics**).

Describe any therapeutic measures used to promote appropriate parenting. State their effectiveness.

RELATED NURSING DIAGNOSES

Aspiration: High Risk *related to*

exposed nasal cavities and a direct pathway created by the cleft to the nasopharynx

Infection: High Risk *related to*

insufficient drainage of the middle ear secondary to the cleft defect

Anxiety: Parental *related to*

a. upcoming surgery
b. unknown outcomes of upcoming surgery

Knowledge Deficit: Parental *related to*

a. feeding techniques
b. origin of defect
c. surgical procedure

POSTOPERATIVE NURSING CARE PLAN

NURSING DIAGNOSIS

Impaired Skin Integrity

DEFINITION   Interruption in integrity of the skin

POSSIBLY RELATED TO

Surgical closure of cleft lip and/or cleft palate
Strain of sutures on repaired lip or palate
Trauma to sutures of repaired lip or palate

CHARACTERISTICS

Nonapproximated edges of suture line
Suture line with redness, edema, or drainage

EXPECTED OUTCOMES   Infant will be free of signs/symptoms of impaired skin integrity as evidenced by intact incision with well-approximated edges. lack of

> redness.
> edema.
> drainage.

POSSIBLE NURSING INTERVENTIONS

Assess and record any signs/symptoms of impaired skin integrity (such as those listed under **Characteristics**).

When indicated, use a medicine dropper or Asepto syringe to feed the infant. Place the dropper or syringe in the mouth from the side to avoid the suture line. Older children may be fed with a spoon, but avoid using straws. Infants with palate repairs should not be tube-, syringe-, or fork-fed.

Burp the infant in a sitting position. Avoid placing the infant over the shoulder.

Prevent the infant from sucking. Until sufficient healing has taken place, do not allow use of a pacifier.

Apply elbow/arm restraints to prevent infant from traumatizing the suture line by trying to put fingers or objects into the mouth. Remove restraints every 2 hours and PRN to exercise infant's arms, provide skin care, and play.

Position the infant on the side or back, keeping the head of the bed elevated, or use an infant seat. When indicated, apply a jacket restraint to prevent the infant from rolling onto the abdomen and rubbing the face on the bed.

Position the infant so that the lip cannot rub against anything.

Provide suture line care as indicated.

> Clean the suture line on schedule and per institutional policy. A solution of 1:2 hydrogen peroxide and saline (or water) applied with a cotton-tipped applicator may be used.
> Apply an antibiotic ointment on schedule.
> After feedings, rinse the infant's mouth with water to remove any milk residue.

If a Logan clamp has been applied, maintain its placement.

Handle the child gently.

🏠 Assess and record family's knowledge of and participation in care regarding

feeding technique.
positioning.
use of restraints.
suture line.
identification of signs/symptoms of impaired skin integrity (such as those listed under **Characteristics**).

🏠 Instruct family in any areas needing improvement. Record results.

EVALUATION FOR CHARTING

Describe any signs/symptoms of impaired skin integrity noted (such as those listed under **Characteristics**).

Describe any therapeutic measures used to prevent impaired skin integrity. State their effectiveness.

🏠 Describe family's knowledge of and participation in care related to preventing impaired skin integrity. State any areas needing improvement and information provided. Describe family's response.

NURSING DIAGNOSIS
Infection: High Risk

DEFINITION   Condition in which the body is at risk for being invaded by microorganisms

POSSIBLY RELATED TO

Surgical repair of cleft lip and/or cleft palate
Residual of formula on the surgical site providing a medium for the growth of pathogens
Aspiration of secretions or formula

CHARACTERISTICS

Fever
Redness, edema, or drainage at suture line
Altered white blood cell count (WBC)
Tachycardia
Tachypnea
Abnormal breath sounds

EXPECTED OUTCOMES   Child will be free of infection as
evidenced by

> body temperature within acceptable range of 36.5°C to
>   37.2°C.
> clean and intact incision.
> WBC within acceptable limits (state specific highest and
>   lowest counts for each child).
> heart rate within acceptable range (state specific highest and
>   lowest rates for each child).
> respiratory rate within acceptable range (state specific highest
>   and lowest rates for each child).
> clear and equal breath sounds bilaterally.

POSSIBLE NURSING INTERVENTIONS
Assess and record the following every 4 hours and PRN:

> temperature, heart rate, and respiratory rate
> breath sounds
> condition of incision
> any signs/symptoms of infection (such as those listed
>   under **Characteristics**)

Maintain good hand-washing technique.

Provide suture line care as indicated

> Clean the suture line on schedule and per institutional
>   policy. A solution of 1:2 hydrogen peroxide and saline
>   (or water) applied with a cotton-tipped applicator may
>   be used.
> Apply an antibiotic ointment on schedule.
> After feedings, rinse the infant's mouth with water to
>   remove any milk residue.

When indicated, place the infant in a partial-side-lying
position to facilitate the drainage of copious serosanguineous
secretions. After cleft palate repair, the infant may require
gentle oral suctioning PRN to prevent aspiration.

Check and record results of complete blood count (CBC).
Notify the physician if CBC results are out of the acceptable
range.

When indicated, administer antibiotics on schedule and

antipyretics PRN. Assess and record effectiveness and any side effects (e.g., rash, diarrhea).

🏠 Assess and record child's/family's knowledge of and participation in care regarding

incision site.
hand washing.
positioning and/or suctioning.
medication administration.
identification of any signs/symptoms of infection (such as those listed under **Characteristics**).

🏠 Instruct child/family in any areas needing improvement. Record results.

EVALUATION FOR CHARTING

State ranges of temperature, heart rate, and respiratory rate.

Describe breath sounds.

Describe incision site.

Describe any signs/symptoms of infection noted (such as those listed under **Characteristics**).

State results of CBC.

State whether antibiotics and antipyretics were administered on schedule. Describe effectiveness and any side effects noted.

Describe any measures used to prevent infection. State their effectiveness.

🏠 Describe family's knowledge of and participation in care related to preventing infection. State any areas needing improvement and information provided. Describe family's response.

RELATED NURSING DIAGNOSES

Pain *related to*
surgical correction of the cleft

Anxiety: Infant *related to*
a. restrained arms and/or body
b. inability to suck or to have pacifier
c. inability to get hands to mouth

Anxiety: Parental *related to*
  a. outcome of surgery
  b. potential for future surgery
  c. home care
  d. potential for child to have speech defects, hearing loss, or dental decay

Knowledge Deficit: Parental *related to*
  home care of infant

Esophageal Atresia and Tracheoesophageal Fistula

PATHOPHYSIOLOGY In esophageal atresia, the embryonic foregut fails to develop, and the esophagus ends in a blind pouch; a tracheoesophageal fistula (TEF, T-E fistula) is a connection (fistula) between the trachea and the esophagus. Normally the foregut lengthens and separates to form two parallel channels (the esophagus and the trachea) during the fourth and fifth weeks of gestation. If there is defective separation or altered cellular growth during this separation, anomalies involving the esophagus and the trachea (such as TEF) result. The five most frequently seen forms of esophageal atresia and TEF are Type A, esophageal atresia; Type B, esophageal atresia and proximal TEF; Type C, esophageal atresia and distal TEF (85% to 90% of all cases); Type D, esophageal atresia with proximal and distal TEF; and Type E, TEF with no esophageal atresia (also called H type).

Diagnosis is established by gently passing a catheter into the esophagus until resistance is met. Attempts to aspirate gastric contents and to auscultate introduced air into the stomach will be unsuccessful when esophageal atresia is present. Fluoroscopic studies and bronchoscopy are necessary to determine the extent of the defect and the location of the fistula(s).

Esophageal atresia and TEF are rare malformations that can occur as separate entities or together. The incidence of these defects is estimated at one in every three thousand to four thousand live births. There is no sex difference in occurrence, and heredity has not been implicated as a factor. Approximately one-third of affected infants are premature, and more than one-fourth also have other congenital anomalies, such as cardiac, anorectal, genitourinary, and/or vertebral defects. A history of polyhydramnios prenatally is common due to the inability of the amniotic fluid to reach the gastrointestinal tract.

The rest of this discussion and the preoperative and postoperative nursing care plans are related to Type C, esophageal atresia and distal TEF, the most common form of the defect. Major clinical manifestations include excessive pharyngeal secretions, drooling, bubbling from the mouth and nose, coughing, choking, and cyanosis. The cyanosis results from laryngospasms, which occur as a compensatory mechanism to try to prevent aspiration of the overflow secretions from the esophageal blind pouch into the trachea. Abdominal distention is present due to air shunting across the fistula.

Treatment is aimed at preventing aspiration pneumonia until surgical repair of the defect is completed. Sometimes the malformation can be corrected in one operation, but at other times it requires two or more procedures. If it can be repaired in one procedure, a thoracotomy is done with TEF ligation and an end-to-end anastomosis of the esophagus. When staged operations are necessary (due to prematurity, multiple anomalies, poor condition of the infant, or insufficient length of the two segments of the esophagus), palliative measures used include ligation of the TEF, a gastrostomy for gastric decompression and feedings, and a cervical esophagostomy to allow for drainage of oral secretions. The major complication following reconstructive surgery is stricture of the esophageal anastomosis site. Infants need periodic esophageal dilatation following corrective surgery.

PREOPERATIVE NURSING CARE PLAN

PRIMARY NURSING DIAGNOSIS
Aspiration: High Risk

DEFINITION   State in which an individual is at risk for entry of extraneous secretions, foods, fluids, or foreign bodies into the tracheobronchial passages

POSSIBLY RELATED TO
>Overflow of saliva from the proximal esophageal pouch
>Reflux of gastric secretions up the distal esophagus into the trachea via the fistula

CHARACTERISTICS
>Diminished breath sounds
>Excessive pharyngeal secretions
>Drooling
>Bubbling from the mouth and nose
>Coughing

Choking
Cyanosis
Abdominal distention with air
Intraabdominal pressure (usually resulting from crying)

EXPECTED OUTCOMES   Infant will be free of signs/symptoms of aspiration as evidenced by

clear and equal breath sounds bilaterally.
lack of

excessive secretions.
drooling.
bubbling from the mouth and nose.
coughing.
choking.
cyanosis.
abdominal distention and intraabdominal pressure.

POSSIBLE NURSING INTERVENTIONS

Assess and record the following every 4 hours and PRN:

breath sounds
any signs/symptoms of aspiration (such as those listed
under **Characteristics**)

Position infant supine with head elevated at least 30° in order to minimize reflux of gastric secretions into the trachea.

Suction (either continuously or intermittently) esophageal blind pouch. Ensure that catheter is changed daily. Record the amount and characteristics of secretions.

If a gastrostomy tube is in place, connect it to gravity drainage so that air can escape from the abdomen.

Keep infant NPO. Assess and record IV fluids and condition of IV site every hour.

Keep accurate record of intake and output.

If indicated, administer antibiotics on schedule. Assess and record any side effects (e.g., rash, diarrhea).

When indicated, ensure that oxygen is administered in the correct amount and route. Assess and record effectiveness of therapy.

🏠 Assess and record family's knowledge of and participation in care regarding

> positioning of infant.
> monitoring of intake and output.
> identification of any signs/symptoms of aspiration (such as those listed under **Characteristics**).

🏠 Instruct family in any areas needing improvement.
Record results.

EVALUATION FOR CHARTING

Describe breath sounds.

Describe condition of IV site.

Describe any signs/symptoms of aspiration noted (such as those listed under **Characteristics**).

Describe any therapeutic measures used to decrease chance of aspiration. State their effectiveness.

State intake and output.

State whether medications were administered on schedule. Describe any side effects noted.

State whether oxygen was administered and state the amount and route of delivery. Describe effectiveness.

🏠 Describe family's knowledge of and participation in care related to decreasing chance for aspiration. State any areas needing improvement and information provided. Describe family's response.

NURSING DIAGNOSIS
Knowledge Deficit: Parental

DEFINITION   Lack of information concerning the infant's disease and care

POSSIBLY RELATED TO
Infant's disease state
Cause of defect
Home care of infant
Sensory overload
Cognitive or cultural-language limitations

CHARACTERISTICS

Verbalization by parents indicating lack of knowledge
Relation of incorrect information to members of the health
   care team
Requests for information

EXPECTED OUTCOMES   Parents will have an adequate
knowledge base concerning the infant's disease state and care as
evidenced by

ability to correctly state information previously taught
   regarding home care.
relation of appropriate information to the health care team.

POSSIBLE NURSING INTERVENTIONS

Listen to parents' concerns and fears.

Assess and record parents' knowledge concerning the disease
state and care of the infant.

🏠 Provide parents with information about the disease state,
including

definition and etiology.
treatment and prognosis.
time frame for surgical correction; whether it can be done
   in one operation or must be staged in two or more
   procedures. Give rationale.

Use pictures as necessary to facilitate teaching.

🏠 Provide parents with any available literature or booklets
concerning esophageal atresia and TEF.

🏠 Instruct parents in home care regarding

positioning of infant.
gastrostomy feedings, if indicated.
skin around cervical esophagostomy.
esophagostomy.
incisions.

When indicated, obtain an interpreter.

Dispel any incorrect information.

EVALUATION FOR CHARTING

State whether parents verbalized a knowledge deficit.

☗ State whether parents were able to repeat information correctly.

☗ State whether parents were able to perform skills previously taught. Describe ability.

Describe any measures used to facilitate parent teaching.

RELATED NURSING DIAGNOSES

Ineffective Breathing Pattern *related to*
  aspiration

Infection: High Risk *related to*
  a. possibility of aspiration
  b. invasive procedures

Fear: Parental *related to*
  a. impending surgery for infant
  b. outcome of surgery

Compromised Family Coping *related to*
  a. birth of imperfect infant
  b. need for the infant to have surgery

POSTOPERATIVE NURSING CARE PLAN

PRIMARY NURSING DIAGNOSIS

Ineffective Airway Clearance

DEFINITION   Condition in which secretions cannot adequately be cleared from the airways

POSSIBLY RELATED TO
  Excessive secretions
  Postoperative complications

CHARACTERISTICS
  Tachypnea
  Diminished breath sounds
  Retractions
  Pallor
  Cyanosis

EXPECTED OUTCOMES   Infant will have adequate airway clearance as evidenced by

> respiratory rate from 30 to 60 breaths/minute.
> clear and equal breath sounds bilaterally.
> lack of
>
>> retractions.
>> pallor.
>> cyanosis.

POSSIBLE NURSING INTERVENTIONS

Assess and record the following every 4 hours and PRN:

> respiratory rate
> breath sounds
> any signs/symptoms of ineffective airway clearance (such as those listed under **Characteristics**)

Suction infant PRN. Ensure that suction catheters are marked and that catheters are not passed farther than a point just above the anastomosis site. Assess and record amount and characteristics of secretions.

Position infant with head slightly elevated. Ensure that infant does not hyperextend the neck and pull on the sutured esophagus. Change infant from the back to either side every two hours.

When indicated, ensure that chest physiotherapy (vibration over the suture line) is performed on schedule. Assess and record effectiveness of treatments.

Ensure that chest tube system is intact and that negative pressure is maintained. Milk chest tube to maintain patency, as indicated. Record chest tube site. Assess and record amount and characteristics of any drainage.

Assess and record family's knowledge of and participation in care regarding

> positioning of the infant.
> identification of any signs/symptoms of ineffective airway clearance (such as those listed under **Characteristics**).

Instruct child/family in any areas needing improvement. Record results.

EVALUATION FOR CHARTING

State highest and lowest respiratory rates.

Describe breath sounds.

Describe any signs/symptoms of ineffective airway clearance noted (such as those listed under **Characteristics**).

Describe amount and characteristics of secretions.

Indicate whether infant was maintained in head-elevated position and how often infant was changed from back to side.

Indicate whether chest physiotherapy was done on schedule. Describe how infant tolerated procedure. State effectiveness of procedure.

Describe amount and characteristics of chest tube drainage.

Describe any therapeutic measure used to improve airway clearance. State their effectiveness.

Describe family's knowledge of and participation in care related to improving airway clearance. State any areas needing improvement and information provided. Describe family's response.

NURSING DIAGNOSIS

Altered Nutrition: Less than Body Requirements

DEFINITION   Insufficient nutrients to meet body requirements

POSSIBLY RELATED TO
Inability to tolerate PO fluids

CHARACTERISTICS
Failure to gain weight
Intolerance of gastrostomy feedings

EXPECTED OUTCOMES   Infant will be adequately nourished as evidenced by

adequate caloric intake, via IV initially, then gastrostomy tube feeding, and eventually PO (state specific amount for each infant).
steady weight gain or lack of weight loss.

POSSIBLE NURSING INTERVENTIONS

Keep accurate record of intake and output.

Assess and record every 4 hours and PRN for any signs/symptoms of altered nutrition (such as those listed under **Characteristics**).

Weigh child on same scale at same time each day. Record results.

Keep infant NPO initially. When indicated, begin feedings. If gastrostomy tube is in place, it is usually connected to gravity drainage for the first two to three days post-operatively. When gastrostomy feedings are begun, they are cautiously increased in volume and strength. When oral feedings are begun (usually 10 to 14 days after total correction) the infant should be fed slowly and given time to swallow.

🏠 Assess and record family's knowledge of and participation in care regarding

> positioning of infant.
> feeding techniques (gastrostomy feedings, if indicated).
> monitoring of intake and output.
> identification of any signs/symptoms of altered nutrition
> (such as those listed under **Characteristics**).

🏠 Instruct family in any areas needing improvement.

EVALUATION FOR CHARTING

State intake and output.

Describe any signs/symptoms of altered nutrition noted (such as those listed under **Characteristics**).

State infant's current weight and determine whether it has increased or decreased since previous weighing.

Describe any therapeutic measures used to maintain adequate nutrition. State their effectiveness.

🏠 Describe family's knowledge of and participation in care related to maintaining adequate nutrition. State any areas needing improvement and information provided. Describe infant's/family's responses.

RELATED NURSING DIAGNOSES

Pain *related to*
   surgical incision

Fluid Volume Deficit *related to*
   a. inability to tolerate oral fluids
   b. high risk for respiratory difficulty

Infection: High Risk *related to*
   a. surgical procedure
   b. invasive procedures (e.g., IV, and chest tubes)

Compromised Family Coping *related to*
   a. hospitalization of infant
   b. home care of infant

MEDICAL DIAGNOSIS
Gastroenteritis

PATHOPHYSIOLOGY Gastroenteritis is an inflammation of the lining of the stomach and intestines. In acute infectious gastroenteritis, the etiology is a microorganism—either viral, bacterial, or, rarely, protozoal. Transmission of these organisms can be direct person-to-person contact (as with *Shigella* and *Giardia*), through contaminated food or water (as with *Salmonella, Escherichia coli,* and Norwalk-like virus), or through contact with family pets (as with *Yersinia enterocolitica* and *Salmonella*). The means of transmission is usually fecal-oral.

Viral infections damage and destroy the epithelial cells that line the intestinal tract. Bacterial infections can damage the intestinal mucosa in one of three ways: (1) the organism multiplies and adheres to the mucosa, producing an enterotoxin that interacts with the bowel mucosa and causes active water and electrolyte secretion; (2) through an inflammatory process, organisms invade the cells in the epithelium; or (3) organisms multiply intracellularly and penetrate the gut wall. Imbalance of the normal flora in the gastrointestinal tract can also cause gastroenteritis. Traveler's diarrhea is most often caused by enterotoxigenic *E. coli*.

PRIMARY NURSING DIAGNOSIS
Fluid Volume Deficit

DEFINITION Decrease in the amount of circulating fluid volume

POSSIBLY RELATED TO
Inflammation of the lining of the stomach and intestine
Invasion of the stomach and intestine by a microorganism
  (specify when indicated: viral, bacterial, or protozoal)

CHARACTERISTICS
Diarrhea (may contain mucus, pus, blood and/or sugar)
Nausea/vomiting

Abdominal cramping
Abdominal distention
Hyperactive bowel sounds
Weight loss
Sunken fontanel
Sunken eyeballs
Dry mucous membranes
Poor skin turgor
Decreased urine output
Fever

EXPECTED OUTCOMES   Child will have an adequate fluid
volume as evidenced by

adequate fluid intake, IV and/or oral (state specific amount
of intake needed for each child).
absence of

diarrhea.
mucus, pus, blood, and sugar in stool.
nausea/vomiting.
abdominal cramping and distention.

normal activity of bowel sounds (one every 10 to 30
seconds).
regaining of weight lost during illness.
flat fontanel.
adequate urine output (state specific highest and lowest
outputs for each child, minimum 1 to 2 ml/kg/hr).
urine specific gravity from 1.008 to 1.020.
temperature within acceptable range of 36.5°C to 37.2°C.

POSSIBLE NURSING INTERVENTIONS
Keep accurate record of intake and output. Weigh diapers
for urine and stool output. Record frequency, color, odor,
and consistency of stool. Measure and record amount and
characteristics of any vomitus. If indicated, offer fluids by
mouth. Record amount taken and child's tolerance of it.

Assess and record

IV fluids and condition of IV site every hour.
bowel sounds every shift and PRN.
temperature every 4 hours and PRN.
signs/symptoms of fluid volume deficit (such as those listed
under **Characteristics**) every 4 hours and PRN.

Weigh child on same scale at same time each day without clothes.

Give mouth care every 4 hours and PRN.

Check and record urine specific gravity every 4 hours or as directed.

Report any of the following to the physician:

> frequent stooling (more than three times/shift)
> large amounts of vomitus
> IV fluids infiltrated and unable to restart

Assess and record family's knowledge of and participation in care regarding

> child's need for appropriate fluids, when indicated.
> need to offer child a pacifier for comfort, if indicated.
> follow-up diet at home; when to reintroduce milk and solid foods.
> monitoring of intake and output.
> identification of any signs/symptoms of fluid volume deficit (such as those listed under **Characteristics**).

Instruct child/family in any areas needing improvement. Record results.

EVALUATION FOR CHARTING

State intake and output.

Describe condition of IV site.

State highest and lowest temperatures.

Describe any signs/symptoms of fluid volume deficit noted (such as those listed under **Characteristics**).

State highest and lowest of urine specific gravity values.

Describe any therapeutic measures used to improve fluid volume deficit. State their effectiveness.

Describe child's/family's knowledge of and participation in care related to improving fluid volume. State any areas needing improvement and information provided. Describe child's/family's responses.

NURSING DIAGNOSIS
High Risk for Spread of Infection*

DEFINITION Condition in which the body is invaded by microorganisms that can be transmitted by direct contact

POSSIBLY RELATED TO
Direct person-to-person contact with infected individual
Centers that care for children in diapers (e.g., day cares, pediatric units)

CHARACTERISTICS
Diarrhea
Vomiting
Fever

EXPECTED OUTCOMES
Child's infection will not spread to others.

POSSIBLE NURSING INTERVENTIONS
Maintain good hand-washing technique.

🏠 Assess and record family's knowledge of hand-washing technique; correct as needed.

Maintain contact and enteric isolation, if indicated.

🏠 Assess and record family's description of living conditions of child/family and of home circumstances. Instruct child/family in any areas needing improvement. Record results. Refer family for follow-up home care, if indicated.

EVALUATION FOR CHARTING
State whether good hand-washing technique was maintained.

🏠 State whether family demonstrated correct hand-washing technique.

If isolation was necessary, describe type.

Describe any other measures used to decrease spread of infection. State their effectiveness.

🏠 Describe living conditions of child/family and of home circumstances. State any areas needing improvement and information provided. Describe child's/family's responses.

---

*Non-NANDA diagnosis.

RELATED NURSING DIAGNOSES

Electrolyte Imbalance: Sodium Losses and Potassium Losses* related to
   a. diarrhea
   b. vomiting

Altered Nutrition: Less than Body Requirements related to
   a. diarrhea
   b. vomiting

Altered Comfort* related to
   a. abdominal cramping
   b. abdominal distention
   c. impaired skin integrity secondary to frequent perineal contact with acid stools

Compromised Family Coping related to
   hospitalization of child

---

*Non-NANDA diagnosis.

Gastroesophageal Reflux

PATHOPHYSIOLOGY   Gastroesophageal reflux (GER, chalasia) occurs when relaxation or incompetence of the lower esophageal sphincter (also called the cardiac sphincter) allows frequent reflux of gastric contents into the esophagus. The exact cause is unknown, but the delay in maturation of neuromuscular control of the gastroesophageal sphincter is thought to be responsible. A hiatal hernia may or may not be present with this disorder.

Some reflux of stomach contents is normal in otherwise healthy individuals. The occurrence of GER in newborns is due to immature neuromuscular control of the gastroesophageal sphincter. If reflux continues to occur beyond the newborn period, however, and if the infant becomes symptomatic, intervention is required. Diagnosis is established by taking a health history, observing the infant's eating habits, and conducting several diagnostic tests, including a barium esophagram, a manometry to measure esophageal sphincter pressure, and an acid reflux (Tuttle) test, which measures the pH of the distal esophagus.

Treatment consists of thickening formula with cereal; giving small, frequent feedings and burping frequently; avoiding overfeeding; and placing the infant in an elevated (30° to 45°), prone position. Medications that promote gastric emptying and/or relax the pyloric sphincter, such as metoclopramide (Reglan), and medications that neutralize gastric acid and decrease production of hydrochloric acid, such as ranitidine (Zantac) or cimetidine (Tagamet), have been used with some success. Most infants outgrow GER by 18 months of age. Infants that do not respond to medical management may need surgical intervention to prevent complications such as aspiration pneumonia, prolonged esophagitis (which can lead to blood loss and anemia), and weight loss (which may lead to failure to thrive). The Nissen fundoplication is the most commonly performed surgical procedure. In it, the fundus of the stomach is wrapped around the distal esophagus and secured with plicating sutures to create a tighter gastroesophageal junction.

137

PRIMARY NURSING DIAGNOSIS

Altered Nutrition: Less than Body Requirements

DEFINITION   Insufficient nutrients to meet body requirements

POSSIBLY RELATED TO
Chronic vomiting or regurgitation

CHARACTERISTICS
Excessive vomiting
Infant readily eating again after vomiting
Vomitus not containing bile
Weight loss or failure to gain weight
Complaint of heartburn from an older child

EXPECTED OUTCOMES   Infant will be adequately nourished as evidenced by

adequate amount of calories absorbed (state specific amount for each infant).

steady weight gain or lack of weight loss.

decreased incidence of vomiting.

POSSIBLE NURSING INTERVENTIONS
Keep accurate record of intake and output. Record emesis: amount, frequency, characteristics, and relationship to feeding.

Assess and record any signs/symptoms of altered nutrition (such as those listed under **Characteristics**) every 4 hours and PRN.

Weigh infant on same scale at same time each day without clothes. Record results and compare to previous weight.

Ensure that infant receives small, frequent feedings (every 2 to 3 hours). Thicken formula with rice cereal (this is somewhat controversial; research has shown that this does not decrease reflux in all infants). The nipple opening may need to be enlarged for easier sucking. Keep infant in an upright position during feeding, feed slowly, and burp often (after every ounce or 30 ml).

Organize nursing care so that medications and baths are given, vital signs checked, etc., prior to feeding.

Position infant prone with head elevated at a 30° to 45° angle for at least 1 hour after feeding.

Administer medication (Reglan and/or Zantac) on schedule. Assess and record effectiveness and side effects (e.g., confusion, agitation, headache, nausea).

⌂ Assess and record family's knowledge of and participation in care regarding

feeding schedule and method of feeding.
positioning of infant.
medication administration.
organization of care so infant is not disturbed after feedings.
identification of any signs/symptoms of altered nutrition (such as those listed under **Characteristics**).

⌂ Instruct family in any areas needing improvement.
Record results.

EVALUATION FOR CHARTING

State intake and output.

Describe amount, frequency, relationship to feedings, and characteristics of any vomitus.

Describe any signs/symptoms of altered nutrition noted (such as those listed under **Characteristics**).

State infant's current weight and determine whether it has increased or decreased since previous weighing.

Describe how infant tolerated feedings. State effectiveness of feedings and positioning in decreasing reflux.

State whether medications were administered on schedule. Describe effectiveness and any side effects noted.

⌂ Describe family's knowledge of and participation in care related to improving nutritional status. State any areas needing improvement and information provided. Describe family's response.

NURSING DIAGNOSIS
Aspiration: High Risk

DEFINITION   State in which an individual is at risk for entry of extraneous secretions, foods, fluids, or foreign bodies into the tracheobronchial passages

POSSIBLY RELATED TO
Excessive vomiting
Reflux of gastric contents into the esophagus

CHARACTERISTICS
Recurrent upper respiratory infections
Bradycardia
Unequal breath sounds
Apnea
Dyspnea
Coughing

EXPECTED OUTCOMES   Infant will be free of signs/symptoms of aspiration as evidenced by

absence of respiratory infection.
heart rate and respiratory rate within acceptable ranges (state specific highest and lowest rates for each infant).
clear and equal breath sounds bilaterally.
lack of

apnea.
dyspnea.
coughing.

POSSIBLE NURSING INTERVENTIONS
Assess and record the following every 4 hours and PRN:

heart rate, respiratory rate, and breath sounds
any signs/symptoms of aspiration (such as those listed under **Characteristics**)

Ensure that infant receives small, frequent feedings (every 2 to 3 hours). Thicken formula with rice cereal (this is somewhat controversial; research has shown that this does not decrease reflux in all infants). The nipple opening may need to be enlarged for easier sucking. Keep infant in upright position during feeding, feed slowly, and burp often (after every ounce or 30 ml).

Organize nursing care so that medications and baths are given, vital signs taken, etc., prior to feeding.

Position infant prone with the head elevated at a 30° to 45° angle for at least 1 hour after feeding.

Administer medication (Reglan and/or Zantac) on schedule. Assess and record effectiveness and side effects (e.g., confusion, agitation, headache, nausea).

Assess and record family's knowledge of and participation in care regarding

> feeding schedule and method of feeding.
> positioning of infant.
> medication administration.
> organization of care so infant is not disturbed after feedings.
> identification of any signs/symptoms of aspiration (such as those listed under **Characteristics**).

Instruct family in any areas needing improvement. Record results.

EVALUATION FOR CHARTING

State highest and lowest heart rates and respiratory rates.

Describe breath sounds.

Describe any signs/symptoms of aspiration noted (such as those listed under **Characteristics**).

Describe any therapeutic measures used to decrease the chance of aspiration. State their effectiveness.

Describe how infant tolerated feedings. State effectiveness of feedings and positioning in decreasing reflux.

State whether medications were administered on schedule. Describe effectiveness and any side effects noted.

Describe family's knowledge of and participation in care related to decreasing chance for aspiration. State any areas needing improvement and information provided. Describe family's response.

NURSING DIAGNOSIS
Altered Development: Motor

DEFINITION   Failure to progress in expected tasks and skills according to chronologic age

POSSIBLY RELATED TO
>Confinement to head-elevated prone position
>Reduced stimulation secondary to prolonged or frequent hospitalization

CHARACTERISTICS
>Vary with age and state of development for each infant. For example, a 4-month-old infant would have a delay in the ability to grasp toys and bring them to the mouth.
>bring hands together to midline.
>use both hands when attempting to pick up an object.
>pull to a sitting position with little head lag.
>possibly roll over.

EXPECTED OUTCOMES   Infant will progress developmentally as evidenced by

>lack of markedly regressed behavior.
>attainment of developmental milestones according to age.

POSSIBLE NURSING INTERVENTIONS
Assess and record developmental progression of infant. Provide adequate stimulation for infants when they are confined to the head-elevated prone position. Place bright and colorful objects (e.g., mobiles) within reach.

Talk to infant with direct eye contact during feeding and diapering.

Touch and stroke infant while in the head-elevated prone position.

Hold and cuddle infant in an upright position with the infant's head and chest higher than the stomach.

🏠 Assess and record family's knowledge of and participation in care regarding

>infant's need for assistance with developmental progression by adequate stimulation.
>positioning of infant while holding.

identification of any signs/symptoms of altered development (such as those listed under **Characteristics**).

Instruct family in any areas needing improvement. Record results.

EVALUATION FOR CHARTING

Describe any altered development or regressed behavior.

Describe infant's level of developmental tasks and skills attainment.

Describe any successful measures used to help infant attain developmental milestones.

Describe family's knowledge of and participation in care related to sustaining developmental progression. State any areas needing improvement and information provided. Describe family's response.

RELATED NURSING DIAGNOSES

Infection: High Risk *related to*
inflammation of the esophagus secondary to presence of acid gastric contents in the esophagus

Anxiety: Parental *related to*
a. infant's failure to gain weight
b. feeding schedule
c. positioning of infant
d. possibility of aspiration

Knowledge Deficit: Parental *related to*
a. disease state
b. care of infant, including feeding schedule, positioning, and appropriate stimulation

7

MEDICAL DIAGNOSIS
Hirschsprung Disease

PATHOPHYSIOLOGY Hirschsprung disease, or aganglionic megacolon, a congenital anomaly, occurs when there is absence or scarcity of autonomic parasympathetic ganglion cells of the submucosal (Meissner's) and myenteric (Auerbach's) plexuses in a segment of the bowel wall. The defect is probably caused by a lack of parasympathetic ganglion cell precursor migration during fetal development. The aganglionic portion results in absence of peristalsis, which causes accumulation of fecal material, obstruction, and distention of the bowel proximal to the defect. In addition, the rectal sphincter is unable to relax, preventing evacuation of solids, liquids, or gas.

The length of aganglionic segment of the bowel can vary from a small area (like the internal anal sphincter) to the entire colon. In the majority of affected children (approximately 80%), the aganglionic segment involves only the rectosigmoid colon. The defect is diagnosed by abdominal radiographic studies that reveal a distended colon and an unexpanded rectum. Rectal biopsy indicating aganglionic bowel segments confirms the diagnosis.

The severity of bowel involvement and the age of the child at the time of diagnosis determine the clinical manifestations. The chief signs and symptoms in a newborn are failure to pass meconium within 24 to 48 hours after birth, a decreased desire to ingest fluids, abdominal distention, and, possibly, bile-stained vomitus. Older infants may present with failure to thrive, constipation, overflow diarrhea, vomiting, and abdominal distention. When the disease goes undiagnosed until childhood, the symptoms include malnutrition, lethargy, muscle wasting, a protuberant abdomen, chronic constipation, and passage of ribbonlike stools.

Therapeutic management usually includes a temporary colostomy in a part of the bowel with normal innervation. Definitive corrective surgery (a pull-through procedure) is done when the child is 8 to 12 months of age and weighs approximately 20 lb (9 kg). Generally the colostomy is left in place until the definitive surgery completely heals. Colostomy closure is usually possible 3 months after the pull-through procedure.

NURSING CARE PLAN AT TIME OF DIAGNOSIS

PRIMARY NURSING DIAGNOSIS
Fluid Volume Deficit

DEFINITION   Decrease in the amount of circulating fluid volume

POSSIBLY RELATED TO
Decreased desire for fluids
Vomiting

CHARACTERISTICS
Failure to pass meconium within 24 to 48 hours of birth
(newborn)
Feeding problems
Vomiting (vomitus may include bile or fecal material)
Hypoproteinemia
Constipation
Passage of ribbonlike, foul-smelling stools
Overflow diarrhea
Abdominal distention
Dry mucous membranes
Decreased urine output

EXPECTED OUTCOMES   Child will have an adequate fluid volume as evidenced by

adequate fluid intake, IV or oral (state specific amount of
intake needed for each child).
absence of

vomiting.
overflow diarrhea.
hypoproteinemia.
abdominal distention.

moist mucous membranes.
adequate urine output (state specific highest and lowest
outputs for each child, minimum 1 to 2 ml/kg/hr).
urine specific gravity from 1.008 to 1.020.

POSSIBLE NURSING INTERVENTIONS

Keep accurate record of intake and output. Record amount and characteristics of any vomitus.

Assess and record

> IV fluids and condition of IV site every hour.
> signs/symptoms of fluid volume deficit (such as those listed under **Characteristics**) every 4 hours and PRN.

Check and record urine specific gravity every 4 hours or as directed.

🏠 Assess and record family's knowledge of and participation in care regarding

> child's need for appropriate fluids, when indicated.
> monitoring of intake and output.
> identification of any signs/symptoms of fluid volume deficit (such as those listed under **Characteristics**).

🏠 Instruct child/family in any areas needing improvement. Record results.

EVALUATION FOR CHARTING

State intake and output. Describe amount and characteristics of any vomitus.

Describe condition of IV site.

Describe any signs/symptoms of fluid volume deficit noted (such as those listed under **Characteristics**).

State highest and lowest urine specific gravity values.

🏠 Describe family's knowledge of and participation in care related to improving fluid volume. State any areas needing improvement and information provided. Describe family's response.

NURSING DIAGNOSIS
Knowledge Deficit: Parental

DEFINITION Lack of information concerning the child's disease and care

POSSIBLY RELATED TO

Disease state
Cause of defect

Home care of child, including colostomy care
Sensory overload
Cognitive or cultural-language limitations

CHARACTERISTICS

Verbalization by parents indicating lack of knowledge
Relation of incorrect information to members of the health
    care team
Requests for information

EXPECTED OUTCOMES Parents will have an adequate
knowledge base concerning the child's disease state and care as
evidenced by

ability to correctly state information previously taught
    regarding disease process and home care, including
    colostomy care.
ability to relate appropriate information to the health
    care team.

POSSIBLE NURSING INTERVENTIONS

Listen to parents' concerns and fears.

Assess and record parents' knowledge concerning the disease
state and care of the child.

Provide parents with information about the disease state,
including

definition and etiology.
treatment and prognosis.
time frame for three-part correction of the defect
    (colostomy, pull-through procedure, colostomy closure).

Use pictures as necessary to facilitate teaching.

Provide parents with any available literature or booklets
concerning Hirschsprung disease.

Instruct parents in the following home care:

colostomy care, including appliance application, skin
    barrier application, cleaning the skin area, emptying the
    pouch, and controlling odor
need to dress the child in loose-fitting clothing that does
    not press on the colostomy
need to notify health care team of bleeding from the
    stoma, bleeding from the skin around the stoma, a

change in bowel pattern, and/or a temperature above 38.0°C

🏠 Have enterostomal therapist, if available, assist in planning home care and teaching.

Assign a primary nurse as usual spokesperson to parents.

When indicated, obtain an interpreter.

Dispel any incorrect information.

EVALUATION FOR CHARTING
State whether parents verbalized a knowledge deficit.

🏠 State whether parents were able to repeat information correctly.

🏠 Describe parents' ability to perform skills previously taught (such as colostomy care).

Describe any measures used to facilitate parent teaching.

RELATED NURSING DIAGNOSES

Anxiety: Parental *related to*
a. hospitalization of child
b. altered home care
c. long-term prognosis

Altered Nutrition: Less than Body Requirements
related to
a. poor feeding
b. vomiting

Altered Comfort* *related to*
a. constipation
b. hunger

Compromised Family Coping *related to*
a. impending surgery
b. colostomy care
c. long-term prognosis

---

*Non-NANDA diagnosis.

PREOPERATIVE NURSING CARE PLAN FOR PULL-THROUGH PROCEDURE

PRIMARY NURSING DIAGNOSIS

Anxiety: Parental

DEFINITION   Feeling of apprehension resulting from an unknown cause

POSSIBLY RELATED TO
Outcome of surgery
Hospitalization of child
Treatments and procedures for child

CHARACTERISTICS
Verbalization of apprehension or nervousness
Inability to relax
Anticipation of misfortune for child during surgery
Inappropriate or hostile behavior toward health care team
Inability to concentrate
Reports of somatic discomfort

EXPECTED OUTCOMES   Parents will demonstrate decreased anxiety as evidenced by

verbalization of decreased anxiety.
ability to relax.
lack of statements indicating anticipated misfortune for child.
lack of inappropriate or hostile behavior.
ability to concentrate.
decreased reports of somatic discomfort.

POSSIBLE NURSING INTERVENTIONS
Listen to parents' concerns and complaints. Encourage expression of feelings to health care team regarding the surgery and its implications.

Explain the surgical procedure and give postoperative home care instructions to the parents. Keep the explanations simple and concise. Use illustrations. Repeat explanations as necessary.

Answer any questions the parents may have regarding the procedure, child's care, and/or child's condition.

Dispel any misinformation.

Remove excess stimulation from the environment.

Record interactions with parents.

EVALUATION FOR CHARTING
Describe parents' behavior and level of anxiety.

⌂ State whether parents were able to understand explanations regarding the surgical procedure, child's care, and child's condition.

Describe any successful measures used to decrease the parents' anxiety.

NURSING DIAGNOSIS
Knowledge Deficit: Parental

DEFINITION   Lack of information concerning the child's disease and care

POSSIBLY RELATED TO
Fear of surgical procedure
Fear of outcome of surgery
Misconceptions or inaccurate information concerning
    surgical procedure and outcome
Sensory overload
Cognitive or cultural-language limitations

CHARACTERISTICS
Verbalization by parents indicating lack of knowledge
Relation of incorrect information to members of the health
    care team
Requests for information

EXPECTED OUTCOMES   Parents will have an adequate knowledge base concerning the child's impending surgery and care as evidenced by

ability to correctly state information previously taught
    regarding the surgical procedure and home care.
ability to relate appropriate information to the health
    care team.

POSSIBLE NURSING INTERVENTIONS
Listen to parents' concerns and fears.

Assess and record parents' knowledge concerning the impending surgery.

Provide parents with information about the impending surgery, including

> preoperative medication.
> bowel preparation.
> explanation and rationale for the postoperative equipment child will need, such as a nasogastric (NG) tube, foley catheter, an IV, a Penrose drain, and dressings over incisions.
> time frame for the surgery.
> child's care after the procedure, including obtainment of vital signs *(no rectal temperatures)*, irrigation of NG tube, NPO status, dressing changes, record of intake and output, chest physiotherapy, and nasopharyngeal suctioning.

Use pictures as necessary to facilitate teaching.

Provide parents with any available literature or booklets concerning surgical procedure.

Assign a primary nurse as usual spokesperson to parents.

When indicated, obtain an interpreter.

Dispel any incorrect information.

👪 Instruct parents in home care of

> colostomy, including skin around the colostomy.
> incision site.
> skin integrity in the diaper area.

EVALUATION FOR CHARTING
State whether parents verbalized a knowledge deficit.

👪 State whether parents were able to repeat information correctly.

Describe any measures used to facilitate parent teaching.

RELATED NURSING DIAGNOSES

Fear: Child *related to*
a. impending surgery
b. hospitalization
c. unfamiliar surroundings
d. forced contact with strangers
e. treatments and procedures

Fear: Family *related to*
a. impending surgery
b. outcome of surgery

Compromised Family Coping *related to*
a. impending surgery
b. hospitalization of child

Altered Parenting *related to*
repeated hospitalization of child

POSTOPERATIVE NURSING CARE PLAN

PRIMARY NURSING DIAGNOSIS
Infection: High Risk

DEFINITION   Condition in which the body is at risk for being invaded by microorganisms

POSSIBLY RELATED TO
Surgical wound(s)
Spread of organisms from bowel

CHARACTERISTICS
Fever
Redness
Swelling
Purulent wound drainage
Foul odor
Lethargy
Irritability
Altered white blood cell count (WBC)
Tachycardia

EXPECTED OUTCOMES   Child will be free of infection as evidenced by

axillary temperature within acceptable range of 36.5°C to 37.2°C.
clean wound site(s) with minimal clear to serosanguineous drainage.
WBC within acceptable range (state specific highest and lowest counts for each child).
heart rate within acceptable range (state specific highest and lowest rates for each child).

lack of signs/symptoms of infection (such as those listed under **Characteristics**).

POSSIBLE NURSING INTERVENTIONS

Assess and record the following every 4 hours and PRN:

axillary temperature *(no rectal temperatures)* and heart rate

any signs/symptoms of infection (such as those listed under **Characteristics**)

Maintain good hand-washing technique.

Ensure that aseptic technique is used for wound care. Assess and record amount and characteristics of drainage.

Obtain culture specimens (wound, blood), if indicated. Check results and notify physician of any abnormalities.

Check and record results of complete blood count (CBC). Notify physician if CBC results are out of the acceptable range.

Reposition child every 2 hours.

Ensure that chest physiotherapy is performed on schedule, if indicated. Record effectiveness and child's response to treatments.

Administer antibiotics on schedule and antipyretics PRN. Assess and record effectiveness and any side effects (e.g., rash, diarrhea).

Assess and record family's knowledge of and participation in care regarding

medication administration. (The child may be sent home on antibiotics.)

incision site(s).

skin around colostomy and perineal area.

identification of any signs/symptoms of infection (such as those listed under **Characteristics**).

Instruct family in any areas needing improvement. Record results.

EVALUATION FOR CHARTING

State ranges of axillary temperature and heart rate.

Describe any signs/symptoms of infection noted (such as those listed under **Characteristics**).

Describe wound site(s) and amount and characteristics of any drainage.

State results of any cultures and/or CBCs, if available.

State how often child was repositioned.

Indicate whether chest physiotherapy was performed on schedule. Describe how child tolerated the procedure. State its effectiveness.

State whether antibiotics and antipyretics were administered on schedule. Describe effectiveness and any side effects noted.

Describe family's knowledge of and participation in care related to decreasing chance for infection. State any areas needing improvement and information provided. Describe family's response.

NURSING DIAGNOSIS
Fluid Volume Deficit

DEFINITION   Decrease in the amount of circulating fluid volume

POSSIBLY RELATED TO
Inability to tolerate PO fluids
Nasogastric suctioning

CHARACTERISTICS
Tachycardia
Hypotension
Abdominal distention
Nausea/vomiting
Dry mucous membranes
Poor skin turgor
Decreased urine output
Increased urine specific gravity

EXPECTED OUTCOMES   Child will have adequate fluid volume as evidenced by

adequate IV fluid intake (state specific amount of intake needed for each child).
heart rate and blood pressure within acceptable ranges (state specific highest and lowest parameters for each child).
nondistended abdomen.
absence of nausea/vomiting.
moist mucous membranes.
rapid skin recoil.
adequate urine output (state specific highest and lowest outputs for each child, minimum 1 to 2 ml/kg/hr).
urine specific gravity from 1.008 to 1.020.

POSSIBLE NURSING INTERVENTIONS

Keep accurate record of intake and output.

Keep child NPO. If indicated, offer oral fluids when tolerated and when bowel sounds have returned.

Assess and record

IV fluids and condition of IV site every hour.
heart rate and blood pressure every 4 hours and PRN.
bowel sounds every 4 hours and PRN.
any signs/symptoms of fluid volume deficit (such as those listed under **Characteristics**) every 4 hours and PRN.

If indicated, measure and record abdominal girth every shift.

Ensure that nasogastric tube is patent and connected to low intermittent suction. Irrigate with air or saline every 4 hours.

Ensure that Foley catheter is in place and draining properly and that a sterile closed drainage system is maintained. Administer catheter care according to institutional policy.

Check and record urine specific gravity every 4 hours or as indicated.

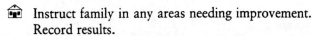 Assess and record family's knowledge of and participation in care regarding

child's need for fluids, when indicated.
monitoring of intake and output.
identification of any signs/symptoms of fluid volume deficit (such as those listed under **Characteristics**).

Instruct family in any areas needing improvement.
Record results.

EVALUATION FOR CHARTING

State intake and output.

Describe condition of IV site.

State highest and lowest heart rates and blood pressures.

Describe bowel sounds.

Describe any signs/symptoms of fluid volume deficit noted (such as those listed under **Characteristics**).

When indicated, state current abdominal girth and determine whether it has increased since the previous measurement.

Describe amount and characteristics of nasogastric drainage.

State whether Foley catheter was in place and draining properly.

State highest and lowest urine specific gravity values.

🏠 Describe family's knowledge of and participation in care related to improving fluid volume. State any area needing improvement and information provided. Describe family's response.

RELATED NURSING DIAGNOSES

Impaired Skin Integrity *related to*
frequent acidic stools in the perineal area

Pain *related to*
surgical incision site(s)

Altered Comfort* *related to*
invasive procedures

Compromised Family Coping *related to*
a. surgical procedure
b. child's hospitalization

---

*Non-NANDA diagnosis.

8

MEDICAL DIAGNOSIS

Inflammatory Bowel Disease

PATHOPHYSIOLOGY Inflammatory bowel disease (IBD) is used to describe both ulcerative colitis and Crohn's disease, two chronic intestinal disorders. These two diseases have similar epidemiologic, immunologic, and clinical features, but Crohn's disease can be more disabling and severe than ulcerative colitis. Although the causes of IBD are unknown, many infectious, nutritional, immunologic, and psychogenic factors have been proposed. Psychological factors, such as stress, may accentuate the symptoms and severity of a relapse but do not contribute to the pathogenesis.

Pharmacologic therapy is palliative, not curative, for both ulcerative colitis and Crohn's disease. If remission is not attainable with medications, total parenteral nutrition (TPN) and/or an elemental diet may be used in an effort to alleviate symptoms. Surgical intervention to remove affected bowel may be indicated for both diseases. A total colectomy with ileostomy may be performed in a child with ulcerative colitis when there is profuse hemorrhage, perforation, toxic megacolon, malignancy, or severe growth retardation. Children with Crohn's disease may need to have obstructed, narrowed bowel or fistulous tracks surgically excised.

Supportive measures are important to the child and family adjusting to IBD. Consultation with psychotherapists and stomal therapists may be beneficial. The National Foundation for Ileitis and Colitis, the United Ostomy Association, and local peer support groups can provide additional support and information.

Ulcerative Colitis

Ulcerative colitis is characterized by mucosal ulcerations and diffuse inflammation of the large intestine. The lesion is continuous, spreading to adjacent areas without skipping healthy bowel, but it rarely extends deeper than the submucosa. Thickening of the bowel results from the colonic edema and inflammation. The damaged bowel is ineffective in reabsorbing nutrients, fluid, and electrolytes.

The onset of ulcerative colitis is usually gradual. The child experiences chronic bloody, mucusy diarrhea; fecal urgency; pain; and lower abdominal cramps, especially before defecation. Anorexia with weight loss develops as the diarrhea persists over time. The bowel also takes on a lead-pipe appearance, with shortening of the colon, loss of mucosal and haustral folds, and the development of fibrous tissue and linear strictures. The onset of ulcerative colitis can also be fulminant, with the child experiencing explosive, bloody diarrhea; high fever; and possibly peritonitis and perforation.

Persisting symptoms of ulcerative colitis can delay growth and development. Extraintestinal symptoms, such as skin rash, arthritis, and iritis, are rare in children but more common in adolescents and young adults.

Crohn's Disease

Crohn's disease can involve one or more segments of the gut from the mouth to the anus; most often it affects the distal ileum and colon. Diseased bowel is usually separated by healthy bowel (skip lesion), and the lesion is transmural (involving all layers of the bowel). Edema and inflammation contribute to a thickened intestinal wall. Fistulas and fissures can develop between loops of bowel or to other structures, such as the skin or urinary tract, but the inflammation and engorgement on the serosal surface inhibit perforation or spillage of intestinal contents into the peritoneal cavity. Crypt abscesses and granulomas develop, as does regional lymphatic involvement. Over time, scar tissue and fibrotic strictures form, which can eventually lead to bowel obstruction.

The onset of Crohn's disease is subtle. The child will present with crampy, abdominal pain; diarrhea; fever; malaise; anorexia; and pain localized periumbilically or in the right lower quadrant. Perianal lesions are also common. Persisting symptoms of Crohn's disease delay growth and development. Extraintestinal symptoms often accompany Crohn's disease and include mouth ulcers, iritis, arthritis, arthralgia, and skin rashes.

PRIMARY NURSING DIAGNOSIS
Fluid Volume Deficit

DEFINITION   Decrease in the amount of circulating fluid volume

POSSIBLY RELATED TO
  Diarrhea
  Vomiting

CHARACTERISTICS

Severe diarrhea, with frequent loose, watery stools, which
may contain blood, pus, and/or mucus

Vomiting

Weight loss

Anorexia

Abdominal cramping

Abdominal distention

Hyperactive bowel sounds

Poor skin turgor

Dry mucous membranes

Decreased urine output

For Crohn's disease: fever

EXPECTED OUTCOMES   Child will have an adequate fluid
volume as evidenced by

adequate fluid intake, IV and/or oral (state specific amount
of intake needed for each child).

absence of

diarrhea.

mucus, pus, or blood in stool.

vomiting.

abdominal cramping and distention.

decreased number and frequency of stools.

normal activity of bowel sounds (one every 10 to 30
seconds).

regaining of weight lost during exacerbation.

adequate urine output (state specific highest and lowest
outputs for each child, minimum 1 to 2 ml/kg/hr).

urine specific gravity from 1.008 to 1.020.

moist mucous membranes.

return of appetite.

rapid skin recoil.

temperature within acceptable range of 36.5°C to 37.2°C.

POSSIBLE NURSING INTERVENTIONS

Keep accurate record of intake and output. Record
frequency, characteristics, and consistency of stools. Measure
and record amount and characteristics of any emesis.

Assess and record

IV fluids and condition of IV site every hour.

bowel sounds every shift and PRN.
temperature every 4 hours and PRN.
signs/symptoms of fluid volume deficit (such as those listed under **Characteristics**) every 4 hours and PRN.

Weigh child on same scale at same time each day without clothes.

Give mouth care every 4 hours and PRN.

Check and record urine specific gravity every void or as indicated.

Administer medications (e.g., sulfasalazine, corticosteroids, metronidazole) on schedule. Assess and record effectiveness and any side effects (e.g., neutropenia, hypersensitivity reactions, moon facies, acne).

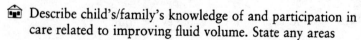 Assess and record child's/family's knowledge of and participation in care regarding

intake of appropriate fluids.
monitoring of intake and output.
identification of any signs/symptoms of fluid volume deficit (such as those listed under **Characteristics**).
medication administration.

 Instruct child/family in any areas needing improvement. Record results.

EVALUATION FOR CHARTING

State intake and output.

Describe condition of IV site.

Describe any signs/symptoms of fluid volume deficit noted (such as those listed under **Characteristics**).

State highest and lowest urine specific gravity values.

State highest and lowest temperatures.

Indicate whether medications were administered on schedule. Describe effectiveness and any side effects noted.

Describe any therapeutic measures used to improve fluid volume. State their effectiveness.

 Describe child's/family's knowledge of and participation in care related to improving fluid volume. State any areas

needing improvement and information provided. Describe child's/family's responses.

NURSING DIAGNOSIS
Pain

DEFINITION   Condition in which an individual experiences severe discomfort

POSSIBLY RELATED TO
>   Abdominal cramping secondary to inflammation and
>   ulceration of the bowel
>   Perianal fistulas and abscesses

CHARACTERISTICS
>   Verbal communication of pain
>   Crying or moaning
>   Facial grimacing
>   For ulcerative colitis: tender abdomen, tenderness upon rectal
>   examination, and lower abdominal pain
>   For Crohn's disease: periumbilical pain and/or pain in the
>   right lower quadrant and excoriated skin around the anus
>   Rebound tenderness
>   Decreased activity, self-imposed
>   Physical signs/symptoms:
>
>   tachycardia
>   tachypnea/bradypnea
>   increased blood pressure
>   diaphoresis
>
>   Rating of pain on pain-assessment tool

EXPECTED OUTCOMES   Child will have decreased pain or be free of pain as evidenced by

>   verbal communication of decreased pain or no pain.
>   decrease in or lack of crying, moaning, and facial grimacing.
>   heart rate and respiratory rate within acceptable ranges (state
>   specific highest and lowest rates for each child).
>   blood pressure within acceptable range (state specific highest
>   and lowest pressures for each child).
>   decreased diaphoresis.
>   increased participation in self-care and in age-appropriate
>   play activities.

rating indicating no pain or decreased pain on
pain-assessment tool.

POSSIBLE NURSING INTERVENTIONS

Assess and record any signs/symptoms of pain (such as those
listed under **Characteristics**) every 2 hours and PRN. Use
age-appropriate pain-assessment tool.

Handle child gently.

Encourage family members to stay and comfort child when
possible.

Allow family members to participate in care of the child
when possible.

If age-appropriate, allow the child to participate in planning
self-care. Encourage to increase participation in self-care as
pain decreases.

Administer analgesics on schedule. Assess and record
effectiveness.

Institute additional pain relief measures, such as relaxation.
Assess and record effectiveness.

⌂ Assess and record child's/family's knowledge of and
participation in care regarding pain relief.

⌂ Instruct child/family in any areas needing improvement.

EVALUATION FOR CHARTING

State range of vital signs.

Describe characteristics of pain.

Describe any therapeutic measures used to decrease or
eliminate pain. State their effectiveness.

⌂ Describe child's/family's knowledge of and participation in
care. State any areas needing improvement and information
provided. Describe child's/family's responses.

RELATED NURSING DIAGNOSES

Altered Nutrition: Less than Body Requirements
related to

impaired ability to absorb nutrients

Body Image Disturbance *related to*
   a. disease symptoms
   b. medication use, especially steroids
   c. colectomy or colostomy
   d. altered growth and development

Altered Growth and Development *related to*
   a. impaired ability to absorb nutrients
   b. large doses of corticosteroids

Compromised Family Coping *related to*
   child's chronic illness

MEDICAL DIAGNOSIS
Pyloric Stenosis

PATHOPHYSIOLOGY   The pylorus is the opening that allows passage of food from the stomach to the duodenum. Hypertrophic pyloric stenosis is a thickening of the muscular ring (pyloric sphincter) that surrounds the pylorus. Spasms of the muscle lead to hypertrophy and eventual obstruction of the opening, thus causing the condition. Because of the obstruction, food is unable to pass out of the stomach and the infant vomits. The obstruction may also lead to prolonged stasis of gastric fluids, which may cause gastritis.

Clinical manifestations of pyloric stenosis vary somewhat, but typically the cardinal sign is vomiting beginning when the infant is about 3 weeks of age, starting with the regurgitation of small amounts of milk immediately after a feeding and progressing to projectile vomiting (may be 2 to 4 feet) within a week or so. Vomiting can occur during a feeding, immediately after a feeding, or several hours later. The infant will be hungry following the vomiting episode and will eagerly accept a second feeding. Emesis may be blood tinged due to gastritis but will not contain bile. Prolonged vomiting can result in decreased serum levels of both sodium and potassium, a striking decrease in serum chloride levels, and increases in pH and carbon dioxide content (bicarbonate), characterizing hypochloremic alkalosis. Other clinical manifestations include failure to gain weight (or even weight loss); signs and symptoms of dehydration; a distended upper abdomen; a palpable, olive-shaped mass (distended pylorus); and visible peristaltic waves that move from left to right.

Treatment is surgical correction to open the pylorus (pyloromyotomy). If the infant is dehydrated, that condition is corrected prior to surgery. The surgical procedure has a high success rate and a low mortality rate (only 1%).

Pyloric stenosis is one of the most common surgical disorders of early infancy. Although the exact etiology is unknown, there is a family history of the problem in about 15% of all cases. The condition is thought to occur five times more often in males than in females, is rare in black and Asian infants, and is most likely to affect full-term infants.

PREOPERATIVE NURSING CARE PLAN

PRIMARY NURSING DIAGNOSIS

Altered Nutrition: Less than Body Requirements

DEFINITION   Insufficient nutrients to meet body requirements

POSSIBLY RELATED TO
> Vomiting secondary to thickening of the circular muscle of the pylorus
> Vomiting secondary to obstruction of the opening between the stomach and duodenum

CHARACTERISTICS
> Projectile vomiting
> Lack of bile in emesis
> Visible peristaltic waves that move from left to right
> Palpable, olive-shaped mass in pyloric region
> Distended upper abdomen
> Failure to gain weight, or weight loss

EXPECTED OUTCOMES   Infant will be adequately nourished as evidenced by

> sufficient caloric consumption (state range of calories needed for each infant).
> lack of vomiting.
> stable weight or lack of weight loss.
> lack of signs/symptoms of altered nutrition (such as those listed under **Characteristics**).

POSSIBLE NURSING INTERVENTIONS
> Keep accurate record of intake and output. Record emesis: frequency, characteristics, and relationship to feeding.

> Assess and record any signs/symptoms of altered nutrition (such as those listed under **Characteristics**) every 4 hours and PRN.

If indicated, maintain NPO status and administer mouth care PRN. Assess and record for patency and condition of IV site every hour.

If oral feedings are ordered, feed infant slowly with small, frequent feedings. Place in a semierect position. Bubble before and frequently during feedings. After feedings, place on right side in the head-elevated position. Encourage family to participate.

Organize care in order to decrease disturbing and handling infant after feedings.

Weigh infant on same scale at same time each day without clothes. Record results.

🏠 Assess and record family's knowledge of and participation in care regarding

monitoring of intake and output.
feeding schedule and method of feeding.
positioning of infant.
organization of care so infant is not disturbed after feedings.
identification of any signs/symptoms of altered nutrition (such as those listed under **Characteristics**).

🏠 Instruct family in any areas needing improvement. Record results.

EVALUATION FOR CHARTING

State intake and output.

Describe amount, frequency, relationship to feedings, and characteristics of any emesis.

Describe any signs/symptoms of altered nutrition noted (such as those listed under **Characteristics**).

If indicated, state whether NPO status was maintained.

Describe condition of IV site.

If indicated, describe how infant tolerated feedings. State effectiveness of feedings and positioning in decreasing vomiting.

State infant's current weight and determine whether it has increased or decreased since previous weighing.

Describe family's knowledge of and participation in care related to improving infant's nutritional status. State any areas needing improvement and information provided. Describe family's response.

NURSING DIAGNOSIS
Fluid Volume Deficit

DEFINITION   Decrease in the amount of circulating fluid volume

POSSIBLY RELATED TO
Vomiting
Dehydration

CHARACTERISTICS
Projectile vomiting
Abdominal distention
Tachycardia
Hypotension
Dry mucous membranes
Poor skin turgor
Sunken fontanel
Sunken eyeballs
Decreased urine output
Increased urine specific gravity

EXPECTED OUTCOMES   Infant will have adequate fluid volume as evidenced by

absence of vomiting.
adequate fluid intake, PO or IV (state specific amount of intake needed for each child).
nondistended abdomen.
heart rate and blood pressure within acceptable ranges (state specific highest and lowest parameters for each child).
moist mucous membranes.
flat fontanel.
lack of sunken eyeballs.
adequate urine output (state specific highest and lowest outputs for each infant, minimum of 1 to 2 ml/kg/hr).
urine specific gravity from 1.008 to 1.020.

POSSIBLE NURSING INTERVENTIONS

Keep accurate record of intake and output. Record emesis: frequency, characteristics, and relationship to feeding.

Assess and record the following every 4 hours and PRN:

heart rate and blood pressure
any signs/symptoms of fluid volume deficit (such as those listed under **Characteristics**)

If indicated, maintain NPO status and administer mouth care every 4 hours and PRN. Assess and record for patency and note the condition of IV site every hour.

If oral feedings are ordered, feed infant slowly with small, frequent feedings. Place in a semierect position. Bubble before and frequently during feedings. After feedings, place on right side in the head-elevated position. Encourage family to participate.

Organize care in order to decrease disturbing and handling of infant after feedings.

Check and record urine specific gravity every 4 hours or as directed.

Assess and record family's knowledge of and participation in care regarding

monitoring of intake and output.
feeding schedule and method of feeding.
positioning of infant.
organization of care so infant is not disturbed after feedings.
identification of any signs/symptoms of fluid volume deficit (such as those listed under **Characteristics**).

Instruct family in any areas needing improvement. Record results.

EVALUATION FOR CHARTING

State intake and output.

Describe amount, frequency, relationship to feedings, and characteristics of any emesis.

State highest and lowest heart rates and blood pressures.

Describe any signs/symptoms of fluid volume deficit (such as those listed under **Characteristics**).

If indicated, state whether NPO status was maintained.

Describe condition of IV site.

If indicated, describe how infant tolerated effectiveness of feedings and positioning in decreasing vomiting.

State highest and lowest urine specific gravity values.

Describe family's knowledge of and participation in care related to improving fluid balance. State any areas needing improvement and information provided. Describe family's response.

RELATED NURSING DIAGNOSES

Electrolyte Imbalance: Sodium Losses and Potassium Losses* *related to*
a. vomiting
b. dehydration

Knowledge Deficit: Parental *related to*
a. disease state
b. surgical correction
c. postoperative home management

Altered Comfort* *related to*
a. hunger
b. vomiting

Compromised Family Coping *related to*
a. hospitalization of infant
b. impending surgery for infant
c. knowledge deficit about medical diagnosis

---

*Non-NANDA diagnosis.

POSTOPERATIVE NURSING CARE PLAN

PRIMARY NURSING DIAGNOSIS

Altered Nutrition: Less than Body Requirements

DEFINITION   Insufficient nutrients to meet body requirements

POSSIBLY RELATED TO

Postoperative vomiting

CHARACTERISTICS

Failure of bowel sounds to return
Inability to tolerate oral feedings

EXPECTED OUTCOMES   Infant will be adequately nourished as evidenced by

patent IV line that will deliver the ordered amount of IV
fluids (state specific amount for each infant).
sufficient calorie consumption (state range of calories needed
for each infant).
absence of

weight loss.
vomiting when oral feedings are started.

POSSIBLE NURSING INTERVENTIONS

Keep accurate record of intake and output. Record emesis:
frequency, characteristics, and relationship to feeding. Assess
and record for patency and condition of IV site every hour.

Assess and record any signs/symptoms of altered nutrition
(such as those listed under **Characteristics**).

When indicated, feed infant slowly with small, frequent
feedings. Advance amount and type of feedings as indicated.
Place in a semierect position. Bubble before and frequently
during feedings. After feedings, place on right side in the
head-elevated position. Encourage family to participate.

Organize care in order to decrease disturbance and handling
of infant after feedings.

🏠 Assess and record family's knowledge of and participation in
care regarding

monitoring of intake and output.

feeding schedule and method of feeding.

positioning of infant.

organization of care so infant is not disturbed after
feedings.

identification of any signs/symptoms of altered nutrition
(such as those listed under **Characteristics**).

 Instruct family in any areas needing improvement.
Record results.

EVALUATION FOR CHARTING

State intake and output.

Describe amount, frequency, relationship to feedings, and
characteristics of any emesis.

Describe condition of IV site.

Describe any signs/symptoms of altered nutrition (such as
those listed under **Characteristics**).

If indicated, describe how the infant tolerated feedings. State
effectiveness of feedings and positioning in decreasing
vomiting.

 Describe family's knowledge of and participation in care
related to improving nutritional status. State any areas
needing improvement and information provided. Describe
family's response.

NURSING DIAGNOSIS
Infection: High Risk

DEFINITION   Condition in which the body is at risk for being
invaded by microorganisms

POSSIBLY RELATED TO

Surgical incision

Young age of patient

Invasive procedures (IV)

CHARACTERISTICS

Fever

Redness

Swelling

Purulent wound drainage
Foul odor
Lethargy
Irritability
Altered white blood cell count (WBC)
Tachycardia

EXPECTED OUTCOMES   Infant will be free of infection as evidenced by

body temperature within the acceptable range of 36.5°C to 37.2°C.

clean wound site with minimal clear to serosanguineous drainage.

WBC within acceptable range (state specific highest and lowest counts for each infant).

heart rate within acceptable range (state specific highest and lowest rates for each child).

lack of signs/symptoms of infection (such as those listed under **Characteristics**).

POSSIBLE NURSING INTERVENTIONS

Assess and record the following every 4 hours and PRN:

temperature and heart rate
any signs/symptoms of infection (such as those listed under **Characteristics**)

Ensure that aseptic technique is used when caring for the incision. Assess and record amount and characteristics of drainage.

Obtain culture specimens (wound) if indicated. Check and record results. Notify physician of any abnormalities.

Check and record results of complete blood count (CBC). Notify physician if CBC results are out of the acceptable range.

Assess and record family's knowledge of and participation in care regarding

incision site.
identification of any signs/symptoms of infection (such as those listed under **Characteristics**).

Instruct family in any areas needing improvement. Record
Record results.

EVALUATION FOR CHARTING
State ranges of temperature and heart rate.

Describe wound site and amount and characteristics of any drainage.

State results of any cultures and/or CBCs, if available.

Describe any signs/symptoms of infection noted (such as those listed under **Characteristics**).

RELATED NURSING DIAGNOSES

Fluid Volume Deficit *related to*
  a. vomiting
  b. dehydration

Pain *related to*
  a. surgical incision
  b. hunger
  c. vomiting and effect on the operative site

Knowledge Deficit: Parental *related to*
  a. incision care
  b. feeding technique and schedule

Compromised Family Coping *related to*
  a. fear of surgery not being successful
  b. apprehension and hesitance secondary to prior feeding experience with infant

Short-Bowel Syndrome (Short-Gut Syndrome)

PATHOPHYSIOLOGY   Short-bowel syndrome, also called short-gut syndrome, is the condition in which there is loss of massive amounts of intestine, affecting the ability of the child to digest and absorb a regular diet. Short-bowel syndrome may be congenital or acquired.

Congenital short-bowel syndrome is often associated with intestinal malrotation or atresia, with diarrhea and malabsorption beginning at birth if the disease is severe. In acquired short-bowel syndrome, massive resection of the small intestine during the neonatal period may be required secondary to necrotizing enterocolitis, gastroschisis, or multiple intestinal atresias. Acquired short-bowel syndrome also occurs when massive amounts of the small intestine are removed because of acute gastrointestinal illnesses. In older infants and children, resectioning may be necessary because of Crohn's disease or intussusception with gangrenous bowel.

The remaining intestines of most infants with short-bowel syndrome usually adapt to assume the function of the jejunal mucosa within the first year after surgery. Various problems with malabsorption can result, though, especially if more than 75% of the small bowel has been removed. Malabsorption of vitamin B12, bile salts, iron, calcium, folic acid, or fat-soluble vitamins may occur. The production of lactase, sucrase, and maltase may also decrease. When the ileocecal valve is left in place, it helps regulate transit time and protects against bacterial contamination of the small bowel so that the body can better tolerate the removal of large amounts of bowel. Overgrowth of bacteria can cause increased intestinal gas and diarrhea.

Treatment of infants and children with short-bowel syndrome focuses on promoting adequate nutrition, using elemental formulas, and preventing complications. Complications such as fluid and electrolyte imbalance, infection, and perianal skin excoriation due to diarrhea and the excretion of bile acids and enzymes are common.

PRIMARY NURSING DIAGNOSIS

Altered Nutrition: Less than Body Requirements

DEFINITION   Insufficient nutrients to meet body requirements

POSSIBLY RELATED TO
Malabsorption
Diarrhea
Vomiting

CHARACTERISTICS
Diarrhea
Vomiting
Malabsorption of vitamins, fat-soluble vitamins, calcium, and iron
Decreased enzymes
Inadequate weight gain
Weight loss

EXPECTED OUTCOMES   Child will be adequately nourished as evidenced by

sufficient caloric consumption—parenterally, orally, or via gastrostomy tube (state specific amount for each child).
lack of

vomiting.
diarrhea.

steady weight gain or lack of weight loss.
lack of vitamin and/or mineral deficiencies.

POSSIBLE NURSING INTERVENTIONS
Keep accurate record of intake and output. Note which elemental formula is being used.

Assess and record signs/symptoms of altered nutrition (such as those listed under **Characteristics**).

Weigh child on same scale at same time each day.

Maintain and record caloric count, as indicated.

Organize care to conserve energy.

Administer gastrostomy tube feedings on schedule, as indicated. Follow institutional policy for care of the gastrostomy tube and site. Note which elemental formula is being used.

When indicated, administer total parental nutrition (TPN) and intralipids. Follow hospital policy for maintenance of TPN and intralipid line and site. Assess and record urine glucose, protein, ketones, and pH every 4 to 8 hours and PRN. Check and record serum glucose and lipid levels, as indicated.

Administer medications (vitamins, oral antibiotics, antireflux medications) on schedule. Assess and record effectiveness and any side effects (e.g., rash, diarrhea, nausea, irritability).

Initiate and maintain consultation with dietitian and visiting nurses.

Assess and record child's/family's knowledge of and participation in care regarding

> type and amount of feedings.
> monitoring of child's weight gain and caloric consumption.
> medication administration.
> gastrostomy tube and site, as indicated.
> identification of signs/symptoms of altered nutrition (such as those listed under **Characteristics**).

Instruct child/family in any areas needing improvement. Record results.

EVALUATION FOR CHARTING

State intake and output.

State caloric intake, when indicated.

Describe any signs/symptoms of altered nutrition noted (such as those listed under **Characteristics**).

Describe type and amount of feedings and how child tolerated feedings.

State child's current weight and determine whether it has increased or decreased since previous weighing.

State whether medications were administered on schedule. Describe effectiveness and any side effects.

📷 Describe any therapeutic measures used to maintain adequate nutrition. State their effectiveness.

📷 Describe child's/family's knowledge of and participation in care related to improving nutritional status. State any areas needing improvement and information provided. Describe child's/family's responses.

NURSING DIAGNOSIS
Fluid Volume Deficit

DEFINITION   Decrease in the amount of circulating fluid volume

POSSIBLY RELATED TO
> Vomiting
> Diarrhea
> Insufficient free water in feedings

CHARACTERISTICS
> Vomiting
> Frequent liquid stools
> Weight loss
> Poor skin turgor
> Dry mucous membranes
> Decreased urine output
> Increase in urine specific gravity
> Absence of tears

EXPECTED OUTCOMES   Child will have an adequate fluid volume as evidenced by

> adequate fluid intake—oral or via IV or gastrostomy tube (state specific amount of fluid intake needed for each child).
> absence of

>> diarrhea.
>> vomiting.

> adequate urine output (state specific highest and lowest outputs for each child, minimum 1 to 2 ml/kg/hr).
> urine specific gravity from 1.008 to 1.020.
> moist mucous membranes.

rapid skin recoil.
tears present when crying.

POSSIBLE NURSING INTERVENTIONS

Keep accurate record of intake and output. Record emesis and diarrhea, including frequency, amount, and characteristics (including consistency, color, pH, and reducing substances).

Assess and record

IV fluids given and condition of IV site every hour.
signs/symptoms of fluid volume deficit (such as those listed under **Characteristics**) every 4 hours and PRN.

Check and record urine specific gravity every void or as indicated.

Weigh child on same scale at same time each day without clothes.

Give mouth care every 4 hours and PRN.

⌂ Assess and record child's/family's knowledge of and participation in care regarding

monitoring of intake and output.
identification of any signs/symptoms of fluid volume deficit (such as those listed under **Characteristics**).

⌂ Instruct child/family in any areas needing improvement. Record results.

EVALUATION FOR CHARTING

State intake and output.

Describe condition of IV site.

Describe any sign/symptoms of fluid volume deficit noted (such as those listed under **Characteristics**).

State highest and lowest urine specific gravity values.

Describe any therapeutic measures used to improve fluid volume. State their effectiveness.

⌂ Describe child's/family's knowledge of and participation in care related to improving fluid volume. State any areas needing improvement and information provided. Describe child's/family's responses.

Impaired Skin Integrity

DEFINITION   Interruption in integrity of the skin

POSSIBLY RELATED TO
Irritation of skin by bile salts and enzymes in stools
Caustic diarrhea

CHARACTERISTICS
Frequent stools that are loose, pasty, or watery
Red, excoriated perianal tissue

EXPECTED OUTCOMES   Child will be free of signs/symptoms
of impaired skin integrity as evidenced by

clean, intact skin.
natural skin color.
lack of

redness.
excoriation.
lesions.

POSSIBLE NURSING INTERVENTIONS
Assess and record skin condition every shift.

Handle child gently.

Bathe child daily (or as indicated) with water. Use a
nonirritating soap, when indicated.

Keep the perianal area clean and dry by

changing diaper and linens as soon as possible after
elimination or soiling.
using cloth diapers.
using cotton underwear.
keeping open to air, when possible.

When indicated, allow child to take sitz baths.

Apply topical medications on schedule. Assess and record
effectiveness.

Use a barrier cream or ointment on schedule, as indicated.

🏠 Assess and record child's/family's knowledge of and
participation in care regarding

measures related to preventing or correcting impaired skin integrity.

medication administration.

🏠 Instruct child/family in any areas needing improvement. Record results.

EVALUATION FOR CHARTING

Describe any potential or actual areas of skin breakdown.

Describe any therapeutic measures used to prevent or correct impaired skin integrity.

🏠 Describe child's/family's knowledge of and participation in care related to preventing or correcting impaired skin integrity. State any areas needing improvement and information provided. Describe child's/family's responses.

RELATED NURSING DIAGNOSES

Altered Growth and Development *related to*
   a. malabsorption
   b. nonoral feeding methods
   c. restricted mobility
   d. frequent hospitalizations

Electrolyte Imbalance: (Specify)* *related to*
   a. vomiting
   b. diarrhea
   c. malabsorption

Knowledge Deficit: Parental *related to*
   home management

---

*Non-NANDA diagnosis.

Five

CARE OF CHILDREN WITH HEMOPOIETIC DYSFUNCTION AND NEOPLASMS

MEDICAL DIAGNOSIS
Hemophilia

PATHOPHYSIOLOGY Hemophilia is the term used to describe a group of hereditary bleeding disorders in which one of the factors needed for blood coagulation is deficient. This deficiency leads to repeated bleeding into soft tissues, muscles, and joint capsules. Approximately 80% of affected individuals have hemophilia A, which results from a deficiency of factor VIII. Next most common is hemophilia B (also known as Christmas disease), which results from a factor IX deficiency. Hemophilia is an X-linked recessive disorder and primarily affects males. It is transmitted about 60% to 70% of the time by an unaffected female carrier to male offsprings. It can also result from a spontaneous genetic mutation. Approximately one-third of all individuals affected with hemophilia have no family history of the disease.

Individuals with hemophilia can be classified into three groups according to the severity of the factor deficiency. Those who are mildly affected have 5% to 50% of the functioning factor present, moderately affected individuals have 1% to 5% present, and severely affected individuals have less than 1% of the functioning factor present. The severe form can result in spontaneous bleeding without any precipitous trauma. Approximately 60% to 70% of children with hemophilia are diagnosed with the severe form of the disease. Laboratory findings that are positive for hemophilia include a prolonged partial thromboplastin time (PTT), a normal prothrombin time (PT), a normal bleeding time, a normal platelet count, and low levels of factor VIII or IX coagulant levels.

The classic sign of hemophilia is prolonged bleeding anywhere in the body. Most children do not begin bleeding episodes until early childhood, when they become active. Bleeding is likely to occur after minor falls or bumps, loss of deciduous teeth, or immunizations. Hemarthrosis (bleeding into a joint cavity) can occur in joints such as the knee, elbow, or ankle. The bleeding can cause joint swelling, tenderness, and pain; repeated bleeds can result in destruction of the joint. Trauma to the head is dangerous and can lead to bleeding in the central nervous system and death.

Therapeutic management consists of prevention and early treatment of bleeding, local control measures such as pressure and application of cold, and, when indicated, replacement of the deficient factor. Three types of plasma products used to treat hemophilia are fresh-frozen plasma, cryoprecipitate, and lyophilized concentrate. All are usually expensive. Comfort measures, such as immobilization and analgesics (non-aspirin-containing drugs), are also used, when indicated. Special efforts are needed to ensure a safe environment, such as padding the crib and playpen for infants and young children. Older children should be encouraged to participate in noncontact sports such as swimming; active hemophiliac children seem to bleed less than those who are sedentary.

Because part of the treatment for hemophilia is administration of blood products, the child is at risk for allergic reactions (rare with cryoprecipitates or factor concentrates), hepatitis, and acquired immune deficiency syndrome (AiDS). Improved processing and donor screening have significantly decreased the risk of disease transmission. Since the discovery of factor concentrates, home management is now possible. The parent/child are taught to do venipuncture and to administer antihemophilic factor concentrates.

PRIMARY NURSING DIAGNOSIS
Injury: High Risk

DEFINITION Situation in which the child is at risk for sustaining damage or harm

POSSIBLY RELATED TO
Hemorrhage secondary to decrease in clotting factor VIII or IX

CHARACTERISTICS
Mild/moderate/severe/frequent/spontaneous bleeding episodes of

skin
mucous membranes
joints (causing warmth, redness, swelling, pain, stiffness, tingling, and/or loss of movement)
viscera (causing hematuria and/or black, tarry stools)

central nervous system (causing headache, slurred speech, and/or loss of consciousness)

Prolonged PTT

Low levels of factor VIII or IX coagulant levels

EXPECTED OUTCOMES   Child will be free of injury that might result in further bleeding as evidenced by

lack of new areas of bleeding.

elevation of deficient clotting factor to desired level (specify).

POSSIBLE NURSING INTERVENTIONS

Assess and record any signs/symptoms of injury (new areas of bleeding) every 4 hours and PRN. If bleeding has occurred, assess and record heart rate and blood pressure every 1 to 2 hours and PRN.

Handle child gently.

Assist child in limiting activity by providing diversional activities (e.g., television, books).

Immobilize and elevate any affected joints.

Check and record results of PTT. Notify physician if results are more prolonged than previous results.

When indicated, perform passive range-of-motion exercises after bleeding has stopped.

Administer fresh-frozen plasma, cryoprecipitate, or lyophilized concentrate, as indicated. Adhere to institutional policy and current guidelines for administration of blood products. Assess and record effectiveness and any side effects such as transfusion reactions (e.g., chills, fever, shaking, urticaria, flushing, nausea/vomiting).

Administer other drugs, such as steroids (used to reduce inflammation in the joints) and epsilon-aminocaproic acid (applied locally to prevent clot destruction), as indicated. Assess and record effectiveness and any side effects (such as gastrointestinal distress and electrolyte imbalance).

 Assess and record child's/family's knowledge of and participation in care regarding

identification of any signs/symptoms of injury (such as those listed under **Characteristics**).

protection of child from injury by providing a safe environment (padded sides of crib and playpen, use of car seats in automobiles, etc.).

recognition and management of bleeding episodes by
• applying pressure to area for 10 to 15 minutes.
• immobilizing and elevating the area above the level of the heart.
• applying cold to promote vasoconstriction.

prevention of joint degeneration by
• elevating and immobilizing the joint.
• performing passive range-of-motion exercises after the bleeding has stopped.
• assisting with physical therapy, when indicated.

venipuncture technique and medication administration, when indicated, by
• assessing for transfusion reactions (e.g., chills, fever, shaking, urticaria, flushing, nausea/vomiting).

fostering of child's independence when child is ready. (Adolescents can usually perform their own venipunctures.)

having child wear Medic Alert identification.

encouraging child to participate in noncontact sports such as swimming.

encouraging child to establish good oral hygiene routine, including use of a soft-bristle toothbrush.

Instruct child/family in any areas needing improvement. Record results.

EVALUATION FOR CHARTING

Describe any signs/symptoms of injury noted (such as those listed under **Characteristics**). If bleeding has occurred, state ranges of heart rate and blood pressure.

Describe any interventions and their effectiveness in preventing injury and further bleeding.

State results of PTT and clotting factor tests. Indicate whether they have increased or decreased from previous results.

Describe effectiveness of medications and any side effects noted.

🏠 Describe child's/family's knowledge of and participation in care related to preventing injury. State any areas needing improvement and information provided. Describe child's/family's responses.

NURSING DIAGNOSIS
Pain

DEFINITION   Condition in which an individual experiences severe discomfort

POSSIBLY RELATED TO

Pressure in a joint or muscle spasms secondary to bleeding into a joint cavity resulting from factor deficiency

CHARACTERISTICS

Inability to move affected joint
Severe discomfort on movement of involved joint
Swelling and redness of affected area
Local increase in skin temperature
Crying or moaning
Facial grimacing
Verbal expression of pain
Restlessness
Physical signs/symptoms:

tachycardia
tachypnea/bradypnea
increased blood pressure
diaphoresis

EXPECTED OUTCOMES   Child will be free of extreme pain as evidenced by

decreased swelling and redness of the affected joint.
decreased skin temperature of the affected joint.
lack of constant crying or moaning.
verbal communication of decreased pain.
lack of facial grimacing and restlessness.
heart rate, respiratory rate, and blood pressure within acceptable ranges (state specific highest and lowest parameters for each child).
decreased diaphoresis.

POSSIBLE NURSING INTERVENTIONS

Assess and record the following every 2 to 4 hours and PRN:

vital signs
signs/symptoms of pain (such as those listed under
  Characteristics)

Handle child gently.

Apply cold packs to help alleviate the pain.

Assist child in limiting activity by providing diversional
activities (e.g., television, books).

Immobilize and elevate any affected joints.

When indicated, perform passive range-of-motion exercise
after the bleeding has stopped.

Administer non-aspirin-containing analgesics and/or narcotics
on schedule. Assess and record effectiveness.

Administer fresh-frozen plasma, cryoprecipitate, or
lyophilized concentrate, as indicated. Adhere to institutional
policy and current guidelines for administration of blood
products. Assess and record effectiveness and any side effects
such as transfusion reactions (e.g., chills, fever, shaking,
urticaria, flushing, nausea/vomiting).

Assess and record child's/family's knowledge of and
participation in care regarding

identification of any signs/symptoms of pain (such as those
  listed under **Characteristics**).
protection of child from injury by providing a safe
  environment (e.g., padded sides of crib and playpen,
  use of car seats in automobiles, etc.).
recognition and management of bleeding episodes by
  • applying pressure to the area for 10 to 15 minutes.
  • immobilizing and elevating the area above the level of
    the heart.
  • applying cold to promote vasoconstriction.
prevention of joint degeneration by
  • elevating and immobilizing the joint.
  • performing passive range-of-motion exercises after the
    bleeding has stopped.
  • assisting with physical therapy, when indicated.

medication administration (non-aspirin-containing analgesics).

venipuncture technique and medication administration, when indicated, by

* assessing for transfusion reactions (e.g., chills, fever, shaking, urticaria, flushing, nausea/vomiting).

🏠 Instruct child/family in any areas needing improvement. Record results.

EVALUATION FOR CHARTING

Describe any signs/symptoms of pain noted (such as those listed under **Characteristics**).

State ranges of vital signs.

Describe effectiveness of analgesics and/or narcotics.

Describe any successful measures used to reduce or eliminate pain.

🏠 Describe child's/family's knowledge of and participation in care regarding reduction of pain. State any areas needing improvement and information provided. Describe child's/family's responses.

RELATED NURSING DIAGNOSES

Impaired Physical Mobility *related to*
a. joint pain
b. joint swelling
c. bleeding episodes

Knowledge Deficit: Child/Family *related to*
a. home management
b. disease state

Fluid Volume Deficit *related to*
blood loss out of vascular system

Compromised Family Coping *related to*
a. home management
b. child's activity restriction
c. genetic nature of disorder

MEDICAL DIAGNOSIS

Idiopathic Thrombocytopenia Purpura

PATHOPHYSIOLOGY Idiopathic thrombocytopenia purpura (ITP), an acquired hemorrhagic disorder characterized by a marked decrease in circulating platelets, is the most common type of childhood thrombocytopenia. Its primary cause is unknown, but it is believed to be due to an autoimmune phenomenon in which platelets become coated with an antiplatelet antibody, which alters the surface of the platelets so they become antigenic and are subsequently destroyed by the reticuloendothelial system in the spleen.

Idiopathic thrombocytopenia purpura can be acute, which is usually self-limiting, or chronic, which is interspersed with periods of remission. The acute form often follows an upper respiratory infection or a common childhood illness such as measles, rubella, mumps, or chickenpox. The most common clinical manifestations of either type include a sudden onset of easy bruising and randomly distributed petechiae and ecchymoses all over the body. Other signs and symptoms include bleeding from mucous membranes (e.g., epistaxis) and internal hemorrhage manifested by hematuria, bloody stools, and menorrhagia. The platelet count is usually reduced to below 30,000 mm^3/dL. Bone marrow aspiration is useful to rule out aplastic anemia or leukemia; in cases of ITP, numbers of megakaryocytes usually increase, and there is little or no evidence of platelet formation. Among other laboratory findings: (1) red and white blood cells are normal, (2) bleeding time is prolonged, (3) the tourniquet test (that demonstrates capillary fragility) is positive, (4) partial thromboplastin time (PTT) is normal, and (5) prothrombin time (PT) is normal.

Treatment of ITP varies. Activity is usually limited to try to prevent further petechiae and ecchymoses, and aspirin-containing drugs are eliminated. Some physicians do not prescribe any medications and allow the disease to run its course. Others prescribe a short course (usually 2 weeks) of corticosteroid therapy to suppress antibody response. Platelet transfusions are not useful because the transfused platelets become coated with the antiplatelet antibody and are destroyed in the spleen. Intravenous immunoglobulins (Sandoglobulin, Gammagard, and Gamimune) have recently been used successfully to increase platelet count. Splenectomy is usually reserved for children over 5 years of age who have recurrent or chronic ITP and who have refractory thrombocytopenia. After a splenectomy, 70% to 90% of children are free of signs and symptoms of ITP. The prognosis for acute ITP is excellent, and children usually recover in 6 months.

PRIMARY NURSING DIAGNOSIS
Injury: High Risk

DEFINITION   Situation in which the child is at risk for sustaining damage or harm

POSSIBLY RELATED TO
Decreased number of circulating platelets

CHARACTERISTICS
Petechiae
Ecchymoses
Bleeding from mucous membranes, including

epistaxis
bleeding gums
hematuria
blood in stools
menorrhagia

Platelet count below 30,000 mm^3/dL
Pain

EXPECTED OUTCOMES   Child will be free of injury that might result in further bleeding as evidenced by

lack of new petechiae or ecchymoses.
lack of bleeding from mucous membranes.
platelet count between 150,000 and 400,000 mm^3/dL.
decrease in or absence of pain.

POSSIBLE NURSING INTERVENTIONS
Assess and record any signs/symptoms of injury (new petechiae or ecchymoses) every 4 hours and PRN.

Handle child gently.

Assist child in limiting activity by providing diversional activities (e.g., television, books).

Check and record results of platelet count. Notify physician if results are decreased from previous results.

If indicated, administer corticosteroids and/or IV immunoglobulins on schedule. Assess and record effectiveness and any side effects (e.g., GI distress, electrolyte imbalance).

Assess and record child's/family's knowledge of and participation in care regarding

identification of signs/symptoms of injury (such as those listed under **Characteristics**), including signs/symptoms of CNS hemorrhage, such as headache, diplopia, projectile vomiting, lethargy, or changes in level of consciousness.
avoidance of activities such as contact sports (until the platelet count has returned to normal).
medication administration.
avoidance of all aspirin-containing drugs.
establishment of good oral hygiene routine, including use of a soft-bristle toothbrush.

Instruct child/family in any areas needing improvement. Record results.

EVALUATION FOR CHARTING

Describe any signs/symptoms of injury noted (such as those listed under **Characteristics**).

Describe any interventions implemented to prevent injury. State their effectiveness.

State results of platelet count and indicate any increase or decrease from previous results.

Describe effectiveness of medications and any side effects noted.

Describe child's/family's knowledge of and participation in care related to preventing injury. State any areas needing improvement and information provided. Describe child's/family's responses.

Fear: Child/Family

DEFINITION   Feeling of apprehension resulting from a known cause

POSSIBLY RELATED TO
Knowledge deficit concerning disease state
Unfamiliar surroundings
Forced contact with strangers
Treatments and procedures
Body image disturbance secondary to ecchymoses and petechiae

CHARACTERISTICS
Uncooperativeness
Hostile behavior
Restlessness
Inability to recall previously taught information
Decreased communication
Decreased attention span

EXPECTED OUTCOMES   Child/family will exhibit only a minimal amount of fear as evidenced by

ability to appropriately relate to family members.
lack of hostile behavior.
ability to rest and sleep, when indicated.
ability to restate information previously taught.
ability to participate in care.
ability to separate for short periods, when indicated.
expression of fear to members of the health care team.

POSSIBLE NURSING INTERVENTIONS
Assess and record any signs/symptoms of fear demonstrated by the child/family (such as those listed under **Characteristics**) every 8 hours and PRN.

Decrease child's/family's fear when possible by

encouraging family members to stay with child.
encouraging child/family members to participate in care.
assigning same staff members to provide care for child.
spending extra time with child when family members are unable to be present.

Encourage child/family to express fears to members of the health care team.

Assist and encourage child/family to meet basic needs, such as eating and resting appropriately.

EVALUATION FOR CHARTING

Describe any signs/symptoms of fear manifested by the child/family (such as those listed under **Characteristics**).

Describe any measures used to help alleviate fear. State their effectiveness.

RELATED NURSING DIAGNOSES

Temporary Impaired Physical Mobility *related to* decreased circulating platelets

Knowledge Deficit: Child/Family *related to*
a. disease state
b. home management

Fluid Volume Deficit *related to* blood loss

Compromised Family Coping *related to*
a. knowledge deficit of disease state
b. home management
c. child's activity restrictions
d. uncertainty of disease course (will child need a splenectomy in the future)

Neoplasms

PATHOPHYSIOLOGY

Acute Lymphocytic Leukemia Leukemia is a primary malignancy of the bone marrow, a proliferation of abnormal white blood cells of the body, and the most common childhood malignancy. Of the childhood leukemias, the majority are acute lymphocytic (lymphoblastic) leukemia (ALL).

Acute lymphocytic leukemia results from malignant changes of the lymphocyte or its precursor and is acute at onset. The condition can be further subdivided according to the morphologic and immunologic features of lymphoblasts (immature white blood cells) and according to the clinical presentation of the child. The subdivisions (determined by cell membrane markers) include T lymphocyte (thymus derived), B lymphocyte (bone marrow derived), and null cell (non-T non-B cell).

Non-T non-B cell leukemia is the most common form of ALL. It also is the most responsive to therapy and has the best prognosis. In non-T non-B cell leukemia, leukemic blasts appear to represent an early stage in the development of lymphocytes, lacking B and T cell markers, surface membrane immunoglobulin, sheep erythrocyte receptors, and T cell specific antigens. The lymphocytes do have the common ALL antigen and the immune-associated (Ia) antigen, both of which are usually lost with T cell maturation.

In T cell leukemia, the cell of origin is a lymphocyte that has developed within the thymus. The ability to spontaneously form heat-stable rosettes with sheep erythrocytes distinguishes these cells. They also lack surface membrane immunoglobulins and the common ALL antigen. Infiltration of the central nervous system, liver, spleen, lymph, and mediastinum is more common in T cell leukemia than in other forms. Males are four times as likely to get this form as females. The prognosis is not as good as that for null cell leukemia.

B cell leukemia is the rarest form of ALL. These blast cells contain surface membrane immunoglobulin, as do mature B cells, but they are negative for the sheep erythrocyte receptor found on T cells. The central nervous system is usually involved, but lymphadenopathy is uncommon, and mediastinal masses rare. B cell leukemia is the most refractory to treatment.

The clinical presentation of children with ALL is fairly consistent. Most of the signs and symptoms are a result of leukemic cells replacing bone marrow components or invading extramedullary sites. Signs and symptoms usually have been in existence for less than 6 weeks prior to diagnosis and are nonspecific. Early manifestations can include anorexia, irritability, lethargy, fever, pallor, bruising, and bleeding. There may be a history of a viral respiratory infection without full recovery.

The goals for treatment of ALL include elimination of the disease and long-term survival. Remission induction, consolidation, central nervous system prophylaxis, and maintenance are the phases of the treatment regimen. Multiple-drug therapy is preferred to the use of a single agent.

Hodgkin's Disease   Hodgkin's disease is a malignancy of the lymphoid system. Histology, cell lineage, clinical behavior, and response to treatment differentiate Hodgkin's lymphoma from other lymphomas. Hodgkin's lymphoma arises in a single lymph node or anatomic group of nodes and follows a predictable pattern of progression. The pattern begins with painless regional nodal enlargement, followed by extension to adjacent nodes and, without treatment, extranodal involvement of the spleen, liver, lungs, and/or bone marrow.

Reed-Sternberg cells, giant, multinucleated cells, are diagnostic of Hodgkin's disease when associated with certain cellular and architectural-type lesions. There are four subtypes of Hodgkin's disease. The lymphocytic-predominant variety, in which almost all cells are mature lymphocytes or a mixture of lymphocytes and benign histiocytes, with only an occasional Reed-Sternberg cell, affects 10% to 20% of patients. This type has the best prognosis. The most common form, affecting 50% of patients, is the nodular-sclerosing variety. In this type, the involved lymph node is divided into nodular cellular areas by broad bands of collagen and a variant of the Reed-Sternberg cell called a lacunar cell. Hodgkin's disease of mixed-cellular variety is characterized by the accumulation of lymphocytes, plasma cells, eosinophil, histocytes, malignant reticular cells, and Reed-Sternberg cells. This is the second most common form, affecting 40% to 50% of patients, and often has extranodal involvement. The lymphocytic-depletion variety, the least common and least favorable form of Hodgkin's disease, has many bizarre malignant reticular cells and Reed-Sternberg cells, with few lymphocytes.

Staging indicates the extent of disease and is as follows: Stage I disease is limited to a single node, a lymph node region, or a single extranodal organ. Stage II disease involves two or more lymph node regions on the same side of the diaphragm. Stage III disease involves lymph node regions on both sides of the diaphragm and involvement of an extranodal organ, usually the spleen. Stage IV disease has diffuse or disseminated involvement of one or more extralymphatic organ. The stages can be further subdivided by the absence (A) or presence (B) of systemic signs and symptoms such as fever, night sweats, and weight loss of greater than 10%.

Painless, enlarged cervical lymph nodes are the most common presenting feature. Regional inflammation can rarely be found to explain the lymphadenopathy. The patient has few if any systemic symptoms other than anorexia, malaise, and lassitude.

Hodgkin's disease is a treatable tumor with a good prognosis. Radiation therapy and chemotherapy, each alone or in combination, are highly effective. Surgery is confined to biopsy procedures. The intensity of treatment varies with disease presentation, histology, and stage.

Hodgkin's disease peaks from age 15 to 34 and again after age 50 and is twice as common in males as in females.

Neuroblastoma Neuroblastoma is a malignant tumor arising from sympathetic ganglion cells or the adrenal medulla. The sympathetic chain extends from the posterior cranial fossa to the coccyx, and the tumor may arise from any site where neuroblast cells are present. The abdomen, adrenal glands, and posterior mediastinum are common sites. Neuroblastoma is usually a firm, gray mass. If hemorrhaging into this vascular neoplasm has occurred, the tumor may impart a maroon color. Most neuroblastomas consist primarily of neuroblastoma cells with little evidence of differentiation. The tumor can invade adjacent tissue, making surgical excision difficult. Neuroblastoma may also extend to the regional lymph nodes via lymphatics. Hematogenous spread usually involves the liver, bones, and bone marrow.

Staging of neuroblastoma indicates the extent of disease. Stage I, a localized primary tumor, can be completely resected. Stage II disease extends beyond the primary tissue and is grossly resectable but does not cross the midline. Stage III disease extends across the midline. Stage IV involves distant metastases. Stage IV-S is a special stage in which metastatic disease is limited to the bone marrow, liver, or skin, which are favorably responsive to either chemotherapy or radiotherapy.

The clinical manifestations of neuroblastoma vary according to the site of the primary tumor. An abdominal mass, fever, irritability, pain from bone metastases, and orbital ecchymoses or proptosis from skull metastases may be present. A history of altered bowel and bladder patterns, anorexia, weight loss, difficulty sleeping, neurological changes, and pain contribute to the diagnosis of neuroblastoma.

Treatment of neuroblastoma involves a variety of combinations of surgery, chemotherapy, and radiation therapy, depending on the stage of disease and the age of the child. The child's prognosis depends on the age of the child at diagnosis and the stage of the disease.

Neuroblastoma is the second most common solid tumor of childhood. Diagnosis is almost always made before the child is 4 years old and often before the age of 2.

Osteogenic Sarcoma   Osteogenic sarcoma, or osteosarcoma, is defined as a primary malignant bone tumor, the neoplastic cells of which produce osteoid and osseous tissue. The tumor usually arises in the metaphyseal of the long bones, the points of most active growth, but it can also occur in the diaphysis. The tumor arises in the medullary canal of the shaft and breaks through the cortex of the bone to form a soft tissue mass. A single tumor may be the site of diverse differentiating cells, including osteosarcomatous, fibrosarcomatous, and chondrosarcomatous elements. Osteosarcoma can occur in any bone, but the distal femur is the most common site. The proximal tibia and the proximal humerus are other common sites. Metastasis to the lungs frequently occurs.

The most common initial findings of osteogenic sarcoma are pain and, sometimes, swelling at the tumor site. Often these symptoms are attributed to an athletic injury. Later symptoms can include limited movement of the affected extremity, limping or an altered gait, and local erythema and warmth.

Treatment for osteogenic sarcoma is aimed toward local control of the primary tumor and prevention of metastasis. A combination of surgery and chemotherapy is often used. Surgery can include amputation or limb preservation. Because osteosarcoma is relatively radioresistant, radiation is reserved for nonresectable tumors of the ribs, pelvis, or skull or for controlling metastatic disease. Prognosis is best when the tumors have low metastatic potential.

Osteogenic sarcoma is the most frequently diagnosed malignant primary tumor of the bone. Its onset is most common during the adolescent growth spurt. After age 13, boys have a higher rate of incidence than girls.

Rhabdomyosarcoma Rhabdomyosarcoma is a malignant tumor of striated muscle cells. Four major histologic types exist: embryonal, alveolar, pleomorphic, and mixed. The rhabdomyoblasts in the embryonal variety resemble fetal cells at 6 to 8 weeks of development. The botryoid type of the embryonal form appears as a cluster of grapes presenting in a body cavity such as the bladder, vagina, uterus, nasopharynx, or middle ear. Embryonal rhabdomyosarcoma has the best prognosis of the four histologic varieties. The rhabdomyoblasts of alveolar rhabdomyosarcoma resemble fetal cells at 10 to 12 weeks of development and occur most often in the trunk and extremities. This variety, seen more commonly in older children and adolescents, has the poorest prognosis. The pleomorphic type is rare in childhood. Mixed rhabdomyosarcoma contains more than one of the histologic types.

Staging indicates the extent of the disease. Group I disease is localized, completely removable, with no involvement of regional nodes. Group II involves regional lymph nodes or microscopic residual disease. Group III is indicated by gross residual disease. Group IV has distant metastatic disease at the time of diagnosis.

Rhabdomyosarcoma can present anywhere in the body, causing a variety of symptoms. Children with the condition usually present with a mass, which can be painful. These tumors are often misdiagnosed, delaying referral and treatment.

Treatment can involve a combination of surgery, chemotherapy, and radiation, depending on the location and stage of the tumor.

Rhabdomyosarcoma accounts for most soft-tissue tumors in childhood. Peak incidence is from 2 to 6 years of age, with a second peak during the adolescent years of 15 to 19.

Wilms Tumor Wilms tumor, or nephroblastoma, is an embryonal tumor of the kidney that originates from immature renoblast cells. The tumor often extends from the kidney parenchyma into the renal cavity, distorting the renal outline as the residual normal kidney is compressed into a thin rim around the tumor. Wilms tumors are sharply demarcated and variably encapsulated. The tumor is vascular and lends itself to hematogenous spread. The abdomen should not be palpated once Wilms tumor has been diagnosed as the tumor may rupture if manipulated, causing its cells to spread throughout the peritoneal cavity.

Treatment protocols are based on the clinical stage and histologic pattern and can include various combinations of surgery, chemotherapy, and radiation. Staging of the tumor is performed during surgery. Stage I tumors are limited to the kidney and can be totally resected. Stage II tumors extend beyond the kidney but can still be completely resected. Stage III tumors leave residual nonhematogenous tumor in the abdomen after surgery. Stage IV indicates hematogenous metastases, usually to the lungs, bone, liver, and/or brain. Stage V tumors have bilateral renal involvement.

The most common presenting sign is an abdominal mass, which is characteristically firm and smooth and is usually asymptomatic. Some children also present with abdominal pain, vomiting, hematuria, dysuria, frequency, anorexia, weight loss, and malaise. Hypertension can also occur, possibly due to pressure on the renal artery, renal ischemia, or increased renin secretion.

Wilms tumor is the most common type of childhood renal neoplasm. It occurs in both sexes and in all races with approximately equal frequency. Most children are between 1 and 5 years of age when diagnosed. Congenital abnormalities, such as hemihypertrophy, aniridia, and other genitourinary anomalies, can be associated with Wilms tumor. Wilms tumor is one of the most curable childhood tumors. Prognosis is influenced by the specific histology, the stage of the tumor, and the age of the child at the time of diagnosis.

NURSING CARE PLAN FOR THE CHILD RECEIVING CHEMOTHERAPY

PRIMARY NURSING DIAGNOSIS
Infection: High Risk

DEFINITION   Condition in which the body is at risk for being invaded by microorganisms

POSSIBLY RELATED TO
Leukopenia
Neutropenia
Side effects of chemotherapeutic agents

CHARACTERISTICS
Fever or drop in temperature
Decreased white blood cell count (WBC)
Positive culture results
Lethargy
Chills
Diaphoresis
Ashen color
Weak, rapid pulse
Hypotension
Decreased urine output
Prolonged capillary refill
Signs/symptoms from various body systems:

thrush
mouth ulcerations
runny nose
sore throat
reddened and/or edematous puncture sites
anal fissures or skin breakdown
decreased breath sounds
changes in rate and depth of respirations
dysuria
cloudy or foul-smelling urine
headache

EXPECTED OUTCOMES   Child will have decreased symptoms
or be free of infection as evidenced by

body temperature within acceptable range of 36.5°C to
37.2°C.
lack of signs/symptoms of being at risk for infection, such as
those listed under Characteristics.
WBC within normal limits (state specific highest and lowest
counts for each child).

POSSIBLE NURSING INTERVENTIONS
Assess and record the following every 2 to 4 hours and PRN:

>   vital signs
>   signs/symptoms of being at risk for infection (such as
>   those listed under **Characteristics**)
>   IV fluids and condition of IV site every hour

Maintain good handwashing technique.

When indicated, obtain cultures (blood, throat, urine).

Check and record results of complete blood count (CBC),
chest x-ray, and any cultures. Notify physician of any
abnormalities.

Administer antibiotics and antifungals on schedule and
antipyretics PRN. Assess and record effectiveness and any
side effects (e.g., rash, diarrhea).

When indicated, use tepid sponge baths to decrease fever.

Ensure that child has a private room and that no ill family
members, friends, or health care or institution employees
visit child.

Use aseptic technique for all procedures.

Keep accurate record of intake and output.

⌂ Assess and record child's/family's knowledge of and
participation in care regarding

>   handwashing technique.
>   medication administration.
>   identification of any signs/symptoms of being at risk for
>   infection (such as those listed under **Characteristics**).
>   adequate nutrition (well-balanced diet, consumption of
>   sufficient calories).
>   avoidance of crowds and ill friends and family members.

⌂ Instruct child/family in any areas needing improvement.
Record results.

EVALUATION FOR CHARTING
State highest and lowest temperatures.

Describe any signs/symptoms of being at risk for infection
(such as those listed under **Characteristics**).

State results of current CBC, chest x-ray, and culture.

State whether medications were administered on schedule. Describe effectiveness and any side effects noted.

State intake and output.

Describe any therapeutic measures used to prevent or treat infection. State their effectiveness.

⌂ Describe child's/family's knowledge of and participation in care regarding the prevention or treatment of infection. State any areas needing improvement and information provided. Describe child's/family's responses.

NURSING DIAGNOSIS
Injury: High Risk

DEFINITION   Situation in which the child is at risk for sustaining damage or harm

POSSIBLY RELATED TO
    Decreased number of circulating platelets
    Increased fragility of mucous membranes or skin
    Side effects of chemotherapeutic agents

CHARACTERISTICS
    Anemia (decreased hemoglobin)
    Thrombocytopenia
    Cutaneous bruises
    Purpura
    Petechiae
    Hematomas
    Epistaxis
    Melena
    Gingival bleeding
    Streaks of blood observable in stool, sputum, or emesis
    Hemorrhage
    Prolonged prothrombin time (PT) and partial thromboplastin time (PTT)
    Hypovolemia (accompanied by tachycardia, hypotension, pallor, diaphoresis, decreased urine output, and/or restlessness or confusion)
    Hemarthrosis
    Indication of potential intracranial bleeding (e.g., headache, changes in mental status, decreased level of consciousness)

EXPECTED OUTCOMES   Child will have minimal injury or be free of injury that might result in bleeding as evidenced by

> lack of signs/symptoms of bleeding such as those listed under **Characteristics**.
>
> improved platelet count for child (state specific values for each child).
>
> improved PT and PTT for child (state specific values for each child).

POSSIBLE NURSING INTERVENTIONS

Assess and record any signs/symptoms of injury (new areas of bleeding and status of old areas) every 4 hours and PRN.

Handle child gently.

Assist child in limiting activity by providing diversional activities (e.g., television, books).

Provide alternate method for child to brush teeth (such as by using a soft toothbrush or toothette).

Ensure that child does not use a straw when drinking.

When checking child's blood pressure, avoid overinflation of the cuff.

Avoid injections, when possible.

Avoid using rectal thermometers.

Ensure that no aspirin or nonsteroidal antiinflammatory drugs (antiplatelet drugs) are administered to the child.

Apply gentle pressure at puncture sites for 5 to 10 minutes.

Check urine, stools, and emesis for blood each shift. Record results.

Ensure that child does not forcefully blow nose. If epistaxis occurs, set child up and hold bridge of nose for 10 minutes.

When indicated, administer stool softeners.

When antiemetic suppositories are indicated, lubricate them well and insert gently.

Check and record results of platelet count, hematocrit, PT, and PTT. Notify physician of any abnormalities.

Administer platelets, as indicated. Adhere to institutional and current guidelines for administration of blood products. Assess and record effectiveness and any side effects such as transfusion reactions (e.g., chills, fever, shaking, urticaria, flushing, nausea/vomiting).

Implement safety precautions: keep child away from sharp toys and furniture, keep bed in lowest position, protect head from injury, etc.

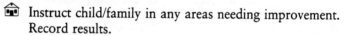 Assess and record child's/family's knowledge of and participation in care regarding

identification of signs/symptoms of injury (such as those listed under **Characteristics**).
all safety measures to be used in the hospital and at home.
any activity restrictions at school.

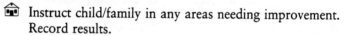 Instruct child/family in any areas needing improvement. Record results.

EVALUATION FOR CHARTING

Describe any interventions implemented to prevent injury. State their effectiveness.

Describe any signs/symptoms of injury noted (such as those listed under **Characteristics**).

State current lab results and indicate if there has been a change from previous results.

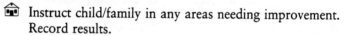 Describe child's/family's knowledge of and participation in care related to minimizing and/or treating injury. State any areas needing improvement and information provided. Describe child's/family's responses.

NURSING DIAGNOSIS
Anticipatory Grieving: Family

DEFINITION   Feelings of deep sadness and distress

POSSIBLY RELATED TO
Perceived potential loss of

child

part or limb of child
various body functions of child

Disfigurement of child

CHARACTERISTICS
Verbal expression of grief by the family
Sadness
Crying, screaming
Hysteria
Inability to carry on with activities of daily living at
optimal level
Need for repeated explanations and reassurance
Passivity

EXPECTED OUTCOMES   Family will grieve appropriately as
evidenced by

crying.
talking and asking questions about the infant/child.
seeking help, support, and advice appropriately.
performing activities of daily living.
discussing feelings, fears, and concerns about the
perceived loss.
using available resources.

POSSIBLE NURSING INTERVENTIONS
Allow family members to grieve in their own way. Give
support.

Encourage family to spend time with the infant or child if
doing so seems to help the grieving process.

If possible, have the same nurse(s) care for infant or child
from day to day to provide consistent feedback for family.

Allow family to participate in care of infant or child when
possible (dressing changes, bath, baptism, diaper changing,
feeding, etc.).

Allow family to spend time alone at the infant or child's
bedside, if possible.

Spend time with the family when possible.

Keep family up to date on the condition of the infant
or child.

When possible, have family members tape their voices to be played for the infant or child.

Allow family to photograph the infant or child, when appropriate.

Allow time for expression of feelings, fears, and concerns.

Assist family, as needed, in planning care of the infant or child.

If family requests, provide access to resources (e.g., social, spiritual, financial) and support groups.

Clarify any misperceptions for family.

EVALUATION FOR CHARTING

State whether family verbalized any feelings of grief.

Describe any signs/symptoms of grief displayed by the family (such as those listed under **Characteristics**).

State whether family was able to carry on with activities of daily living.

Describe any successful measures used to help family cope with grief.

RELATED NURSING DIAGNOSES

Altered Nutrition: Less than Body Requirements
related to
a. dysphagia secondary to stomatitis
b. increased metabolic rate
c. insufficient nutrients available for normal cells due to malignant cell utilization of nutrients
d. anorexia
e. vomiting

Knowledge Deficit: Child/Parental *related to*
a. disease process
b. effects and side effects of chemotherapy
c. procedures

Body Image Disturbance *related to*
a. alopecia
b. cushingoid features
c. weight loss

Sickle Cell Disease

PATHOPHYSIOLOGY   Sickle cell disease is the term applied to a group of inherited (autosomal recessive) hemoglobinopathies. These diseases are characterized by the production of the hemoglobin variant, hemoglobin S (Hb S), in place of the normal adult hemoglobin A (Hb A). The most common forms of sickle cell disease include sickle cell anemia (Hb SS), sickle hemoglobin C disease (Hb SC), and the hemoglobin S beta thalassemia syndromes (Hb S beta thal). Chronic hemolytic anemia and vaso-occlusion resulting in ischemic tissue injury of various organs are the two cardinal pathophysiological features of sickle cell disease.

Red blood cells contain hemoglobin, which binds to oxygen and then releases it at a tissue site. Hemoglobin is a complex protein made up of globin molecules and heme (iron-containing) molecules. Oxygenated hemoglobin is bright red in color, giving arterial blood its color.

In Hb S, valine replaces glutamic acid in the sixth position of the amino acid beta chain. This substitution reduces the solubility of the deoxygenated Hb S molecule within the red cell. *Sickling* is the term used to describe the change of the normally round red blood cells into crescent, or half-moon–shaped, cells as the Hb S polymerizes and forms tactoids. Sickling can occur in the red blood cells of children with sickle cell anemia when oxygen tension is reduced or as a result of other forms of stress, such as acidosis, infection, dehydration, vigorous exercise, and high altitudes. Usually, a red cell can initially resume the round shape upon reoxygenation. After repeated episodes of sickling, however, these normally pliable red cells undergo membrane changes, become irreversibly sickled, and are destroyed. The red cell life span in individuals with sickle cell disease is reduced from the normal length of 120 days to 15 to 60 days.

Hypoxia usually produces acute and chronic tissue injury and may eventually lead to organ failure. The hypoxia is secondary to obstruction of blood vessels by an accumulation of the sickled red cells. Although no organ is spared, the organs at greatest risk are those with limited terminal arterial blood supply (e.g., the eye, the head of the femur) or with venous sinuses, where blood flow is slow and oxygen tension and pH are low (e.g., the spleen, the kidney, and bone marrow). The ischemic tissue injury resulting from the obstruction of blood flow is believed to be the cause of painful episodes.

Children with sickle cell disease can experience a number of complications, including the following:

infections, especially with *Streptococcus pneumoniae* and *Haemophilus influenzae*

dactylitis (hand and foot syndrome), characterized by swelling of the soft tissues over the metacarpals or metatarsals and the proximal phalanges of the hands and feet

splenic sequestration, a sudden pooling of blood in the spleen when sickled cells totally occlude venous outflow. The spleen often becomes dysfunctional in young children. Splenectomy is indicated when the anemia, neutropenia, or thrombocytopenia is severe

acute chest syndrome, characterized by chest pain, fever, prostration, and pulmonary infiltrates (usually infectious) as seen on chest x-ray

stroke

aplastic crisis, a decrease in hemoglobin associated with reticulocytopenia

retinopathy

gallstones secondary to increased bilirubin production.

jaundice

aseptic necrosis

acute or chronic liver disease

leg ulcers

hyposthenuria, the inability of the kidney to maximally concentrate urine

priapism

pallor

altered growth and development

delayed sexual maturation

increased risk of perioperative complications

Although sickle cell disease has no cure, comprehensive management can greatly improve a child's prognosis. Treatment involves child/parent education to avoid the triggers of sickling episodes (infection, dehydration, hypoxia, high altitude, vigorous exercise, and emotional stress); management of vaso-occlusive episodes, including hydration and effective analgesia; and treatment of the anemia with transfusions of packed red blood cells. Children with sickle cell disease should start on oral penicillin twice a day from age 2 months. Along with standard immunizations, pneumococcal and flu vaccines should also be administered. Due to the risk for eye complications, retinal examinations should be performed at regular intervals by an ophthalmologist.

The sickle cell disorders can be found in people of African, Mediterranean, Indian, Caribbean, Asian, and Middle Eastern heritage. Genetic counseling is recommended for individuals and families who have sickle cell disease or trait.

NURSING DIAGNOSIS
Pain

DEFINITION   Condition in which an individual experiences severe discomfort

POSSIBLY RELATED TO
Ischemic tissue secondary to vascular occlusion precipitated by hypoxia, infection, fever, acidosis, dehydration, exposure to extreme cold, emotional stress, and/or unknown etiologies

CHARACTERISTICS
Crying or moaning
Facial grimacing
Verbal expression of pain
Restlessness
Guarding or protective behavior of the painful site (often the abdomen or musculoskeletal areas)
Physical signs/symptoms of:

tachycardia
tachypnea
increased blood pressure

Altered muscle tone (tense or listless)
Irritability
Refusal to walk
Rating of pain on pain assessment tool

EXPECTED OUTCOMES   Child will be free of pain as evidenced by
> lack of

> > crying or moaning.
> > facial grimacing
> > restlessness.
> > guarding or protective behavior of painful site.
> > signs/symptoms of pain (such as those listed under **Characteristics**).

> heart rate, respiratory rate, and blood pressure within acceptable ranges (state specific highest and lowest parameters for each child).
> verbal communication of comfort.
> rating of no pain on pain assessment tool.

POSSIBLE NURSING INTERVENTIONS

Assess and record any signs/symptoms of pain (such as those listed under **Characteristics**) every 2 to 4 hours. Use an age-appropriate pain assessment tool.

Handle child gently. Reposition, immobilize, or elevate the painful area, as indicated.

When indicated, ensure that bedrest is maintained.

Administer analgesics and/or narcotics on schedule (usually at regular intervals, as opposed to PRN). Assess and record their effectiveness.

Monitor patient-controlled analgesia (PCA).

Administer fluids, as indicated, both oral and parenteral (usually 1½ times the normal maintenance). Keep accurate record of intake and output.

If age-appropriate, explain all procedures beforehand.

If age-appropriate, allow child to participate in planning self-care. Encourage child to practice self-care. Encourage family members to stay and comfort the child, when possible.

Allow family members to participate in care of the child, when possible.

When indicated, institute additional pain relief measures, such as application of moist heat (warm packs, warm tub baths, or whirlpool), massage, relaxation, hypnosis, guided imagery, and music. Assess and record effectiveness.

Use diversional activities and distraction measures (e.g., toys, play activities, television, radio), when appropriate.

Consult with a pain management team, if available.

☗ Assess and record child's/family's knowledge of and participation in care regarding

> pain assessment.
> identification of potential triggers of pain events.
> use of additional pain relief measures, especially massage and application of moist heat.
> protection against exposure to cold.
> oral hydration.
> administration of analgesics/narcotics.

☗ Instruct child/family in any areas needing improvement. Record results.

EVALUATION FOR CHARTING
Describe any signs/symptoms of pain noted (such as those listed under **Characteristics**).

State ranges of vital signs.

Describe any successful measures used to reduce or eliminate pain.

Describe effectiveness of analgesics and/or narcotics.

☗ Describe child's/family's knowledge of and participation in care related to child's pain. State any areas needing improvement and information provided. Describe child's/family's responses.

NURSING DIAGNOSIS
Actual Infection*

DEFINITION   Condition in which microorganisms have invaded the body

---
*Non-NANDA diagnosis.

POSSIBLY RELATED TO

Bacterial, viral, granulomatous, or parasitic invasion of any organ or body system, especially the blood, lungs, meninges, throat, ears, urinary tract, bone, or gall bladder

CHARACTERISTICS

Fever

Localized tenderness, redness, and swelling; increased warmth over involved area

Irritability

Restlessness

Pain on movement of involved area

Elevated white blood cell count (WBC)

Elevated erythrocyte sedimentation rate

Positive cultures (sputum, cerebral spinal fluid, blood, urine, throat, stool, other)

Infiltrates or pleural effusion revealed on chest x-ray

Diarrhea

EXPECTED OUTCOMES   Child will be free of infection as evidenced by

body temperature between 36.5°C and 37.2°C.

lack of extreme irritability and restlessness.

lack of the following to the affected area:

tenderness
redness
swelling
increased warmth

freedom from pain on movement of the involved area.

WBC within acceptable range (state specific highest and lowest counts for each child).

erythrocyte sedimentation rate from 0 to 13 mm/hr.

negative culture results.

clear chest x-ray.

absence of diarrhea.

POSSIBLE NURSING INTERVENTIONS

Assess and record

temperature every 4 hours and PRN.

IV fluids and condition of IV site every hour.

signs/symptoms of infection (such as those listed under **Characteristics**) every 4 hours and PRN.

Administer antibiotics on schedule. Administer antipyretics and analgesics PRN. Assess and record their effectiveness and any side effects, (e.g., rash, diarrhea).

Maintain good handwashing technique. If an open wound is present, maintain wound isolation precautions in accordance with institutional policy.

When indicated, keep involved area immobilized. Assess area for sensation, circulation, pain, color, swelling, heat, and tenderness. Record. Ensure that bedrest is maintained.

Check and record results of any cultures, laboratory tests, and/or chest x-rays. Notify physician of any abnormalities.

🏠 Assess and record child's/family's knowledge of and participation in care regarding

> handwashing technique.
> medication administration.
> activity restrictions, including immobilization and bedrest, when indicated.
> identification of any signs/symptoms of infection (such as those listed under **Characteristics**).
> monitoring of child's temperature, and ability to read the thermometer.
> obtainment of immediate medical attention when a temperature of 38.4°C develops.
> proper administration of antipyretics.
> well child care, including routine immunizations and additional vaccines.
> preventive factors, including adequate nutrition, adequate hydration, rest, as needed, and good hygiene, including oral hygiene.

🏠 Instruct child/family in any areas needing improvement. Record results.

EVALUATION FOR CHARTING

State highest and lowest temperatures.

Describe condition of IV site.

Describe any signs/symptoms of infection (such as those listed under **Characteristics**).

Describe any therapeutic measures used to treat the infection. State their effectiveness in increasing child's level of comfort.

State current results of any cultures, laboratory tests, and/or chest x-rays.

State whether medications were administered on schedule. Describe effectiveness and any side effects noted.

⌂ Describe child's/family's knowledge of and participation in care regarding treatment of infection. State any areas needing improvement and information provided. Describe child's/family's responses.

RELATED NURSING DIAGNOSES

Activity Intolerance *related to*
a. pain
b. fatigue
c. shortness of breath
d. impaired gas exchange

Knowledge Deficit: Parental *related to*
home management of a child with sickle cell disease

Body Image Disturbance *related to*
a. physical restrictions
b. altered growth and development
c. sequelae from strokes

Compromised Family Coping *related to*
a. parental guilt
b. frequent hospitalization of child with sickle cell disease

SIX

CARE OF CHILDREN WITH HEPATIC DYSFUNCTION

MEDICAL DIAGNOSIS
Chronic Liver Failure

PATHOPHYSIOLOGY Liver failure results when the liver is unable to maintain its many functions. With this failure, substances normally produced by the liver are absent and those normally removed by the liver accumulate. In children, liver failure most often occurs with chronic liver disease. Less often, viruses—such as in hepatitis, idiosyncratic reactions to medications, or accidental ingestion of drugs or toxins—cause acute liver failure.

Two common anatomic disorders of the biliary system are biliary atresia and choledochal cysts. Biliary atresia is the complete obstruction of bile flow of the extrahepatic biliary duct system secondary to fibrosis or obliteration, which can progress into the intrahepatic ducts, eventually leading to cirrhosis. Choledochal cysts (congenital cystic dilatation of the common bile duct) may occur at any place along the biliary tree. Complications of these two problems can include cirrhosis, portal hypertension, esophageal varices, hepatic coma, and liver failure.

The liver, one of the most vital organs in the body, performs more than four hundred functions. Briefly, these functions include blood storage and filtration; secretion of bile and bilirubin; metabolism of fat, protein, and carbohydrate; synthesis of blood-clotting components; detoxification of hormones, drugs, and other substances; and storage for glycogen, iron, and vitamins A, D, E, and B12. These functions can be affected by inflammatory, obstructive, or degenerative disorders. When the liver is unable to maintain normal body functions, complications may arise, such as portal hypertension, hepatic encephalopathy, and hepatorenal syndrome.

Liver failure impacts on every organ system.

1. The phagocytic activity of Kupffer's cells is decreased; thus, the blood is inadequately filtered as it passes through the liver, making the patient more susceptible to infections.

2. Inadequate amounts of bile salts are manufactured, resulting in decreased emulsification of fats when insufficient quantities of bile salts reach the small intestine. Fats too large to enter the cir-

culation are lost in the feces (steatorrhea), a source of high calorie loss. Decreased fat intake can contribute to malnutrition. Reduced absorption of fat-soluble vitamins A, D, E, and K can also occur.

The deposit of excessive bile salts in the skin causes pruritus when these salts are inadequately extracted from the portal venous blood by the liver cells in hepatic disorders such as hepatitis, cholestasis, or extrahepatic biliary obstruction.

3. Albumin synthesis is decreased and serum albumin levels fall in proportion to the degree of hepatocellular failure. This state of hypoproteinemia can contribute to the formation of ascites (the accumulation of fluid within the peritoneal cavity), peripheral edema, and malnutrition.

4. The liver's production of blood-clotting factors is decreased. Since fat-soluble vitamin K has limited absorption, the manufacture of vitamin K– dependent clotting factors (factors II, VII, IX, and X) are decreased, resulting in a prolonged prothrombin time, easy bruising, and overt bleeding.

5. The liver is unable to remove activated clotting factors from the serum, contributing to the formation of microthrombi and the consumption of platelets, fibrinogen, and other clotting factors.

6. When hepatic circulatory bypasses exist, blood is shunted around the liver directly into the systemic circulation, and ammonia is not converted to urea. Hyperammonemia contributes to hepatic encephalopathy. (Ammonia is formed in the gastrointestinal tract from amino acids following bacterial and enzymatic breakdown of proteins.)

7. The liver is unable to effectively detoxify certain hormones, harmful compounds, and drugs.

8. Serum glucose levels can drop because gluconeogenesis is not completed by the liver. This can compromise cerebral function since glucose is the brain's major energy source.

9. The release of vasoactive substances into the blood contributes to a hyperkinetic circulation.

10. Jaundice occurs due to staining of elastic tissue by conjugated or unconjugated bilirubin.

11. Sodium and water are retained. Significant intravascular fluid loss secondary to ascites or splanchnic sequestration because of portal hypotension causes the heart, adrenal cortex, and kidneys to perceive a decrease in circulating blood volume, stimulating aldosterone secretion and resulting in renal sodium and water retention.

12. Other common electrolyte imbalances include hypokalemia, due to vomiting, diarrhea, anorexia, hyperaldosteronism, or use of diuretics; hypocalcemia, due to decreased absorption of vitamin D, steatorrhea, and inadequate dietary intake; and hypomagnesemia, due to decreased storage by the liver.

13. The spleen becomes congested and enlarged as increased venous pressures delay blood flow through the splanchnic bed. This hypersplenism can produce thrombocytopenia, anemia, and leukopenia, which in turn can contribute to hypoxemia, increased susceptibility to infection, and increased bleeding tendencies.

14. Ascites elevates the diaphragm and interferes with lung expansion. Intrapulmonary right-to-left shunting can also occur, as can hypoxemia.

15. The hepatic enzymes—serum glutamic-oxaloacetic transaminase (SGOT) (aspartate aminotransferase—AST), serum glutamic-pyruvic, transaminase (SGPT) (alanine aminotransferase—ALT), lactate dehydrogenase (LDH), and creatine phosphokinase (CPK)—are elevated due to their release into the blood with the destruction of liver cells.

PRIMARY NURSING DIAGNOSIS
Altered Metabolic Function*

DEFINITION   Imbalance or altered utilization of specific body biochemicals

POSSIBLY RELATED TO
Hepatic damage

CHARACTERISTICS
Hypoalbuminemia
Hyperammonemia
Prolonged prothrombin time
Increased hepatic enzymes (SGOT, SGPT, LDH, CPK)
Hypoglycemia
Increased total, direct, and indirect bilirubin
Jaundice
Easy bruising, nosebleeds, gingival bleeding, bleeding from
    puncture sights, blood in urine, and/or petechiae
Dark and foamy urine
Hyperaldosteronism

---

*Non-NANDA diagnosis.

EXPECTED OUTCOMES Child will have adequate metabolic function as evidenced by

> ammonia within acceptable range of 15 to 45 μg/dL.
> prothrombin time within acceptable range of 12 to
>   14 seconds.
> SGOT (AST) within acceptable range of 0 to 40 U/L.
> SGPT (ALT) within acceptable range of 5 to 35 U/L.
> LDH within acceptable range of 80 to 120 U/L.
> CPK within acceptable range of 0 to 70 IU/L.
> glucose within acceptable range of 60 to 120 mg/dL.
> direct bilirubin within acceptable range of up to 0.3 mg/dL.
> indirect bilirubin within acceptable range of 0.1 to
>   1.0 mg/dL.
> total bilirubin within acceptable range of 0.2 to 0.8 mg/dL.
> serum albumin within acceptable range of 4.0 to 5.8 g/dL.
> lack of signs/symptoms of metabolic dysfunction (such as
>   those listed under **Characteristics**).

POSSIBLE NURSING INTERVENTIONS
Assess and record

> signs/symptoms of metabolic dysfunction (such as those
>   listed under **Characteristics**) every 4 hours and PRN.
> IV fluids and condition of IV site every hour.
> laboratory values, as indicated. Report abnormalities to
>   the physician.

Administer medications (e.g., lactulose, neomycin, kanamycin, tetracycline, stool softeners) on schedule, as indicated. Assess and record effectiveness and any side effects (e.g., diarrhea, arrhythmias). Monitor drug levels, as indicated, and notify the physician of any abnormalities.

Administer plasma, colloids, and/or diuretics, as indicated. Assess and record effectiveness.

Keep accurate record of intake and output. Record characteristics of all output, as indicated.

Assess and record child's/family's knowledge of and participation in care regarding

> identification of signs/symptoms of metabolic dysfunction
>   (such as those listed under **Characteristics**).
> monitoring of intake and output.
> medication administration.

Instruct child and family in any areas needing improvement. Record results.

EVALUATION FOR CHARTING

State current ranges of laboratory values.

State intake and output. When indicated, describe characteristics of all output.

State whether medications were given on schedule. Describe effectiveness and any side effects noted. State current drug levels, as indicated.

Describe any signs/symptoms of metabolic dysfunction noted (such as those listed under **Characteristics**).

Describe any therapeutic measures used to correct metabolic dysfunction. State their effectiveness.

 Describe child's/family's knowledge of and participation in care related to correcting metabolic dysfunction. State any areas needing improvement and information provided. Describe child's/family's responses.

NURSING DIAGNOSIS

Fluid Imbalance: Deficit (Intravascular) and/or Excess (Extravascular or Intravascular)

DEFINITION   Decrease in the amount of circulating fluid volume *and/or* interstitial fluid overload
or increased intravascular volume (which can eventually lead to interstitial or intracellular fluid overload)

POSSIBLY RELATED TO

Hypoalbuminemia
Peripheral edema
Ascites
Increased serum aldosterone
Increased antidiuretic hormone
Hemorrhage

CHARACTERISTICS

Tachycardia
Dry mucous membranes

Hypotension
Absence of tears
Poor skin turgor
Sunken fontanel
Peripheral edema
Ascites
Decreased urine output
Increased urine specific gravity
Increased weight
Vomiting
Diarrhea
Increased urine osmolality
Increased serum osmolality

EXPECTED OUTCOMES   Child will have improved fluid
balance as evidenced by

adequate fluid intake, PO or IV (state specific amount needed
    for each child).
moist mucous membranes.
flat fontanel.
rapid skin recoil.
lack of

ascites.
peripheral edema.
vomiting.
diarrhea.

adequate urine output (state specific highest and lowest
    outputs for each child, minimum of 1 to 2 ml/kg/hr).
urine specific gravity from 1.008 to 1.020.
heart rate and blood pressure within acceptable ranges (state
    specific parameters for each child).
urine osmolality from 500 to 800 mOsm/L.
serum osmolality from 280 to 295 mOsm/L.

POSSIBLE NURSING INTERVENTIONS
Keep accurate record of intake and output. If indicated,
maintain fluid and sodium restriction.

Assess and record

heart rate and blood pressure every 4 hours and PRN.
any signs/symptoms of fluid imbalance (such as those
    listed under **Characteristics**) every 4 hours and PRN.

IV fluids and condition of IV site every hour.

laboratory values, as indicated. Report abnormalities to
the physician.

Weigh child on same scale at same time each day without
clothes.

Check and record urine specific gravity every 4 hours or as
indicated.

Measure and record abdominal girth every shift and PRN.

Administer plasma, colloids, and/or diuretics, as indicated.
Assess and record effectiveness.

🏠 Assess and record child's/family's knowledge of and
participation in care regarding

monitoring of intake and output.

identification of any signs/symptoms of fluid imbalance
(such as those listed under **Characteristics**).

🏠 Instruct child/family in any areas needing improvement.
Record results.

EVALUATION FOR CHARTING

State intake and output.

Describe condition of IV site.

State highest and lowest heart rates and blood pressures.

Describe any signs/symptoms of fluid imbalance noted (such
as those listed under **Characteristics**).

State current abdominal girth and determine whether it has
increased or decreased since the previous measurement.

State current laboratory values.

Describe any therapeutic measures used to improve fluid
balance. State their effectiveness.

🏠 Describe child's/family's knowledge of and participation in
care related to improving fluid balance. State any areas
needing improvement and information provided. Describe
child's/family's responses.

RELATED NURSING DIAGNOSES

Altered Level of Consciousness* *related to*

   a. increased serum ammonia levels secondary to decreased ammonia excretion and/or reduced conversion to urea
   b. increased circulating nitrogenous wastes secondary to decreased liver detoxification of these wastes
   c. hypoglycemia
   d. decreased storage of vitamins, such as niacin and B vitamins
   e. electrolyte imbalances, such as hypocalcemia
   f. hypoxemia

Altered Nutrition: Less than Body Requirements *related to*

   a. altered metabolism of fats, proteins, and carbohydrates
   b. decreased absorption of fats
   c. decreased storage of vitamins and minerals
   d. anorexia
   e. hypoalbuminemia

Infection: High Risk *related to*

   a. decreased activity of Kupffer cells
   b. malnutrition

Anticipatory Grieving: Family *related to*

   a. severity of illness
   b. change in child's physical appearance
   c. uncertain prognosis
   d. potential of not finding a donor (if needed)

---

*Non-NANDA diagnosis.

SEVEN

CARE OF CHILDREN WITH INFECTIONS

MEDICAL DIAGNOSIS

Acquired Immunodeficiency Syndrome (AIDS)

PATHOPHYSIOLOGY   A child with acquired immunodeficiency syndrome (AIDS) has been infected with the human immunodeficiency virus (HIV), a retrovirus that causes an immune deficiency. HIV selectively infects and destroys certain T cells, which are involved in the mediation of cellular immunity and in the regulation of B cell function (the humoral immune system). The child infected with HIV experiences the destruction and depletion of CD-4 helper/inducer T cells, as well as a reversal of the helper to suppressor T cell ratio, resulting in depression of cellular immunity. The loss of T cell regulation of B cell function leaves the child with AIDS unable to properly respond to new antigens and particularly vulnerable to common bacterial infections. This child also experiences monocyte/macrophage abnormalities, contributing to an increased susceptibility to parasitic and other intracellular infections.

Once HIV enters the child's bloodstream, it becomes attached to CD-4 positive T cells. The external surface antigen of the virus binds to the CD-4 receptor of the cell, and then the virus enters the cell and is uncoated. With the help of the reverse transcriptase enzyme, the retroviral RNA is transcribed into DNA. This newly formed DNA then integrates itself into the cell nucleus (forming a provirus) or remains unintegrated in the cellular cytoplasm. Not only does the provirus affect cellular gene function, but as the infected cells proliferate, a proviral sequence remains in all progeny cells. An infected cell can continue to actively produce HIV or can remain latent until stimulated. Cofactors, stimuli that activate the production of HIV, include cytokines and can include certain other viruses as well. The host cell is usually destroyed once active replication of the virus occurs. After cellular death, viral particles from the cell may be released and lead to the spread of the HIV infection.

Infection by HIV can have a wide spectrum of clinical manifestations varying from no symptoms to severe opportunistic infections, neurological deterioration, pulmonary failure, and/or death. Most children with AIDS present with the triad of failure to thrive, hepatosplenomegaly, and chronic interstitial pneumonitis. Since their bodies lack the appropriate cellular response, many children present with two or more opportunistic infections—most commonly *Pneumocystis carinii* pneumonia, invasive candidal esophagitis, and/or disseminated cytomegalovirus.

Because children with AIDS are unable to respond to new antigens, they can have many bacterial infections, presenting as pneumonia, meningitis, and sepsis, which can be recurrent and life-threatening. Causative organisms include *Haemophilus influenzae, Staphylococcus aureus, Staphylococcus epidermidis, Streptococcus pneumoniae, Streptococcus pyogenes,* and some gram-negative enteric bacteria. A child with AIDS is also susceptible to rare neoplasms.

The majority of pediatric AIDS patients acquire the infection during the perinatal period and have mothers who have HIV infection; for most of these, at least one parent is an intravenous drug user. A small portion of children with AIDS acquire the virus through blood or blood product transfusion. These include children with coagulopathies and infants who received transfusions during the neonatal period.

A multitude of issues exist for children with HIV infection and their families: physical, psychosocial, societal, ethical, and legal. This illness has many implications not only for the child, but for the entire family, requiring compassionate, consistent, and comprehensive care from the health care system and the community.

PRIMARY NURSING DIAGNOSIS

Actual Infection and High Risk for Further Infection*

DEFINITION   Condition in which microorganisms have invaded and threaten to further invade the body

POSSIBLY RELATED TO
Humoral immunosuppression
Depression of cellular immunity
Opportunistic agents
Common bacterial agents
Malnutrition

---

*Non-NANDA diagnosis.

CHARACTERISTICS
Fever
Lymphadenopathy
Diarrhea (often profuse)
Nausea/vomiting
Painful swallowing
Skin rashes and mucous membrane lesions
Cough
Chest pain
Dyspnea
Malaise
Fatigue
Night sweats
Change in the level of consciousness/meningeal signs
Altered complete blood count (CBC) with differential
Poor feeding
Weight loss

EXPECTED OUTCOMES Child will be free of secondary
infection as evidenced by

body temperature within the acceptable range of 36.5°C to
37.2°C.
clear and intact skin and mucous membranes.
alertness when awake.
if age-appropriate, orientation to person, place, and time
(oriented ×3).
lack of signs/symptoms of infection (such as those listed
under **Characteristics**).
CBC within acceptable range (state specific highest and
lowest counts for each child).

POSSIBLE NURSING INTERVENTIONS
Assess and record the following every 4 hours and PRN:

temperature
signs/symptoms of infection (such as those listed under
Characteristics)

Maintain good handwashing technique.

Adhere to Center for Disease Control (CDC) guidelines and/
or institutional policy for current precaution/isolation
techniques.

When indicated, obtain culture specimens (blood, stool, wound, urine, sputum). Check results and notify physician of any abnormalities.

Use tepid baths and cooling blankets, as indicated.

Administer antibiotics, antiviral agents, antiretroviral agents, antifungal agents, steroids, antipyretics, and gamma globulin on schedule. Assess and record effectiveness and any side effects (e.g., rash, diarrhea).

🏠 Assess and record child's/family's knowledge of and participation in care regarding

> identification of any signs/symptoms of infection (such as those listed under **Characteristics**).
> handwashing technique.
> isolation/precaution guidelines.
> maintenance of modified immunization practices.
> medication administration.

🏠 Instruct child/family in any areas needing improvement. Record results.

EVALUATION FOR CHARTING

State highest and lowest temperatures.

Describe any signs/symptoms of infection (such as those listed under **Characteristics**).

Document maintenance of isolation/precaution techniques.

State current results of any cultures and/or CBCs.

State whether medications were administered on schedule. Describe effectiveness and any side effects noted.

Describe any therapeutic measures used to treat the infection and make the child comfortable.

🏠 Describe child's/family's knowledge of and participation in care regarding treatment of infection. State any areas needing improvement and information provided. Describe child's/family's responses.

Altered Nutrition: Less than Body Requirements

DEFINITION   Nutrients insufficient to meet body requirements

POSSIBLY RELATED TO
   Increased metabolic demands secondary to fever, increased
      respiratory rate, and sepsis
   Nausea/vomiting secondary to infection or side effects of
      medications
   Diarrhea secondary to gram-negative enteric microorganisms
   Decreased oral intake secondary to painful oral lesions and
      inflamed esophagus
   Lack of interest in food
   Altered taste sensation

CHARACTERISTICS
   Anorexia
   Weight loss or failure to gain weight
   Vomiting
   Diarrhea
   Abdominal cramping
   Muscle wasting
   Dysphagia
   Oral lesions

EXPECTED OUTCOMES   Child will be adequately nourished
as evidenced by

   sufficient caloric consumption, parenterally and orally (state
      specific amount for each child).
   steady weight gain.
   lack of

      vomiting.
      diarrhea.
      abdominal cramping.
      muscle wasting.
      dysphagia.

POSSIBLE NURSING INTERVENTIONS
   Keep accurate record of intake and output.

Assess and record any signs/symptoms of altered nutrition (such as those listed under **Characteristics**).

Organize care to conserve energy.

Weigh child on the same scale at same time each day.

Maintain and record daily calorie count, as indicated.

Encourage child to eat by assessing likes/dislikes and, when possible, providing foods that the child likes to eat.

Offer small, frequent feedings (six small meals per day).

Provide high-caloric meals, snacks, and supplements.

Initiate a nutritional consultation with a pediatric dietitian who will take into account cultural and social factors.

When indicated, administer tube feedings on schedule. Follow institutional policy for changing and care of the feeding and tube.

When indicated, administer total parenteral nutrition (TPN) and intralipids. Follow institutional policy for maintenance of TPN, intralipid line, and dressing. Monitor and record serum glucose and lipid levels.

Provide good oral hygiene.

Administer antiemetics, antidiarrheals, and oral topical anesthetics on schedule. Assess and record effectiveness and any side effects (such as drowsiness).

When indicated, initiate a social services consultation to facilitate obtainment of groceries or food supplements.

 Assess and record child's/family's knowledge of and participation in care regarding

> monitoring of intake and output.
> identification of any signs/symptoms of altered nutrition (such as those listed under **Characteristics**).
> provision of a nutritious diet.
> maintenance of good oral hygiene, including regular dental visits.

 Instruct family in any areas needing improvement. Record results.

EVALUATION FOR CHARTING

State intake and output.

Describe any signs/symptoms of altered nutrition (such as those listed under Characteristics).

State child's current weight and determine whether it has increased or decreased since previous weighing.

State caloric intake.

Describe any therapeutic measures used to maintain adequate nutrition. State their effectiveness.

State whether medications were administered on schedule. Describe effectiveness and any side effects noted.

🏠 Describe child's/family's knowledge of and participation in care related to improving nutrition. State any areas needing improvement and information provided. Describe child's/family's responses.

NURSING DIAGNOSIS
Compromised Family Coping

DEFINITION   Decreased ability of family members to manage problems and concerns effectively

POSSIBLY RELATED TO

Child's terminal illness
Financial considerations
Inadequate support system
Guilt
Lack of material resources
Social isolation
Grieving
Depression
Fear
Parental drug use

CHARACTERISTICS

Inability to leave the child
Inability to meet basic needs such as eating and sleeping
Inability to ask for and accept outside help
Inappropriate anger toward other family members
Failure to understand repeated explanations regarding the
    child's illness and treatment

EXPECTED OUTCOMES Family will be able to cope effectively as evidenced by

> ability to leave the child for short periods, especially to care for own basic needs such as eating meals and getting rest.
>
> appropriate expression of anger toward staff or others.
>
> requests for outside help or acceptance of outside help when offered.
>
> ability to express fears and concerns to members of the health care team.
>
> participation in the child's care.
>
> verbalization of understanding of explanations regarding the illness and treatment.

POSSIBLE NURSING INTERVENTIONS

> Communicate with family members concerning child's condition at least once/shift and PRN. This may require telephoning family members when they are not able to come to the hospital.
>
> Encourage family members to express feelings, fears, and concerns.
>
> Assist and encourage family members to meet own basic needs, such as eating and resting appropriately.
>
> Explain the course of the illness and treatment to the family. Include reasons for procedures and specific treatments.
>
> Support family's participation in child's care. Record results.

When indicated,

> initiate visiting-nurse consultation.
>
> refer family to social services for assessment of financial status, housing, transportation, clothing, ability to obtain food, and ability to obtain medications.
>
> enroll family in entitlement programs.
>
> collaborate with child's school nurse.
>
> refer family for counseling.

Encourage family to use extended family members, church members, and volunteers to meet their needs.

Assist family members in identifying their strengths and past successful coping strategies.

Encourage family involvement with support groups.

EVALUATION FOR CHARTING

State whether family members were able to leave the child long enough to meet their own basic needs.

Describe any feelings, fears, and concerns expressed by the family.

🏠 State whether the family is willing to accept outside help, as indicated.

🏠 State whether family members were able to understand information given to them about the child's illness.

🏠 State whether family was able to understand the necessity and rationale for procedures and specific treatments.

🏠 State any successful measures used to improve family's coping ability.

🏠 Describe family's participation in child's care.

RELATED NURSING DIAGNOSES

Impaired Gas Exchange *related to*
chronic lung infections

Knowledge Deficit: Child/Family *related to*
a. guilt
b. fear
c. sensory overload
d. misconceptions or inaccurate information
e. cognitive or cultural-language limitations
f. home care

Fear: Child/Parental *related to*
a. terminal illness
b. death
c. social ramifications of illness

MEDICAL DIAGNOSIS
Cellulitis

PATHOPHYSIOLOGY Cellulitis, an inflammation of connective tissue and/or dermis, occurs when bacterial organisms destroy hyaluronic acid, a binding and protective agent known as the cement substance of tissue. In this condition, bacterial organisms produce hyaluronidase (an enzyme that hydrolyzes hyaluronic acid), increasing the permeability of connective tissue and destroying tissue barriers, thus allowing the invasion by and spread of bacteria. The most common bacterial organisms responsible for cellulitis are *Staphylococcus aureus,* beta-hemolytic streptococci, and *Haemophilus influenzae.* The infection can occur at or near an open wound or an intravenous infusion site, or even where there is a vague history of recent trauma to an area.

Clinical manifestations include redness, edema, warmth, and pain in the affected area. Treatment consists of administration of intravenous antibiotics (mild cases can sometimes be treated with oral antibiotics at home), immobilization and elevation of the infected area, and application of warm soaks. Cellulitis is a common occurrence in the pediatric population because of the social nature of young children and their close proximity to other children.

PRIMARY NURSING DIAGNOSIS
Actual Infection*

DEFINITION Condition in which microorganisms have invaded the body

POSSIBLY RELATED TO
Bacterial invasion of cellular or connective tissue

CHARACTERISTICS
Redness

---

*Non-NANDA diagnosis.

Edema
Warm to touch
Red streaks radiating from infected area
Tenderness
Pain
Fever

EXPECTED OUTCOMES Child will be free of infection as evidenced by

lack of the following in the affected area:

redness
edema
warm to touch
red streaks
tenderness
pain

body temperature between 36.5°C and 37.2°C.

POSSIBLE NURSING INTERVENTIONS

Assess and record

temperature every 4 hours and PRN.
IV fluids and condition of IV site every hour.
signs/symptoms of infection (such as those listed under **Characteristics**) every 4 hours and PRN.

Keep accurate record of intake and output.

Maintain good handwashing technique.

Administer antibiotics on schedule and antipyretics PRN. Assess and record effectiveness and any side effects (e.g., rash, diarrhea).

When indicated, immobilize and elevate infected area and apply warm, moist packs, as directed. Assess and record effectiveness in reducing tenderness/pain to infected area. Assess circulation in affected area every 2 to 4 hours. Record every 4 hours and PRN.

Assess and record child's/family's knowledge of and participation in care regarding

handwashing technique.
immobilization and elevation of infected area.

application of warm, moist packs to infected area.

identification of any signs/symptoms of infection (such as those listed under **Characteristics**).

🏠 Instruct child/family in any areas needing improvement. Record results.

EVALUATION FOR CHARTING

State highest and lowest temperatures.

Describe condition of IV site.

Describe any signs/symptoms of infection (such as those listed under **Characteristics**).

State intake and output.

State whether medications were administered on schedule. Describe effectiveness and any side effects noted.

Describe circulation in affected area.

Describe any therapeutic measures used to treat the infection. State their effectiveness in increasing child's level of comfort.

🏠 Describe child's/family's knowledge of and participation in care regarding treatment of infection. State any areas needing improvement and information provided. Describe child's/family's response.

NURSING DIAGNOSIS
Impaired Tissue Integrity

DEFINITION   Interruption of the integrity of or damage to the mucous membrane, integumentary, or subcutaneous tissue

POSSIBLY RELATED TO

Increased permeability of connective tissue and destruction of the tissue barriers secondary to bacterial invasion

CHARACTERISTICS

Redness
Edema
Warm to touch
Red streaks radiating from the infected area
Tenderness
Pain

EXPECTED OUTCOMES   Child will be free of signs/
symptoms of impaired tissue integrity as evidenced by

natural color of the skin tissue.

lack of the following to the infected area:

redness
edema
warm to touch
red streaks
tenderness
pain

POSSIBLE NURSING INTERVENTIONS
Assess and record

condition of tissue surrounding the infected site every 4
hours and PRN.
IV fluids and condition of IV site every hour.
signs/symptoms of impaired tissue integrity (such as those
listed under **Characteristics**) every 4 hours and PRN.

Keep accurate records of intake and output.

Maintain good handwashing technique.

Administer antibiotics on schedule and antipyretics PRN.
Assess and record effectiveness and any side effects (e.g.,
rash, diarrhea).

When indicated, immobilize and elevate infected area and
apply warm, moist packs and/or wound dressing, as directed.
Assess and record effectiveness in reducing tenderness and/or
pain in infected area. Assess circulation in affected area every
2 to 4 hours. Record results every 4 to 8 hours.

 Assess and record child's/family's knowledge of and
participation in care regarding

handwashing technique.
immobilization and elevation of infected area.
application of warm, moist packs to the infected area.
wound care and/or dressing changes, if indicated.
identification of any signs/symptoms of impaired tissue
integrity (such as those listed under **Characteristics**).

Instruct child/family in any areas needing improvement. Record results.

EVALUATION FOR CHARTING

Describe condition of tissue surrounding infected area.

Describe condition of IV site.

Describe any signs/symptoms of impaired tissue integrity (such as those listed under **Characteristics**).

State intake and output.

State whether medications were administered on schedule. Describe effectiveness and any side effects noted.

Describe circulation in the affected area.

Describe any therapeutic measures used to treat the infection. State their effectiveness in increasing child's level of comfort.

 Describe child's/family's knowledge of and participation in care regarding treatment of impaired tissue integrity. State any areas needing improvement and information provided. Describe child's/family's responses.

RELATED NURSING DIAGNOSES

Altered Comfort* *related to*
a. joint involvement
b. bacterial invasion

Activity Intolerance *related to*
a. immobilization of infected area
b. IV fluids
c. warm soaks
d. fever

Fear: Child *related to*
a. hospitalization
b. treatment and procedures
c. altered comfort

Compromised Family Coping *related to*
hospitalization of the child

---

*Non-NANDA diagnosis

EIGHT

CARE OF CHILDREN
WITH
MUSCULOSKELETAL
DYSFUNCTION

MEDICAL DIAGNOSIS

Duchenne Muscular Dystrophy

PATHOPHYSIOLOGY Duchenne muscular dystrophy (DMD), also called pseudohypertrophic muscular dystrophy, is the most common and most severe form of muscular dystrophy in children. Muscular dystrophy is the name of a group of genetically acquired diseases that cause gradual progressive muscle wasting. Duchenne muscular dystrophy is an X-linked recessive disorder primarily affecting boys. Initial muscle weakness and atrophy begins in the proximal muscles, especially of the hips, shoulders, and spine, and presents between the ages of 2 and 4. Eventually it affects all the muscles of the body, including those of the respiratory and cardiovascular systems. Death results between the ages of 15 and 25, often following cardiac and/or respiratory complications.

The muscles of children with DMD undergo several histologic changes: nerve fibers degenerate, fat and connective tissue replace muscle fibers, and there is a variation in fiber size and central nuclei. As a compensatory mechanism, adjacent fibers hypertrophy. All of these processes contribute to the pseudohypertrophy of the calves, thighs, and upper arms. Although the etiology of DMD is unknown, increased levels of serum creatine phosphokinase (CPK) in affected individuals assist in confirming the diagnosis. Additional enzymes also leak from the damaged muscle fibers, resulting in increased serum levels.

Clinical manifestations include the inability to get up from a supine position, difficulty running and jumping, waddling gait, and difficulty climbing stairs. Ambulation becomes impaired, the child has difficulty rising from the sitting position, and severe contractures and joint deformities may develop as the condition progresses. Involvement of the facial muscles, oropharyngeal muscles, diaphragm and respiratory musculature, and myocardium rarely occurs until the final stages of the illness.

The goal of treatment for DMD is to promote optimal functioning. A regular exercise program of stretching and range of motion, aggressive management of respiratory and cardiac problems, the use of adaptive devices to facilitate activities of daily living, and modifications in the home help to assist ambulation and independence as long as possible. The Muscular Dystrophy Association offers support services to these children and their families.

NURSING DIAGNOSIS
Impaired Physical Mobility

DEFINITION   Limited ability of movement

POSSIBLY RELATED TO
　　Muscle weakness
　　Contractures
　　Joint deformities

CHARACTERISTICS
　　Decreased range of motion
　　Contractures
　　Muscle weakness
　　Fatigue
　　Joint deformities
　　Muscle atrophy
　　Clumsiness
　　Falling
　　Waddling gait
　　Difficulty arising from a sitting position
　　Lordosis
　　Difficulty climbing stairs

EXPECTED OUTCOMES   Child will maximize ability of movement as evidenced by (state specific examples for each child).

POSSIBLE NURSING INTERVENTIONS
　　Assess and record child's activity level at least once/shift.

　　Assess and record any signs/symptoms of impaired physical mobility (such as those listed under **Characteristics**).

　　Ensure that child keeps scheduled appointments with occupational therapy and physical therapy, as indicated.

　　Encourage child to participate as much as possible in self-care.

Make available activities within child's limitations (state specific examples for each child).

Allow adequate rest periods (state specific amount of rest needed for each child).

Perform scheduled active and passive range-of-motion exercises (at least every 4 hours).

Reposition child every 1 to 2 hours.

Ensure that child's body stays in proper alignment, whether in bed, chair, or wheelchair.

Encourage use of devices such as handrails, footboards, and rubber-soled shoes to facilitate activities of daily living.

Assist child as necessary with use of braces.

🏠 Initiate referrals to home health agencies, visiting nurses, and social services. Encourage registration with the Muscular Dystrophy Association.

🏠 Assess and record child's/family's knowledge of and participation in care regarding

> identification of any signs/symptoms of impaired physical mobility (such as those listed under **Characteristics**).
> monitoring of activity level and rest periods.
> correct use of adaptive devices and home modifications.
> correct handling and positioning techniques.
> continuation of range-of-motion exercises, bracing, and occupational and/or physical therapy, as indicated.
> appropriate use of resources.

🏠 Instruct child/family in any areas needing improvement. Record results.

EVALUATION FOR CHARTING

Describe child's level of mobility.

Describe any signs/symptoms of impaired physical mobility (such as those listed under **Characteristics**).

State child's ability to participate in self-care.

Describe any therapeutic measures used to improve physical mobility. State their effectiveness.

Describe child's/family's knowledge of and participation in care related to improving physical mobility. State any areas needing improvement and information provided. Describe child's/family's responses.

NURSING DIAGNOSIS
Ineffective Breathing Pattern

DEFINITION   Breathing pattern that results in inadequate oxygen consumption (failure to meet the cellular requirements of the body)

POSSIBLY RELATED TO
Weakness of pulmonary musculature
Scoliosis
Lordosis

CHARACTERISTICS
Shallow respiration
Pooled secretions and/or mucus
Tachypnea
Diaphoresis
Pallor or cyanosis
Crackles and/or rhonchi
Decreased breath sounds
Infiltrates revealed on chest x-ray

EXPECTED OUTCOMES   Child will have an effective breathing pattern as evidenced by

respiratory rate within acceptable range (state highest and lowest rates for each child).
clear and equal breath sounds bilaterally.
absence of

pallor or cyanosis.
crackles and/or rhonchi.
diaphoresis.
pooled secretions and/or mucus.

clear chest x-ray.

POSSIBLE NURSING INTERVENTIONS
Assess and record the following every 4 hours and PRN:

respiratory rate
breath sounds

signs/symptoms of ineffective breathing pattern (such as those listed under **Characteristics**). Notify physician of any abnormalities.

Administer humidified oxygen in correct amount and route of delivery. Record percent of oxygen and route of delivery. Assess and record effectiveness of therapy.

Ensure that chest physiotherapy is done on schedule. Record effectiveness of treatments. Suction child PRN, if child is unable to clear airway. Record characteristics of the secretions and the response of the child.

Elevate head of bed at a 30° angle.

When using a pulse oximeter, record reading every 2 to 4 hours and PRN.

Check and record results of chest x-ray, when indicated.

When indicated, administer antibiotics on schedule. Assess and record effectiveness and any side effects (e.g., rash, diarrhea).

Initiate referrals to home health agencies, visiting nurses, and social services.

Assess and record child's/family's knowledge of and participation in care regarding

identification of any signs/symptoms of ineffective breathing pattern (such as those listed under **Characteristics**).
chest physiotherapy.
suctioning.

Instruct child/family in any areas needing improvement. Record results.

EVALUATION FOR CHARTING
State highest and lowest respiratory rates.

Describe breath sounds.

Describe any signs/symptoms of ineffective breathing pattern noted (such as those listed under **Characteristics**).

State whether oxygen was administered and amount and route of delivery. Describe effectiveness.

Indicate whether chest physiotherapy was done on schedule. Describe child's tolerance of procedure and its effectiveness.

State whether suctioning was needed. If so, describe the amount and characteristics of the secretions and the child's response.

State the results of chest x-ray, when indicated.

State range of oxygen saturation.

State whether head of bed was elevated.

Indicate whether medications were administered on schedule. Describe effectiveness and any side effects noted.

Describe any therapeutic measures used to maintain an effective breathing pattern. State their effectiveness.

Describe child's/family's knowledge of and participation in care related to maintaining an effective breathing pattern. State any areas needing improvement and information provided. Describe child's/family's responses.

RELATED NURSING DIAGNOSES

Body Image Disturbance *related to*
a. chronic illness
b. disabling features of the illness
c. limited physical activity
d. weight gain

Self-Care Deficit: (Specify) *related to*
a. joint contractures and/or deformities
b. muscle weakness

Anticipatory Grieving: Family *related to*
a. child's debilitating chronic illness
b. poor prognosis for child

Compromised Family Coping *related to*
a. child's debilitating chronic illness
b. knowledge deficit
c. necessary home modifications
d. X-linked recessive disorder
e. genetic counseling

MEDICAL DIAGNOSIS
Fractures

DESCRIPTION A fracture is a break in the continuity of the tissue of the bone. Fractures can be complete, with fragments separated, or incomplete, with fragments remaining attached. They can also be classified as simple (closed) or compound, with one or both ends of the broken bone protruding through an open wound.

Common fractures in children include a complete fracture, a buckle fracture, a greenstick fracture, and a spiral fracture. A buckle fracture, also called a torus fracture, occurs when the porous bone is compressed, resulting in a budging projection at the fracture site. A greenstick fracture, the most frequently seen type in children, occurs when the bone is angulated beyond the limits of bending. The fracture is incomplete, and there is a break through the periosteum on the compressed side only. A spiral, or transverse, fracture occurs from a sudden, twisting, violent exertion upon an extremity, resulting in a fracture line across the bone. This type of injury is often seen in physically abused children.

Since a child's skeletal structure is not the same as that of an adult, the management and treatment of fractures in children is different than in adults. Children's bones are more easily injured, and fractures can result from minor falls or twists. In children, bones are more flexible, have decreased density, and have a thicker periosteum. The increased flexibility allows the bone to bend 45° or more before breaking. A break in a young child's bone is more often incomplete due to the decreased density of the bone. The thick periosteum can sometimes serve as a hinge and facilitate closed reduction of a fracture. The epiphyseal growth plate, which serves to absorb shock and protect joint surfaces in children, is the weakest point of long bones and consequently a frequent site of damage during trauma. If the fracture occurs in this portion of the bone and destroys the germinal layer, it can cause shortening and a progressive angular deformity of the affected limb. If the injury stimulates blood supply to the epiphysis, it can lead to overgrowth of the affected bone. Fractures usually heal faster in children than in adults because of the rich blood supply and high osteogenic activity in children. Diagnosis can be made from x-ray films of the injured area.

The management and treatment of fractures involves bringing the fracture fragments into proper alignment. This can be accomplished by open or closed reduction. Closed reduction, the most common method used in children, consists of a combination of manual manipulation and force applied with the hands to push the bone ends into position. Some overriding of the fracture fragments (1 cm) is sometimes desirable in children to allow for the overgrowth that may occur in the injured extremity. After manual manipulation, the fragments are held in place with a cast. When the pull or spasms of muscles close to the fracture make setting difficult, traction or internal or external fixation devices are used to hold the fragments in place. Open reduction, used when alignment cannot be obtained by the closed method, is a surgical procedure and requires general anesthesia. Some type of internal fixation device, such as a rod, screw, or plate, is used to stabilize the fracture.

Complications of fractures include malunion as healing occurs, compartment syndrome (progressive interference of blood flow to an extremity), emboli, and growth disturbance. Nursing care includes frequent neurovascular assessment of the injured area and reduction of pain.

PRIMARY NURSING DIAGNOSIS
Pain

DEFINITION   Condition in which an individual experiences severe discomfort

POSSIBLY RELATED TO
> Break in the continuity of the tissue of the bone
> Muscle spasms

CHARACTERISTICS
> Crying or moaning
> Facial grimacing
> Verbal expression of pain
> Restlessness
> Guarding or protective behavior of the injured site
> Physical signs/symptoms:

tachycardia
tachypnea/bradypnea
increased blood pressure
diaphoresis

EXPECTED OUTCOMES   Child will be free of extreme pain as evidenced by

lack of constant crying or moaning.
verbal communication of decreased pain.
lack of facial grimacing and restlessness.
decreased guarding or protective behavior of the injured site.
heart rate, respiratory rate, and blood pressure within
   acceptable ranges (state specific highest and lowest
   parameters for each child).
decreased diaphoresis.

POSSIBLE NURSING INTERVENTIONS

Assess and record

signs/symptoms of pain (such as those listed under
   Characteristics) every 2 to 4 hours and PRN.
neurovascular status of extremity every 1 to 2 hours and
   PRN.

Administer analgesics and/or narcotics on schedule. Assess and record effectiveness.

Handle injured area with extreme care. Avoid bumping or jarring the bed if the child is in traction. Maintain correct alignment of injured area.

If age-appropriate, explain all procedures beforehand.

Encourage family members to stay and comfort child when possible.

Allow family members to participate in care of the child when possible.

When indicated, institute additional pain relief measures (e.g., relaxation, guided imagery, music.) Assess and record effectiveness.

Use diversional activities and distraction measures (e.g., toys, play activities, television, radio) when appropriate.

Assess and record family's knowledge of and participation in care regarding

> medication administration.
> gentle handling of child.
> correct alignment of injured area.
> additional pain relief measures.
> identification of any signs/symptoms of pain (such as those listed under **Characteristics**).

 Instruct family in any areas needing improvement. Record results.

EVALUATION FOR CHARTING

Describe any signs/symptoms of pain noted (such as those listed under **Characteristics**).

State ranges of vital signs.

Describe neurovascular assessment of extremity.

Describe effectiveness of analgesics and/or narcotics.

Describe any successful measures used to reduce or eliminate pain.

 Describe family's knowledge of and participation in care regarding reduction of pain. State any areas needing improvement and information provided. Describe family's response.

NURSING DIAGNOSIS

Impaired Physical Mobility

DEFINITION   Limited ability of movement

POSSIBLY RELATED TO

Break in continuity of the tissue of the bone
Cast
Traction

CHARACTERISTICS

Restricted movement of part of the body
Decreased range of motion of part of the body
Inability to ambulate
Muscle pull and/or spasms

EXPECTED OUTCOMES   Child will return to preinjury mobility level.

POSSIBLE NURSING INTERVENTIONS

Assess and record any signs/symptoms of impaired physical mobility (such as those listed under **Characteristics**).

Arrange for therapeutic play, occupational therapy, and physical therapy, as indicated.

Encourage child to participate as much as possible in self-care. Provide apparatus, such as overhead trapeze, when indicated.

Make available activities within child's limitations (state specific examples for each child).

Allow adequate rest periods (state specific amount of rest needed for each child).

Perform active and passive range-of-motion exercises every 4 hours.

Ensure that injured area remains in proper alignment at all times. Use footboard to prevent foot drop, when indicated.

If child is in a cast, assess and record the following every 2 hours and PRN:

> neurovascular status of affected area
> warm area on the cast
> swelling
> bleeding on cast. Mark bleeding and record date and time on cast with a ballpoint pen.

Petal cast for added comfort.

 Assess and record child's/family's knowledge of and participation in care regarding

> identification of any signs/symptoms of impaired physical mobility (such as those listed under **Characteristics**).
> monitoring of activity level and rest periods.
> activity restrictions, as indicated.
> continuation of range-of-motion exercises and/or occupational and/or physical therapy, as indicated.
> cast care, including
> • drying and cleaning of cast.

- neurovascular checks of casted extremity.
- petaling of cast.

monitoring for bleeding, swelling, pain, discoloration of exposed portions, lack of warmness, and "hot spots" of casted extremity.

assistance with activities of daily living (may need bedpan and/or urinal if child is in a hip spica).

correct use of crutches, when indicated.

🏠 Instruct child/family in any areas needing improvement. Record results.

EVALUATION FOR CHARTING

Describe child's current level of mobility.

Describe any signs/symptoms of impaired physical mobility (such as those listed under **Characteristics**).

State child's ability to participate in self-care.

Describe any therapeutic measures used to improve physical mobility. State their effectiveness.

If child is casted, describe neurovascular assessment, amount of any bleeding or swelling present, and any warm spots noted.

🏠 Describe child's/family's knowledge of and participation in care related to improving physical mobility. State any areas needing improvement and information provided. Describe child's/family's responses.

RELATED NURSING DIAGNOSES

Impaired Skin Integrity _related to_
   a. immobility
   b. traction
   c. internal or external fixation devices
   d. cast

Fear: Child _related to_
   a. discomfort
   b. procedures and equipment
   c. forced contact with strangers
   d. hospital environment

Self-Care Deficit: (Specify) *related to*
a. immobility
b. traction
c. cast

Infection: High Risk *related to*
a. fixation devices
b. open reduction
c. wound site

MEDICAL DIAGNOSIS

Juvenile Rheumatoid Arthritis

PATHOPHYSIOLOGY Arthritis is defined as joint swelling or restriction of motion with pain, tenderness, and/or heat. Inflammatory arthritis in children is called juvenile rheumatoid arthritis (JRA). Juvenile Rheumatoid Arthritis is a systemic disorder of connective tissue, joints, and viscera. Tissue injury in the joint, possibly from a previous infection, may cause normal immunoglobulins to become antigenic. The body responds by developing rheumatoid factors (RF), autoantibodies anti-IgG and anti-IgM, which lodge in synovial fluid and other tissues and cause inflammation. The inflammatory process thickens the synovial membrane, increases synovial fluid production, and changes the composition of the synovial fluid. Joint effusion (swollen, boggy joints), edema, pain (from pressure on sensory nerves), and limited mobility may result. The child may experience articular erosion and synovitis for long periods before permanent joint damage occurs.

The three types of JRA, each designated by the clinical manifestations present during the first 6 months of illness, are pauciarticular, polyarticular, and systemic. Pauciarticular JRA involves fewer than four joints. Usually, large joints, such as the knees, ankles, or elbows, are affected with joint stiffness, which is greater in the morning and lessens as the day goes on. There are two subtypes of pauciarticular JRA. Type I affects primarily girls under 10 years of age. These children have antinuclear antibody (ANA) positive serum, but they are negative for RF and are at risk for developing inflammation of the iris and ciliary bodies of the eyes. Type II, which may be genetically transmitted, affects boys older than 10 years of age and involves the hip and lower extremity joints.

Polyarticular JRA involves more than four joints, usually the knees, ankles, neck, wrists, and/or elbows. Joint stiffness is worst in the morning or after the child sits for a while. Disability can be mild or severe.

Systemic JRA initially presents with a high fever, sometimes accompanied by a rash on the trunk and extremities, anorexia, and/or weight loss. Later, the disease may involve the joints, as well as carditis, pleurisy, pneumonia, severe anemia, and/or liver enlargement. Disability ranges from mild to severe.

Juvenile Rheumatoid Arthritis is one of the most common chronic illnesses in children. It is characterized by spontaneous exacerbations and remissions, with the prognosis depending on the subtype. Treatment involves attempts to reduce inflammation, relieve pain, and prevent joint contractures and other complications. Pharmacological management includes nonsteroidal antiinflammatory drugs, slower-acting antirheumatic drugs, and, when needed, steroids. Cytotoxic agents may be used for children whose disease process has been unresponsive to other drugs. Exercise, physical therapy, and/or joint immobilization through splinting, casting, or traction are also important.

NURSING DIAGNOSIS
Impaired Physical Mobility

DEFINITION   Limited ability of movement

POSSIBLY RELATED TO
   Pain
   Joint inflammation
   Synovitis

CHARACTERISTICS
   Decreased range of motion
   Contractures
   Arthralgias
   Myalgias
   Fatigue
   Swelling
   Joint stiffness
   Joint destruction

EXPECTED OUTCOMES   Child will maximize ability of movement as evidenced by (state specific examples for each child).

POSSIBLE NURSING INTERVENTIONS
   Assess and record child's activity level at least once per shift.

Assess and record any signs/symptoms of impaired physical mobility (such as those listed under **Characteristics**) every 8 hours and PRN.

Ensure that child keeps scheduled appointments with occupational therapy and physical therapy, as indicated.

Encourage child to participate as much as possible in self-care.

Make available activities within child's limitations (state specific examples for each child).

Allow adequate rest periods (state specific amount of rest needed for each child).

Perform scheduled active and passive range-of-motion exercises at least every 4 hours.

Reposition child every 1 to 2 hours.

Ensure that child's body stays in proper alignment, whether in bed, chair, or wheelchair.

Assist child as necessary with use of splints and other appliances.

Administer analgesics, nonsteroidal antiinflammatory medications, slower-acting antirheumatic medications, steroids, and/or cytotoxic agents on schedule, as indicated. (Medicate with analgesics and antiinflammatory medications 30 to 60 minutes prior to activity, exercises, and getting up in the morning.) Assess and record effectiveness and any side effects (e.g., diarrhea, GI irritation).

Initiate referrals to home health care agencies, visiting nurses, and social services, as indicated.

Assess and record child's/family's knowledge of and participation in care regarding

> identification of any signs/symptoms of impaired physical mobility (such as those listed under **Characteristics**).
> monitoring of activity level and rest periods.
> correct use of appliances.
> correct handling and positioning techniques.
> medication administration.

continuation of range-of-motion exercises, splinting, and/
or occupational and/or physical therapy, as indicated.
appropriate use of resources.

🏠 Instruct child/family in any areas needing improvement.
Record results.

EVALUATION FOR CHARTING

Describe child's level of mobility.

Describe any signs/symptoms of impaired physical mobility
(such as those listed under **Characteristics**).

State child's ability to participate in self-care.

State whether medications were administered on schedule
and describe any side effects noted.

Describe any therapeutic measures used to improve physical
mobility. State their effectiveness.

🏠 Describe child's/family's knowledge of and participation in
care related to improving physical mobility. State any areas
needing improvement and information provided. Describe
child's/family's responses.

NURSING DIAGNOSIS

Self-Care Deficit: (Specify)

DEFINITION   State in which the individual has decreased
ability to complete the activities of daily living for his/her age,
such as feeding, hygiene/bathing, dressing/grooming, and toileting

POSSIBLY RELATED TO

Pain
Joint contractures
Immobility
Decreased range of motion
Visual impairment

CHARACTERISTICS

Self-feeding deficits (e.g., inability to hold utensils or cut
food)
Self-bathing deficits (e.g., inability to get in and out of the
tub)
Self-toileting deficits (e.g., inability to sit on and rise from the
toilet seat)

Self-dressing deficits (e.g., inability to fasten or unfasten clothing or shoes)

Self-hygiene deficits (e.g., inability to hold toothbrush)

EXPECTED OUTCOMES

Child will demonstrate no self-care deficits or will have increased ability to accomplish usual activities of daily living for age (state specific examples for each child).

Child will demonstrate correct use of adaptive devices to accomplish activities of daily living (state specific examples for each child).

POSSIBLE NURSING INTERVENTIONS

Assess and record child's current level of self-care.

Encourage child to have maximum independence in performing activities of daily living. Provide assistance when necessary. Record results.

Initiate consultations with physical therapist and occupational therapist to assist in establishing a self-care program. Be sure to include child when establishing plans and goals.

Advise child/family to allow extra time for activities. Assist in obtaining articles or devising methods to facilitate independent functioning, such as

utensils for eating with large, graspable handles.
toothbrush, comb, and brush with large, graspable handles.
chair or stool in tub or shower.
elevated toilet seat.
handrails in the home (especially in hallways and bathrooms).
clothes that are easy to put on and remove.
dressing aides as needed, such as Velcro fasteners.

Record results of measures attempted to facilitate independent functioning.

Initiate referrals to home health care agencies, visiting nurses, social services, and/or local or national arthritis foundations and clearinghouses.

Assess and record child's/family's knowledge of and participation in care regarding

maximization of child's independent functioning.
correct use of adaptive devices.
maintenance of appropriate amount of rest for child.
appropriate use of resources.

⌂ Instruct child/family in any area needing improvement. Record results.

EVALUATION FOR CHARTING
State child's current level of self-care.

Describe any therapeutic measures used to improve self-care. State their effectiveness.

⌂ Describe child's/family's knowledge of and participation in care related to maximizing self-care. State any areas needing improvement and information provided. Describe child's/family's responses.

RELATED NURSING DIAGNOSES

Pain *related to*
a. inflamed joints
b. joint immobility and stiffness
c. gastric irritation secondary to aspirin use

Body Image Disturbance *related to*
a. chronic illness
b. disabling features of illness
c. side effects of medications

Altered Growth and Development *related to*
a. physical limitations of illness
b. weight loss or inadequate weight gain due to increased metabolic needs
c. weight gain due to decreased mobility
d. irregular school attendance
e. parents with overprotective behavior
f. side effects of medications

Compromised Family Coping *related to*
a. child's debilitating chronic illness
b. knowledge deficit

MEDICAL DIAGNOSIS

Osteomyelitis

PATHOPHYSIOLOGY   Osteomyelitis is an infection of the bone. The most common etiology is a blood-borne infection secondary to an infection elsewhere in the body, referred to as hematogenous sources. Osteomyelitis can also be acquired from exogenous sources, as when it results from an extension of a local infectious process, a contamination of a compound fracture, or introduction of infection during a surgical procedure. The hematogenous origin is the primary type that occurs in children, with the sources of foci including boils, skin abrasions, impetigo, upper respiratory tract infection, acute otitis media, tonsillitis, abscessed teeth, pyelonephritis, and infected burns. *Staphylococcus aureus* is the causative organism in approximately 80% of the cases involving older children, and *Haemophilus influenzae* is the predominate causative organism in younger children.

The infection usually localizes in the bone metaphyses. The infectious process leads to accumulation of pus under the periosteum, causing elevation of the periosteum and compression of medullary circulation, resulting in local bone destruction. In children, the site of infection is often near the epiphyseal plate, which acts to contain the infection by forming new bone (involucrum). The abscess formed exerts pressure because of the rigid, unyielding nature of the bone, resulting in further vascular compromise and necrosis. Eventually the abscess can cause the periosteum to rupture, leading to the release of purulent matter, which can infect the nearest joint. Necrotic bone that is not absorbed continues to produce more intraosseous tension and necrosis, with eventual formation of a sequestrum (granulation around dead bone). Sinuses that occasionally develop between the sequestra and the skin surface or into a joint can lead to septic arthritis. If large areas of sequestrum are present, multiple sinuses can retain infective material and result in chronic osteomyelitis.

Treatment consists of prompt and vigorous antibiotic therapy with immobilization of the extremity. Surgical intervention may be indicated to decrease pressure within the metaphyseal space and allow drainage of the pus.

PRIMARY NURSING DIAGNOSIS
Actual Infection*

DEFINITION Condition in which microorganisms have invaded the body

POSSIBLY RELATED TO
Bacterial invasion of the bone via a hematogenous or exogenous source (specify when possible)

CHARACTERISTICS
Fever
Localized tenderness, redness, and swelling and increased warmth over involved area
Irritability
Restlessness
Pain on movement of involved area
Leukocytosis
Elevated erythrocyte sedimentation rate
Positive blood culture

EXPECTED OUTCOMES Child will be free of infection as evidenced by

body temperature between 36.5°C and 37.2°C.
lack of extreme irritability and restlessness.
lack of the following in the infected area:

tenderness
redness
swelling
increased warmth

freedom from pain on movement of the involved area.
white blood cell count within the acceptable range (state specific highest and lowest counts for each child).
erythrocyte sedimentation rate from 0 to 13 mm/hr.
negative blood culture.

---

*Non-NANDA diagnosis.

POSSIBLE NURSING INTERVENTIONS
Assess and record

> temperature every 4 hours and PRN.
> IV fluids and condition of IV site every hour.
> signs/symptoms of infection (such as those listed under
> **Characteristics**) every 4 hours and PRN.

Keep accurate record of intake and output. If wound is draining, record amount and characteristics of drainage.

Administer antibiotics on schedule. Administer antipyretics and analgesics PRN. Assess and record effectiveness and any side effects (e.g., rash, diarrhea).

Maintain good handwashing technique. If an open wound is present, maintain wound isolation precautions in accordance with institutional policy.

If surgical drainage has been performed, make sure that antibiotic solution is draining properly into involved area and that suction is properly applied to remove drainage.

When indicated, change the dressing on schedule according to institutional protocol. Assess and record characteristics of drainage and wound site every 8 hours and PRN.

Keep involved area immobilized. Assess and record area for sensation, circulation, pain, color, swelling, heat, and tenderness every 4 to 8 hours and PRN. Ensure that bedrest is maintained.

Check and record results of any blood cultures and/or laboratory work. Notify physician if results increase over previous results.

Assess and record child's/family's knowledge of and participation in care regarding

> handwashing technique.
> medication administration.
> dressing change and wound assessment.
> activity restrictions, including avoidance of falls and jerky
> movements; quiet play activities; and immobilization
> and bedrest, when indicated.
> identification of any signs/symptoms of infection (such as
> those listed under **Characteristics**).

preventive factors, including adequate nutrition, rest, and maintenance of skin integrity.

🏠 Instruct child/family in any areas needing improvement. Record results.

EVALUATION FOR CHARTING

State highest and lowest temperatures.

Describe condition of IV site.

Describe any signs/symptoms of infection (such as those listed under **Characteristics**).

State intake and output. Describe characteristics of any drainage.

State whether medications were administered on schedule. Describe effectiveness and any side effects noted.

Describe characteristics of involved area.

Describe characteristics of wound site and any drainage.

Describe any therapeutic measures used to treat the infection. State their effectiveness in increasing the child's level of comfort.

State current results of any blood cultures and/or laboratory work.

🏠 Describe child's/family's knowledge of and participation in care regarding treatment of the infection. State any areas needing improvement and information provided. Describe child's/family's responses.

NURSING DIAGNOSIS

Pain

DEFINITION Condition in which an individual experiences severe discomfort

POSSIBLY RELATED TO

Pressure secondary to bacterial invasion of the bone

CHARACTERISTICS

Verbal communication of pain
Crying unrelieved by usual comfort measures

Hesitation or refusal to use limb
Decreased activity, self-imposed
Severe discomfort on movement of involved area
Physical signs/symptoms:

> tachycardia
> tachypnea/bradypnea
> increased blood pressure
> diaphoresis

EXPECTED OUTCOMES   Child will be free of extreme pain as evidenced by

> verbal communication of decreased pain.
> lack of constant crying.
> heart rate, respiratory rate, and blood pressure within acceptable ranges (state specific parameters for each child).
> decrease in or lack of diaphoresis.
> lack of signs/symptoms of bone pain (such as those listed under **Characteristics**).

POSSIBLE NURSING INTERVENTIONS

Assess and record signs/symptoms of pain (such as those listed under **Characteristics**) every 4 hours and PRN.

Handle child gently. Support and protect involved area when the child is moved. Have two individuals move child, if necessary. Keep involved area immobilized.

Encourage family members to stay and comfort child when possible.

Allow family members to participate in care of the child when possible.

Administer analgesics, as indicated. Assess and record effectiveness.

When indicated, institute additional pain relief measures, such as relaxation and music. Assess and record effectiveness.

Use diversional activities and distraction measures (e.g., toys, play activities, television, radio) when appropriate.

EVALUATION FOR CHARTING

Describe any signs/symptoms of pain noted (such as those listed under **Characteristics**).

State range of vital signs.

Describe any successful measures used to reduce or eliminate pain.

Describe effectiveness of analgesics.

RELATED NURSING DIAGNOSES

Impaired Physical Mobility *related to*
pain on movement of involved area secondary to bacterial invasion of the bone

Knowledge Deficit: Child/Family *related to*
a. disease process and treatment
b. prevention of complications
c. activity restrictions

Noncompliance *related to*
a. bedrest
b. non-weight-bearing on lower extremities

Compromised Family Coping *related to*
a. prolonged hospitalization of child (antibiotic therapy needed for 4 to 6 weeks)
b. complicated home care (if child is sent home with a heparin lock for IV therapy at home)
c. financial considerations
d. interruption of parental work schedule

Scoliosis

PATHOPHYSIOLOGY   Scoliosis is a lateral deviation (generally a right thoracic curvature) of the spine from the midline, usually associated with a rotation of a series of vertebrae. This lateral deviation is a consequence of weakened muscle strength resulting from genetic, environmental, and/or physiological factors. Growth spurts lead to progression of the curvature by exerting pressure on the vertebrae, which causes them to become wedged.

    The two basic types of scoliosis are functional and structural. Functional scoliosis, also called nonstructural or postural scoliosis, is a temporary flexible curvature caused by poor posture, position changes, or some deformity such as unequal leg length. The condition can be corrected by active and passive exercise and correction of any underlying defect.

    Structural scoliosis is an inflexible curve that cannot be voluntarily corrected and is further classified as congenital, neuromuscular, or idiopathic. Congenital scoliosis is an embryonic malformation of the bony vertebral column that occurs during the third to fifth week of gestation. It is not unusual for children with this type of scoliosis to have other anomalies, such as urinary tract and cardiac defects. Early treatment, such as bracing or spinal fusion, is essential to prevent progression of the curve.

    Neuromuscular scoliosis is secondary to neuropathic and myopathic diseases such as poliomyelitis, cerebral palsy, myelomeningocele, and muscular dystrophy. Scoliosis is believed to occur as a result of paralysis of the paraspinal and trunk muscles or of alteration of balance mechanisms. Bracing and spinal fusion are used to stabilize progressive curves.

    Idiopathic scoliosis, the most common form of structural scoliosis, accounts for 70% of cases. The etiology is unknown; however, evidence indicates that it may be genetic, transmitted as an autosomal-dominant trait. Individual types of idiopathic scoliosis include infantile, juvenile, and adolescent. Infantile, which occurs in the first year of life, can resolve spontaneously or may progress and require spinal fusion. Juvenile idiopathic scoliosis, which occurs in the middle childhood years (usually around 6 to 10 years of age), will not resolve spontaneously but responds well to bracing or an Orthoplast jacket. If progression occurs or if the curve is greater than 55° to 60°, spinal fusion is indicated. Adolescent idiopathic scoliosis occurs between 10 years of age and skeletal maturity, usually in females (85% of all cases). It will not resolve spontaneously and requires either bracing and exercise or electrical stimulation. If the curve is greater than 40°, surgical intervention, involving spinal fusion with or without instrumentation, is usually necessary. Since adolescent idiopathic scoliosis is the most prevalent type, the remainder of this discussion will refer to this type of scoliosis.

Diagnosis of scoliosis is made by observation of the child walking, standing erect, and bending forward. Positive findings include scapular prominence, rib hump, shoulder asymmetry, hip asymmetry, uneven waistline, torso malalignment when standing erect, and anterior rib and breast asymmetry. The diagnosis is confirmed by roentgenographies, which also establish the degree of spinal curvature.

Mild to moderate curves can usually be treated with braces (Milwaukee, Orthoplast jacket, Cotrel, or Pasadena) and exercise—with a great deal of cooperation from the child and family. The child must wear the brace 23 hours a day until growth is complete. An alternative method is electrospinal orthosis. The device for this treatment, which is used only at night, sends a low-voltage electrical stimulation to the paraspinal muscles.

For severe or progressive curves, surgical management is usually indicated. The child may need traction (Cotrel, halofemoral, or halopelvic) preoperatively to stretch out soft tissue and assist in straightening the curve. Surgery consists of spinal fusion (arthrodesis) with or without instrumentation (Harrington rods, Lugue wires, and/or Dwyer procedure).

Postoperative care includes monitoring the neurovasular status of the extremities, accurately recording intake and output, having the child cough and deep-breathe, carefully log-rolling the child (or turning on a Stryker frame), and administering antibiotics and analgesics. The child will usually have an indwelling urinary catheter, Hemovac wound drain, nasogastric tube, and intravenous fluids. Depending on the type of surgical instrumentation used, the child may be placed in an immobilizing plaster jacket for 6 months following surgery. When Lugue segmental instrumentation is used, the child does not need to be placed in a plaster jacket and can walk within a few days after surgery. Follow-up management is needed every 3 to 6 months for 3 to 5 years.

POSTOPERATIVE NURSING CARE PLAN

PRIMARY NURSING DIAGNOSIS

Pain

DEFINITION Condition in which an individual experiences severe discomfort

POSSIBLY RELATED TO
Surgical incision and manipulation

CHARACTERISTICS
Verbal communication of pain
Crying
Moaning
Physical signs/symptoms:

tachycardia
tachypnea/bradypnea
increased blood pressure
diaphoresis

Rating of pain on pain assessment tool

EXPECTED OUTCOMES Child will be free of extreme pain as evidenced by

verbal communication of decreased pain.
lack of constant crying and moaning.
heart rate, respiratory rate, and blood pressure within
acceptable ranges (state specific parameters for each child).
decrease in or lack of diaphoresis.
rating of decreased or no pain on pain assessment tool.

POSSIBLE NURSING INTERVENTIONS
Assess and record any signs/symptoms of pain (such as those listed under **Characteristics**) every 2 hours and PRN. Use an age-appropriate pain assessment tool.

Log-roll and handle child gently.

Encourage family members to stay and comfort child when possible.

Allow family members to participate in care of the child when possible.

Administer analgesics and/or narcotics on schedule. Assess and record effectiveness.

Monitor patient-controlled analgesia (PCA).

When indicated, institute additional pain relief measures, such as relaxation and music. Assess and record effectiveness.

Use distraction measures (e.g., television), when appropriate.

Assess and record neurovascular status of extremities every 2 hours and PRN.

🏠 Assess and record child's/family's knowledge of and participation in care regarding

incision site.
daily skin checks for pressure areas.
avoidance of strenuous activity until healing is complete.
avoidance of sitting for long periods of time.
assistance with activities of daily living.

🏠 Instruct child/family in any areas needing improvement. Record results.

EVALUATION FOR CHARTING

Describe any signs/symptoms of pain noted (such as those listed under **Characteristics**).

State range of vital signs.

Describe effectiveness of analgesics and/or narcotics.

Describe any successful measures used to reduce or eliminate pain.

Describe neurovascular status of extremities.

🏠 Describe child's/family's knowledge of and participation in care regarding increasing comfort after discharge. State any areas needing improvement and information provided. Describe child's/family's responses.

NURSING DIAGNOSIS
Fluid Volume Deficit

DEFINITION   Decrease in the amount of circulating fluid volume

POSSIBLY RELATED TO
Blood loss secondary to surgical procedure

CHARACTERISTICS
Dry mucous membranes
Poor skin turgor
Decreased urine output
Increased urine specific gravity
Tachycardia
Hypotension
Diminished or absent bowel sounds

EXPECTED OUTCOMES   Child will have an adequate fluid
volume as evidenced by

adequate IV and/or PO fluid intake (state specific amount of
fluid needed for each child).
moist mucous membranes.
rapid skin recoil.
adequate urine output (state specific highest and lowest
outputs for each child, minimum 1 to 2 ml/kg/hr).
urine specific gravity from 1.008 to 1.020.
heart rate and blood pressure within acceptable ranges (state
specific highest and lowest parameters for each child).
presence of bowel sounds.

POSSIBLE NURSING INTERVENTIONS
Keep accurate record of intake and output. Child will have
an indwelling urinary catheter, a nasogastric tube, and
possibly a Hemovac wound drain in the immediate
postoperative period. Measure the output from each and
record characteristics of the drainage.

Keep NPO in the immediate postoperative period. Ensure
that nasogastric tube is patent and connected to low
intermittent suction. Irrigate to maintain patency, as
indicated.

Assess and record

IV fluids and condition of IV site every hour.
heart rate and blood pressure every 4 hours and PRN.
bowel sounds every 4 hours and PRN. (Paralytic ileus
following surgery may be a problem.)
any signs/symptoms of fluid volume deficit (such as those
listed under **Characteristics**) every 4 hours and PRN.

Check and record urine specific gravity every 4 hours and PRN.

EVALUATION FOR CHARTING

State intake and output.

Describe amount and characteristics of nasogastric and Hemovac drainage.

Describe condition of IV site.

State highest and lowest heart rates and blood pressures.

Describe any signs/symptoms of fluid volume deficit noted (such as those listed under **Characteristics**).

State highest and lowest urine specific gravity values.

Describe bowel sounds.

Describe any therapeutic measures to promote adequate fluid volume. State their effectiveness.

RELATED NURSING DIAGNOSES

Knowledge Deficit: Child/Family _related to_
a. surgical procedure
b. immediate postoperative care
c. home care

Body Image Disturbance _related to_
wearing of a cast and/or brace postoperatively

Self-Care Deficit (Specify Bathing/Hygiene, Dressing/Grooming, and/or Toileting) _related to_
mobility restrictions and pain

Compromised Family Coping _related to_
a. assisting child in accepting a postoperative period of casting and/or bracing and activity restriction
b. assisting child in choosing appropriate clothing to wear over cast and/or brace
c. long-term follow-up care (may need assistance from home health agencies)

MEDICAL DIAGNOSIS
Septic Arthritis

PATHOPHYSIOLOGY Septic arthritis, also called suppurative arthritis, is an infection of the joint. The source of the infection is usually by hematogenous dissemination. It can also occur by direct extension of a soft tissue infection, such as osteomyelitis, or a direct inoculation from organisms into the joint space via a wound. The usual causative organisms are *Staphylococcus aureus,* group A beta-hemolytic streptococci, and *Haemophilus influenzae.* Large joints, such as the hip, knee, and shoulder, are most commonly affected.

The synovial membrane of the joint produces increased amounts of synovial fluid in response to the presence of infection. Pus begins to accumulate, leading to destructive and degenerative changes in the articular cartilage. The increased amounts of fluids and pus cause distention, and the joint can eventually dislocate.

Diagnosis is made by roentgenographic studies indicating joint swelling, blood cultures, and joint aspiration of fluid. If the fluid obtained from the joint aspiration contains pus, surgical drainage is usually indicated. Treatment consists of joint immobilization, antibiotic therapy, and, sometimes, surgical opening and drainage of the joint.

PRIMARY NURSING DIAGNOSIS
Actual Infection*

DEFINITION Condition in which microorganisms have invaded the body

POSSIBLY RELATED TO
Bacterial invasion of the joint

---

*Non-NANDA diagnosis.

CHARACTERISTICS

Fever

Localized tenderness, redness, swelling, and increased
warmth over involved joint

Pain on movement of affected joint

Limited range of motion of affected joint

Muscular rigidity

Limping or refusal to walk (if lower extremities are affected)

Leukocytosis

Elevated erythrocyte sedimentation rate

Joint swelling revealed on x-rays

Increased uptake of radioisotope in the infected areas, as
shown on a bone scan

Joint aspiration containing pus

EXPECTED OUTCOMES   Child will be free of infection as
evidenced by

body temperature between 36.5°C and 37.2°C.

lack of the following to the affected joint:

tenderness
redness
swelling
increased warmth

adequate range of motion of affected joint.

freedom from pain on movement of affected joint.

white blood cell count within acceptable range (state specific
highest and lowest counts for each child).

erythrocyte sedimentation rate from 0 to 13 mm/hr.

lack of signs/symptoms of joint infection (such as those listed
under **Characteristics**).

POSSIBLE NURSING INTERVENTIONS

Assess and record

temperature every 4 hours and PRN.

IV fluids and condition of IV site every hour.

signs/symptoms of infection (such as those listed under
Characteristics) every 4 hours and PRN.

Keep accurate record of intake and output.

Administer antibiotics on schedule. Administer antipyretics
and analgesics PRN. Assess and record effectiveness and any
side effects (e.g., rash, diarrhea).

Maintain good handwashing technique.

If surgical drainage has been performed, make sure that antibiotic solution is draining properly into involved area and that suction is properly applied to remove drainage.

Maintain isolation precautions in accordance with institutional policy.

When indicated, change dressing on schedule according to institutional protocol. Assess and record characteristics of drainage and wound site.

Keep involved area immobilized. Begin range-of-motion exercises when indicated. Protect weight-bearing joints from pressure.

Check and record results of any laboratory work or x-rays. Notify physician of any abnormalities.

Assess and record child's/family's knowledge of and participation in care regarding

> handwashing technique.
> medication administration.
> activity restrictions.
> identification of any signs/symptoms of infection (such as those listed under **Characteristics**).

Instruct child/family in any areas needing improvement. Record results.

EVALUATION FOR CHARTING

State highest and lowest temperatures.

Describe condition of IV site.

Describe any signs/symptoms of infection (such as those listed under **Characteristics**).

State whether medications were administered on schedule. Describe effectiveness and any side effects noted.

Describe characteristics of affected joint.

Describe characteristics of wound site and any drainage.

Describe any therapeutic measures used to treat the infection. State their effectiveness in increasing child's level of comfort.

State current results of laboratory work and x-rays.

🏠 Describe child's/family's knowledge of and participation in care regarding treatment of infection. State any areas needing improvement and information provided. Describe child's/family's responses.

NURSING DIAGNOSIS
Pain

DEFINITION   Condition in which an individual experiences severe discomfort

POSSIBLY RELATED TO
>Inflammation and swelling secondary to bacterial invasion of the joint
>Treatment methods (e.g., surgery, exercise)

CHARACTERISTICS
>Verbal communication of pain
>Crying unrelieved by usual comfort measures
>Hesitation or refusal to bear weight on limb
>Decreased activity, self-imposed
>Severe discomfort on movement of affected joint
>Physical signs/symptoms:
>
>>tachycardia
>>tachypnea/bradypnea
>>increased blood pressure
>>diaphoresis

EXPECTED OUTCOMES   Child will be free of extreme pain as evidenced by

>verbal communication of decreased pain.
>lack of constant crying.
>heart rate, respiratory rate, and blood pressure within acceptable ranges (state specific parameters for each child).
>decrease in or lack of diaphoresis.
>lack of signs/symptoms of joint pain (such as those listed under **Characteristics**).

POSSIBLE NURSING INTERVENTIONS
>Assess and record signs/symptoms of pain (such as those listed under **Characteristics**) every 4 hours and PRN.
>
>Handle child gently. Support and protect involved area when

moving the child. Have two individuals move child, if necessary. Keep involved area immobilized.

Encourage family members to stay with and comfort child when possible.

Allow family members to participate in care of the child when possible.

Administer analgesics, as indicated. Assess and record effectiveness.

When indicated, institute additional pain relief measures, such as relaxation and music. Assess and record effectiveness.

Use diversional activities and distraction measures (e.g., toys, play activities, television, radio) when appropriate.

EVALUATION FOR CHARTING
Describe any signs/symptoms of pain noted (such as those listed under **Characteristics**).

State range of vital signs.

Describe any successful measures used to reduce or eliminate pain.

Describe effectiveness of analgesics.

RELATED NURSING DIAGNOSES

Impaired Physical Mobility *related to*
pain on movement of involved area secondary to bacterial invasion of the joint

Knowledge Deficit: Child/Family *related to*
a. disease process and treatment
b. prevention of complications
c. activity restrictions

Impaired Skin Integrity *related to*
a. bedrest
b. surgical wound

Compromised Family Coping *related to*
a. prolonged hospitalization of child (antibiotic therapy needed for 2 to 4 weeks)
b. financial considerations
c. interruption of parental work schedule

NINE

CARE OF CHILDREN WITH NEUROLOGIC/ NEUROMUSCULAR DYSFUNCTION

MEDICAL DIAGNOSIS
Cerebral Palsy

PATHOPHYSIOLOGY   Cerebral palsy is defined as any nonprogressive central motor deficit linked to events in the prenatal, perinatal, or postnatal period that resulted in a central nervous system lesion or in damage to or dysfunction of the central nervous system. The types of movement exhibited by the child differ for the varieties of cerebral palsy and are influenced by muscle tone. Tone describes the state of the muscle at rest: how much it is contracted and how it resists the movement of the limb. Muscle tone is determined by sensory receptors in the muscle and by descending cortical fibers (nerves within the spinal cord that come from the brain). The sensory receptors, also called spindles, attempt to recoil when stretched. Muscles contract when signaled by the nerve cells within the spinal cord after they have received messages sent by the spindles along their sensory fibers. The shortening of the muscle during contraction allows the spindle to recoil. The descending cortical fibers serve two purposes: they control how tightly the spindles are set, and they inhibit the motor neuron's response to incoming signals from the muscle spindles. When the brain suffers an injury, this process is disrupted. Hypertonic muscles have a high degree of tension and can severely limit movement. Hypotonic muscles have low tone and feel limp. A child with cerebral palsy can have both extremes of muscle tone.

There are five types of cerebral palsy: spastic, dyskinetic, ataxic, hypotonic, and mixed. The limb and trunk muscles of a child with spastic cerebral palsy are tight and contract strongly with sudden attempted movements or stretching. Injuries to the cerebral cortex can result in this type of cerebral palsy. The cerebral cortex has nerve fibers that control voluntary muscles and is responsible for learned and purposeful movements. A child with dyskinetic (athetoid) cerebral palsy has uncontrolled and involuntary movements; the limbs have involuntary, purposeless movements and purposeful movements that are contorted. Damage to cells in the basal ganglia can result in dyskinesia. Children with ataxic cerebral palsy have a disturbance in the coordination of voluntary movements. Damage to the cerebellum, which controls balance, equilibrium, and kinesthetic sense, results in ataxia. Children with hypotonic cerebral palsy have fluctuating low muscle tone, which prevents them from maintaining posture and causes difficulty in initiating movement. Children with mixed cerebral palsy exhibit more than one movement disorder.

In addition to nonprogressive motor disability, the child with cerebral palsy may exhibit other manifestations of cerebral dysfunction, such as epilepsy, mental retardation, learning disabilities, poor attention span, easy distractibility, hyperactivity, hearing or visual loss, and/or emotional problems. Additionally, due to oropharyngeal and respiratory muscle impairment, these children are at risk for nutritional deficiencies and respiratory disease. Presentation and clinical manifestations for each child vary depending on limb involvement, type of movement, and other accompanying conditions. A child with severe cerebral palsy can be exceptionally adept in learning, while some mildly physically involved children can be severely mentally retarded, and others can be both mentally and physically debilitated.

The treatment goals for children with cerebral palsy include improving motor function and preventing further disabilities. Comprehensive care can best be provided by a multidisciplinary team. Orthopedic management may include surgery and/or the use of braces, casts, and corrective appliances. Neurosurgical procedures have also been used in the treatment of cerebral palsy. Physical therapy, occupational therapy, and special educational programming are integral to the child's management.

Nursing Diagnosis
Impaired Physical Mobility
Definition   Limited ability of movement

Possibly Related To
> Nonprogressive motor deficits secondary to central nervous system injury
> Status/post orthopedic surgery
> Status/post neurosurgery
> Status/post casting

CHARACTERISTICS
Muscle weakness
Muscle dysfunction
Problems with coordination, balance, and kinesthetic sense
Hypertonic and/or hypotonic muscles
Uncontrolled movements
Involuntary movements
Decreased range of motion
Monoplegia, hemiplegia, paraplegia, diplegia, triplegia,
  or quadriplegia
Contractures

EXPECTED OUTCOMES Child will maximize ability of
movement as evidenced by (state specific examples for each
child).

POSSIBLE NURSING INTERVENTIONS
Assess and record child's activity level at least once/shift.

Assess and record any signs/symptoms of impaired physical
mobility (such as those listed under **Characteristics**).

Ensure that child keeps scheduled appointments with
occupational therapist and physical therapist as indicated.

Encourage child to participate as much as possible in
self-care.

Make available activities within child's limitations (state
specific examples for each child).

Perform scheduled active and passive range-of-motion
exercises (at least every 4 hours).

Reposition child every 1 to 2 hours.

Ensure that child's body stays in proper alignment, whether
in bed, chair, or wheelchair.

Assist child as necessary in using splints, braces, and other
appliances.

When indicated, use Hoyer lift for totally dependent
transfers. Use pivot or two-person transfer, as indicated.

 Initiate referrals to home health agencies, visiting nurses,
orthotics, prosthetics, and social services.

▥ Assess and record child's/family's knowledge of and participation in care regarding

  identification of any signs/symptoms of impaired physical mobility (such as those listed under **Characteristics**).
  monitoring of activity level and rest periods.
  correct use of appliances.
  correct handling and positioning techniques.
  continuation of range-of-motion exercises, splinting, bracing, and occupational and/or physical therapy, as indicated.
  appropriate use of resources.

▥ Instruct child/family in any areas needing improvement. Record results.

EVALUATION FOR CHARTING
Describe child's level of mobility.

Describe any signs/symptoms of impaired physical mobility (such as those listed under **Characteristics**).

State child's ability to participate in self-care.

Describe any therapeutic measures used to improve physical mobility. State their effectiveness.

▥ Describe child's/family's knowledge of and participation in care related to improving physical mobility. State any areas needing improvement and information provided. Describe child's/family's responses.

NURSING DIAGNOSIS
Body Image Disturbance

DEFINITION   Condition in which the child has a negative self-view

POSSIBLY RELATED TO
Spastic or athetoid movements
Physical deformities secondary to spasticity
Altered growth and development
Personal frustration with difficulty in speech, feeding, eating, and motor behaviors

CHARACTERISTICS

Verbalization about displeasure with body
Refusal to look in mirror
Refusal to participate in care or play and social activities
Decreased interest in appearance

EXPECTED OUTCOMES   Child will indicate acceptance of
body image as evidenced by

ability to verbally describe self positively.
ability to look in mirror.
willingness to participate in care.
willingness to participate in play and social activities.
developmentally appropriate interest in appearance.

POSSIBLE NURSING INTERVENTIONS

Assess and record child's/family's ability to accept body
image.

Encourage child to express feelings, fears, or concerns
regarding cerebral palsy and appearance.

Clarify any misconceptions child may express regarding
cerebral palsy and appearance.

Provide child with opportunities for age-appropriate
therapeutic play.

Encourage child to maintain usual state of grooming and
appearance.

🏠 Encourage child to attend camp, ski, and participate in
additional activities with other children with cerebral palsy,
as well as with children without cerebral palsy.

🏠 Assess and record child's/family's knowledge of and
participation in care regarding promoting a positive
self-image.

🏠 Instruct child/family in any area needing improvement.
Record results.

EVALUATION FOR CHARTING

Describe child's/family's ability to accept body image.

Describe any methods successful in helping child/family cope
with child's body image.

State whether child/family participated in care.

State whether child showed appropriate interest in his or her appearance.

🏠 Describe child's/family's knowledge of and participation in care related to promoting a positive self-image. State any areas needing improvement and information provided. Describe child's/family's responses.

RELATED NURSING DIAGNOSES

Altered Nutrition: Less than Body Requirements
related to
- a. increased caloric needs secondary to increased muscle tension and movements
- b. difficulty with chewing and swallowing secondary to muscle weakness and/or dental irregularities
- c. inability to feed self secondary to motor deficits
- d. distractibility

Altered Parenting *related to*
- a. child with a physical dysfunction and possible intellectual impairment
- b. inability of infant to cuddle or mold to caregiver for comfort
- c. frequent hospitalizations of child

Altered Growth and Development *related to*
- a. inadequate caloric intake
- b. lack of muscle strength and coordination to achieve motor milestones and perform skills or activities of daily living
- c. limited social interaction secondary to speech and motor deficits
- d. lack of appropriate stimulation in environment

Impaired Home Maintenance Management *related to*
- a. child's need for assistance with hygiene, feeding, toileting, ambulation, and communication
- b. child's need for equipment
- c. inadequate resources, including relief from care giving
- d. need to change and adapt home environment

MEDICAL DIAGNOSIS

Guillain-Barré Syndrome

PATHOPHYSIOLOGY Guillain-Barré Syndrome (GBS) is a progressive polyneuritis (inflammation of many nerves) thought to be a toxic autoimmune response to a viral agent, although the exact cause is unknown. Sensitized lymphocytes migrate to the peripheral nerves, causing inflammation and demyelinization. As a result, peripheral and/or cranial nerve conduction becomes slower and less intense, leading to a gradual paresis or paralysis, accompanied by loss of sensation.

The progression of muscle weakness and paralysis in GBS may be rapid, but most often it continues for several weeks before reaching a plateau. Symmetrical motor weakness and loss of deep tendon reflexes begin in the lower extremities and advance rapidly upward. These processes are characterized by a prickling sensation in the hands and feet, accompanied by pain, with the eventual development of paralysis. Often the respiratory muscles are affected, resulting in respiratory insufficiency. Severe respiratory insufficiency or failure can progress to the point where the child requires a tracheostomy and/or mechanical ventilation. Cranial nerve paralysis may also appear, presenting as impaired swallowing, impaired gag reflex, and/or facial weakness. Sensory impairment, manifested as paresthesia (numbness or tingling) and/or loss of position sense, may occur as well but is less common. Hypertension, diaphoresis, pupillary changes, postural hypotension, cardiac arrhythmias, and/or urinary retention can also occur if autonomic function is impaired.

An upper respiratory infection or viral illness usually appears 2 to 3 weeks before the onset of GBS. Approximately 4 to 8 weeks after the appearance of symptoms, recovery begins. Treatment is usually supportive, and recovery is generally complete but slow, at times taking up to 2 years. Physiotherapy is helpful during the recovery period. In the pediatric population, GBS most commonly occurs in children ages 4 to 10 years.

PRIMARY NURSING DIAGNOSIS
Ineffective Breathing Pattern

DEFINITION   Breathing pattern that results in inadequate oxygen consumption (failure to meet the cellular requirements of the body)

POSSIBLY RELATED TO
Respiratory insufficiency secondary to intercostal and phrenic nerve paralysis

CHARACTERISTICS
Shallow, irregular respirations
Diminished breath sounds
Decreased chest expansion
Pallor or cyanosis
Breathlessness in vocalizations
Inability to swallow
Inability to clear secretions due to weak cough
Tachypnea
Hypoxia
Hypercarbia
Drowsiness
Confusion
Restlessness

EXPECTED OUTCOMES   Child will have an adequate breathing pattern as evidenced by

respiratory rate within acceptable range (state specific highest and lowest rates for each child).
strong, clear, equal breath sounds bilaterally.
adequate and equal bilateral chest expansion.
clear, audible vocalizations.
ability to swallow secretions.
cough strong enough to clear secretions.
absence of

pallor or cyanosis.
hypercarbia.
drowsiness.
confusion.
restlessness.

oxygen saturation (via pulse oximeter) from 85% to 100%.

POSSIBLE NURSING INTERVENTIONS

Assess and record the following every 4 hours and PRN:

> respiratory rate, rhythm, and depth
> breath sounds
> chest expansion
> color
> status of speech
> ability to swallow or cough
> signs/symptoms of ineffective breathing pattern (such as
> those listed under **Characteristics**)

When using a pulse oximeter, record reading every 2 to 4 hours and PRN.

When indicated, assess and record arterial blood gases. Report any abnormalities to the physician.

Assist child with coughing, deep breathing, and use of incentive spirometry.

Provide gentle oropharyngeal and/or nasotracheal suctioning, as needed.

When indicated, administer oxygen in the correct amount and route. Assess and record effectiveness of therapy.

Keep head of bed elevated at a 30° to 45° angle.

Reposition child every 1 to 2 hours.

When indicated, ensure that chest physiotherapy is done effectively and on schedule.

Assist child as needed with pulmonary function tests.

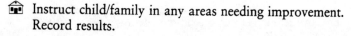 Assess and record the child's/family's knowledge of and participation in care regarding

> identification of any signs/symptoms of ineffective
> breathing pattern (such as those listed under
> **Characteristics**).
> chest physiotherapy.
> effective coughing and deep breathing.
> positioning.

Instruct child/family in any areas needing improvement. Record results.

EVALUATION FOR CHARTING

State highest and lowest respiratory rates.

Describe breath sounds.

Describe any signs/symptoms of ineffective breathing pattern (such as those listed under **Characteristics**).

State whether oxygen was administered. Include amount and route of delivery. Describe effectiveness.

If indicated, state whether chest physiotherapy was done on schedule. Describe child's tolerance of procedure and its effectiveness.

Indicate whether child needed suctioning. If so, state frequency and describe amount and characteristics of secretions.

When indicated, state highest and lowest arterial blood gas values. State ongoing physiological process (e.g., respiratory acidosis).

Describe any therapeutic measures used to maintain an effective breathing pattern. State their effectiveness.

Describe child's/family's knowledge of and participation in care related to maintaining an effective breathing pattern. State any areas needing improvement and information provided. Describe child's/family's responses.

NURSING DIAGNOSIS
Impaired Physical Mobility

DEFINITION   Limited ability of movement

POSSIBLY RELATED TO
Weakness
Paralysis secondary to demyelinization

CHARACTERISTICS
Inability to move part or all of the body
Decreased range of motion
Limited or decreased coordination
Hesitation to walk or run
Reduced muscle tone

Decreased muscle strength, control, and/or mass
Paraparesis
Quadriplegia
Complete areflexia
Contractures

EXPECTED OUTCOMES   Child will return to pre-illness activity level as evidenced by (state specific examples for each child).

POSSIBLE NURSING INTERVENTIONS

Assess and record the child's activity level at least once/shift and PRN.

Assess and record any signs/symptoms of impaired physical mobility (such as those listed under **Characteristics**).

Arrange for therapeutic play, occupational therapy, and physical therapy, as indicated.

Encourage child to participate as much as possible in self-care.

Make available activities within child's limitations (state specific examples for each child).

Allow adequate rest periods (state specific amount of rest needed for each child).

Perform scheduled active and passive range-of-motion exercises (at least every 4 hours).

Reposition child every 1 to 2 hours.

Ensure that child's body stays in proper alignment.

Use footboard, splints, braces, and/or high-top shoes, when indicated.

Assess and record child's/family's knowledge of and participation in care regarding

identification of any signs/symptoms of impaired physical mobility (such as those listed under **Characteristics**).
monitoring of activity level and rest periods.
continuation of range-of-motion exercises, splinting, bracing, and occupational and/or physical therapy, as indicated.

Instruct child/family in any areas needing improvement. Record results.

EVALUATION FOR CHARTING

Describe child's current level of activity.

Describe any signs/symptoms of impaired physical mobility (such as those listed under **Characteristics**).

State child's ability to participate in self-care.

Describe any therapeutic measures used to improve physical mobility. State their effectiveness.

 Describe child's/family's knowledge of and participation in care related to improving physical mobility. State any areas needing improvement and information provided. Describe child's/family's responses.

RELATED NURSING DIAGNOSES

Decreased Cardiac Output *related to*
cardiac arrhythmias, hypotension, or hypertension secondary to autonomic instability

Altered Comfort* *related to*
a. sensitivity to touch
b. cramping muscles
c. prickling sensations
d. paresthesia

Altered Nutrition: Less than Body Requirements
related to
a. paralysis
b. anorexia
c. diarrhea and/or steatorrhea

Fear: Child *related to*
a. paralysis
b. uncertain prognosis
c. procedures/treatments
d. loss of control

---

*Non-NANDA diagnosis.

MEDICAL DIAGNOSIS

Hydrocephalus

PATHOPHYSIOLOGY Hydrocephalus is an abnormal increased accumulation of cerebrospinal fluid (CSF) within the ventricles of the brain. Cerebrospinal fluid, primarily produced in the choroid plexus, normally circulates through the ventricular cavities and subarachnoid space. The rate of production is approximately 200 to 300 ml/day in infants and 700 ml/day in adults. Subarachnoid villi, located in the dural sinuses, reabsorb the CSF.

Hydrocephalus occurs either when reabsorption of CSF in the subarachnoid space is impaired (also called communicating hydrocephalus) or when the flow of CSF from the ventricles of the brain to the subarachnoid space is obstructed (also called noncommunicating hydrocephalus). A less common cause is increased CSF production resulting from a choroid plexus tumor. With an increased amount of CSF, the fluid accumulates in the ventricles, which then begin to dilate and compress the brain against the bony cranium. When this occurs prior to the fusion of the cranial sutures, enlargement of the skull results. As the CSF continues to accumulate, intracranial pressure increases. In communicating hydrocephalus, the CSF pathways are open, but reabsorption is impaired because of occlusion of the subarachnoid cysterns, obliteration of the subarachnoid spaces, or fibrosis of the arachnoid villa (often the result of hemorrhage or infection). Noncommunicating hydrocephalus most often results from developmental malformations such as aqueductal stenosis (narrowing or obstruction of the aqueduct of Sylvius between the third and fourth ventricles), Chiari malformations (defects in the lower brain stem, cerebellum, or fourth ventricle), and Dandy-Walker syndrome (congenital atresia of the fourth ventricle that resembles a cyst). Other causes of noncommunicating hydrocephalus include neoplasms, infection, and trauma.

The age of the child at the onset of hydrocephalus and the degree of increased CSF determine the signs and symptoms. Visible characteristics of children from infancy through 2 years of age include an enlarging head size, bulging fontanels, a prominent forehead, and "sunset sign" (downward rotation of the eyes with sclera visible above the iris). Older children commonly show signs and symptoms of increased intracranial pressure, such as headache, lethargy, vomiting, and diplopia.

Treatment of hydrocephalus is usually surgical intervention to correct an obstruction to CSF and/or to implant a shunting device to divert CSF. When a shunt is implanted, CSF drains from the ventricle into an extracranial body compartment such as the peritoneal cavity (ventriculoperitoneal [VP] shunt) or the right atrium (ventriculoatrial [VA] shunt). Once fluid reaches the extracranial body compartment, it is reabsorbed or excreted in a normal fashion. If the initial shunt is on a young infant (3 to 4 months of age), shunt revisions are usually planned for when the child is 18 to 24 months of age, 4 to 6 years of age, and 10 to 12 years of age. These planned revisions are to accommodate the normal growth of the child. Infection and malfunction are the major complications associated with shunts.

PREOPERATIVE NURSING CARE PLAN

PRIMARY NURSING DIAGNOSIS
Altered Level of Consciousness*

DEFINITION   Reduced or impaired state of awareness, ranging from mild to complete impairment (coma)

POSSIBLY RELATED TO
Increased intracranial pressure secondary to an increased amount of cerebrospinal fluid in the cerebrum as a consequence of obstruction, decreased reabsorption, or increased production

CHARACTERISTICS

FOR INFANTS

Increasing head circumference
Dilated scalp veins; shiny skin on scalp
Separation of sutures
Full or bulging fontanels

---

*Non-NANDA diagnosis.

Bulging eyes with "sunset sign"
High-pitched cry
Vomiting
Poor feeding
Lethargy or irritability
Change in level of consciousness
Seizures
Pupillary changes

FOR OLDER CHILDREN

Headache
Vomiting
Lethargy
Diplopia
Ataxia
Irritability
Decline in school work
Change in level of consciousness
Seizures

EXPECTED OUTCOMES   Child will maintain an appropriate
level of consciousness as evidenced by

stable head circumference.
alertness when awake.
if age-appropriate, orientation to person, place, and time
(oriented ×3).
recognition of family members (if age-appropriate).
age-appropriate response to pain.
strong, equal movements of all extremities.
pupils that are equal and react to light.
decreased signs/symptoms of altered level of consciousness
such as those listed under **Characteristics**).

POSSIBLE NURSING INTERVENTIONS
Assess and record the following every 2 to 4 hours and PRN:

neurological vital signs (e.g., changes in level of
consciousness, orientation to time and place, pupillary
changes, equal movements of extremities)
signs/symptoms of altered level of consciousness and
increased intracranial pressure (such as those listed
under **Characteristics**)

Measure and record head circumference daily (measure the FOC, occipitofrontal circumference).

Keep head in midline position.

Elevate head of bed at 30° angle.

Keep accurate record of intake and output. (Overhydration can cause an increase in intracranial pressure.)

Organize nursing care to allow child uninterrupted rest periods to aid in decreasing intracranial pressure.

Prepare child/family for any treatments or procedures such as ventricular tap or tomography.

⌂ Assess and record child's/family's knowledge of and participation in care regarding preparation for impending surgery aimed at restoring appropriate level of consciousness.

⌂ Instruct child/family in any areas needing improvement. Record results.

EVALUATION FOR CHARTING

Describe neurological signs.

Describe any signs/symptoms of a decreasing level of consciousness or of increased intracranial pressure noted (such as those listed under **Characteristics**).

State current head circumference and determine whether it has increased or decreased since previous measurement.

State intake and output.

Describe any therapeutic measures used to increase level of consciousness and/or decrease intracranial pressure. State their effectiveness.

⌂ Describe child's/family's knowledge of and participation in care related to restoring appropriate level of consciousness. State any areas needing improvement and information provided. Describe child's/family's responses.

NURSING DIAGNOSIS

Altered Nutrition: Less than Body Requirements

DEFINITION　Insufficient nutrients to meet body requirements

POSSIBLY RELATED TO

Altered level of consciousness
Increased intracranial pressure

CHARACTERISTICS

Vomiting
Poor feeding
Lethargy
Change in level of consciousness

EXPECTED OUTCOMES　Child will be adequately nourished as evidenced by

lack of vomiting.
adequate caloric intake (state range of calories needed for each child).

POSSIBLE NURSING INTERVENTIONS

Keep accurate record of intake and output.

Assess and record any signs/symptoms of altered nutrition (such as those listed under **Characteristics**) every 4 hours and PRN.

Offer child small, frequent feedings. Allow extra time for feedings, when indicated.

🏠 Assess and record child's/family's knowledge of and participation in care regarding

feeding techniques.
identification of signs/symptoms of altered nutrition (such as those listed under **Characteristics**).

🏠 Instruct child/family in any areas needing improvement. Record results.

EVALUATION FOR CHARTING

State intake and output.

Describe any signs/symptoms of altered nutrition noted (such as those listed under **Characteristics**).

Describe any therapeutic measures used to improve nutritional status. State their effectiveness.

🏠 Describe child's/family's knowledge of and participation in care related to improving nutritional status. State any areas needing improvement and information provided. Describe child's/family's responses.

RELATED NURSING DIAGNOSES
Impaired Skin Integrity *related to*
a. thin and fragile skin of the head
b. pressure and weight of the head
c. child's inability to move head

Fluid Volume Deficit *related to*
a. vomiting
b. lethargy
c. decreased level of consciousness

Altered Comfort* *related to*
a. headache
b. vomiting

Compromised Family Coping *related to*
a. seriousness of illness
b. child's hospitalization
c. impending surgery
d. possibility of long-term developmental problems of child
e. child's physical appearance

POSTOPERATIVE NURSING CARE PLAN

PRIMARY NURSING DIAGNOSIS
Altered Level of Consciousness*

DEFINITION   Reduced or impaired state of awareness, ranging from mild to complete impairment (coma)

---

*Non-NANDA diagnosis.

POSSIBLY RELATED TO

Increased intracranial pressure secondary to increased amount of cerebrospinal fluid in the cerebrum as a consequence of obstruction, decreased reabsorption, or increased production

CHARACTERISTICS

FOR INFANTS

Increasing head circumference
Dilated scalp veins; shiny skin on scalp
Separation of sutures
Full or bulging fontanels
Bulging eyes with "sunset sign"
High-pitched cry
Vomiting
Poor feeding
Lethargy or irritability
Change in level of consciousness
Seizures
Pupillary changes

FOR OLDER CHILDREN

Headache
Vomiting
Lethargy
Diplopia
Ataxia
Irritability
Decline in school work
Change in level of consciousness
Seizures

EXPECTED OUTCOMES   Child will maintain an appropriate level of consciousness and be free of increased intracranial pressure as evidenced by

stable head circumference.
alertness when awake.
if age-appropriate, orientation to person, place, and time (oriented ×3).
recognition of family members (if age-appropriate).
age-appropriate response to pain.

normal-pitched cry.

strong, equal movements of all extremities.

pupils that are equal and react to light.

absence of signs/symptoms of altered level of consciousness
such as those listed under **Characteristics**).

POSSIBLE NURSING INTERVENTIONS

Assess and record the following every 2 to 4 hours and PRN:

neurological vital signs (e.g., changes in level of
consciousness, orientation to time and place, pupillary
changes, equal movements of extremities)

operative site for signs of bleeding, drainage, swelling,
and/or redness

signs/symptoms of altered level of consciousness and
increased intracranial pressure (such as those listed
under **Characteristics**)

Measure and record head circumference daily (measure the
FOC, occipitofrontal circumference).

Position child on the nonoperative side to prevent pressure
on the operative site and shunt. Sheepskin or a foam donut
may be necessary to prevent skin breakdown. Keep child's
head flat or only slightly elevated to prevent too rapid
reduction in CSF fluid.

Keep accurate record of intake (IV and/or PO) and output.
(Overhydration can cause an increase in intracranial
pressure.)

Organize nursing care to allow child uninterrupted rest
periods to aid in decreasing intracranial pressure.

Assess and record child's/family's knowledge of and
participation in care regarding

identification of signs/symptoms of increased intracranial
pressure (such as those listed under **Characteristics**) that
might be present if the shunt becomes obstructed or
infected.

assessment of surgical incisions for redness, swelling, and/
or drainage.

palpation of the shunt and valve to denote normal
activity.

"pumping" of the shunt to check for patency (although this is usually not done routinely).

avoidance of contact sports.

administration of prophylactic antibiotic therapy prior to dental treatment to reduce the risk of bacteremia.

🏠 Instruct child/family in any areas needing improvement. Record results.

EVALUATION FOR CHARTING

Describe neurological signs.

Describe any signs/symptoms of decreasing level of consciousness or increased intracranial pressure noted (such as those listed under **Characteristics**).

State current head circumference and determine whether it has increased or decreased since previous measurement.

State intake and output.

Describe any therapeutic measures used to increase level of consciousness and/or decrease intracranial pressure. State their effectiveness.

🏠 Describe child's/family's knowledge of and participation in care related to restoring appropriate level of consciousness. State any areas needing improvement and information provided. Describe child's/family's responses.

NURSING DIAGNOSIS

Pain

DEFINITION   Condition in which an individual experiences severe discomfort

POSSIBLY RELATED TO

Surgical incision and manipulation
Headache

CHARACTERISTICS

Crying unrelieved by usual comfort measures
Facial grimacing
Verbal expression of pain
Decreased activity, self-imposed
Restlessness

Physical signs/symptoms:

> tachycardia
> tachypnea/bradypnea
> increased blood pressure
> diaphoresis

EXPECTED OUTCOMES Child will be free of extreme pain as evidenced by

lack of
> constant crying.
> facial grimacing.
> restlessness.
> signs/symptoms of extreme pain (such as those listed under **Characteristics**).

verbal communication of comfort.

heart rate, respiratory rate, and blood pressure within acceptable ranges (state specific highest and lowest parameters for each child).

POSSIBLE NURSING INTERVENTIONS

Assess and record any signs/symptoms of pain (such as those listed under **Characteristics**) every 2 to 4 hours and PRN.

Handle child gently.

Allow family members to stay and comfort child when possible.

Allow family members to participate in care of child when possible.

Administer analgesics (carefully titrated in order to relieve pain and still allow for adequate neurological assessment) on

schedule. Assess and record effectiveness and any side effects (e.g., nausea/vomiting).

When indicated, institute additional pain relief measures, such as relaxation, guided imagery, and music. Assess and record effectiveness.

Use diversional activities and distraction measures (e.g., toys, play activities, television, radio) when appropriate.

🏠 Assess and record family's knowledge of and participation in care regarding

additional pain relief measures.

handling of child.
identification of signs/symptoms of pain (such as those listed under **Characteristics**).

⌂ Instruct family in any areas needing improvement. Record results.

EVALUATION FOR CHARTING

Describe any signs/symptoms of pain noted (such as those listed under **Characteristics**).

State range of vital signs.

Describe any successful measures used to reduce or eliminate pain.

Describe effectiveness of analgesics and any side effect noted.

⌂ Describe family's knowledge of and participation in care related to reducing or eliminating pain. State any areas needing improvement and information provided. Describe family's response.

RELATED NURSING DIAGNOSES

Infection: High Risk *related to*
a. surgical incision
b. foreign body (shunt and catheters) inserted into cranium

Fear: Family *related to*
a. long-term outcome of surgery
b. possible recurrence of child's neurological symptoms

Altered Tissue Perfusion: Cerebral *related to*
possibility of subdural hematoma secondary to shunt complications

Compromised Family Coping *related to*
a. need for repeated surgical procedures in the future
b. possible recurrence of child's neurological symptoms
c. home care of shunt

MEDICAL DIAGNOSIS
Bacterial Meningitis

PATHOPHYSIOLOGY Meningitis is defined as inflammation of the meninges (the protective membrane covering the brain and spinal cord). Bacterial meningitis results when bacteria invade the meninges via the bloodstream from various possible foci of infection. For example, the pathogens responsible for pneumonia, otitis media, and sinusitis can disseminate into the meninges via the bloodstream. Bacterial organisms can also directly invade the meninges after head trauma, penetrating wounds, and neurosurgical procedures.

This bacterial invasion and the spread of the pathogen into the cerebrospinal fluid (CSF) and to the brain parenchyma lead to inflammation. The brain becomes hyperemic and edematous as a purulent exudate forms and cerebral perfusion is compromised. Obstruction of CSF by clumps of purulent exudate at the base of the brain can result in hydrocephalus and cranial nerve palsies. Vasculitis with associated thrombosis can cause infarctions, seizures, and focal deficits. Necrosis of brain cells and hydrocephalus can lead to increased intracranial pressure, permanent neurological damage, and death.

The child with meningitis usually presents with signs of generalized infection, since bacteremia often precedes the meningitis. The child also exhibits signs and symptoms of meningeal irritation such as headache, photophobia, stiff neck, positive Kernig's sign, and positive Brudzinski's sign.

Haemophilus influenzae (Type B), *Neisseria meningitidis* (meningococcus), and *Streptococcus pneumoniae* are the bacterial organisms most likely to cause meningitis in children.

PRIMARY NURSING DIAGNOSIS
Altered Level of Consciousness*

DEFINITION   Reduced or impaired state of awareness, ranging from mild to complete impairment (coma)

POSSIBLY RELATED TO
  Inflammation of the meninges secondary to invasion by a
      bacterial agent (state specific organism, if known)

CHARACTERISTICS
  Fever
  Headache
  Irritability
  Lethargy
  Vomiting
  Bulging fontanel
  Photophobia
  Nuchal and/or spinal rigidity
  Poor feeding
  High-pitched cry
  Pupillary changes
  Positive Kernig's and Brudzinski's signs
  Seizures
  Apnea
  Increased head circumference
  Changed level of consciousness

EXPECTED OUTCOMES   Child will maintain an appropriate level of consciousness and be free of increased intracranial pressure as evidenced by

  pupils that are equal and react to light.
  normal-pitched cry.
  age-appropriate reflexes.
  age-appropriate response to pain.
  alertness when awake.
  if age-appropriate, orientation to person, place, and time
      (oriented ×3).
  recognition of family members (if age-appropriate).

---

*Non-NANDA diagnosis.

strong, equal movements of all extremities.

spontaneous respirations within acceptable range (state specific highest and lowest rates for each child).

temperature within acceptable range of 36.5°C to 37.2°C.

head circumference appropriate for age (per growth chart).

lack of signs/symptoms of altered level of consciousness (such as those listed under **Characteristics**).

POSSIBLE NURSING INTERVENTIONS

Assess and record the following every 2 to 4 hours and PRN:

neurological vital signs (use Glasgow Coma Scale, if available)

respiratory rate and temperature

signs/symptoms of altered level of consciousness (such as those listed under **Characteristics**)

Organize nursing care to minimize disturbance and stimulation of child.

Keep child's environment as quiet as possible.

Elevate head of bed at 30° angle.

Measure and record head circumference daily.

Keep accurate record of intake and output. Restrict fluid intake, as indicated (usually to two-thirds of maintenance).

Maintain child's body temperature between 36.5°C and 37.2°C.

Administer antibiotics, antipyretics, and, when indicated, anticonvulsants on schedule. Assess and record effectiveness and any side effects (e.g., diarrhea, rash, vomiting, sedation).

🏠 Assess and record child's/family's knowledge of and participation in care regarding

identification of signs/symptoms of altered level of consciousness (such as those listed under **Characteristics**).

medication administration.

🏠 Instruct child and family in any areas needing improvement. Record results.

EVALUATION FOR CHARTING

State range of temperature.

Describe neurological signs.

Describe any signs/symptoms of altered level of consciousness (such as those listed under **Characteristics**).

Describe any therapeutic measures used to restore appropriate level of consciousness. State their effectiveness.

State intake and output.

State whether medications were administered on schedule and describe any side effects noted.

Describe child's/family's knowledge of and participation in care related to restoring appropriate level of consciousness. State any areas needing improvement and information provided. Describe child's/family's responses.

NURSING DIAGNOSIS

Pain

DEFINITION Condition in which an individual experiences severe discomfort

POSSIBLY RELATED TO

Headache, nuchal rigidity, and/or fever secondary to inflammation and/or irritation of the meninges
Head trauma
Earache
Invasive procedures (such as blood drawing and lumbar puncture)

CHARACTERISTICS

Verbal communication of pain
Crying unrelieved by usual comfort measures
Facial grimacing
Physical signs/symptoms:

tachycardia
tachypnea/bradypnea
increased blood pressure

diaphoresis
pupillary dilation

Rating of pain on pain assessment tool

EXPECTED OUTCOMES   Child will be free of severe pain as evidenced by

verbal communication of decreased pain.
lack of constant crying.
facial expression free of discomfort.
heart rate, respiratory rate, and blood pressure within
   acceptable ranges (state specific parameters for each child).
decrease in or lack of diaphoresis.
lack of dilated pupils.
rating of decreased or no pain on pain assessment tool.

POSSIBLE NURSING INTERVENTIONS

Assess and record any signs/symptoms of pain (such as those listed under **Characteristics**) every 2 hours and PRN. Use age-appropriate pain assessment tool.

Handle child gently.

Encourage family members to stay and comfort child when possible.

Allow family members to participate in care of the child when possible.

Administer antipyretics, analgesics, and antibiotics on schedule. Assess for effectiveness and any side effects (e.g., rash and diarrhea).

When appropriate, use distraction measures, diversional activities, or additional pain relief measures (e.g., music, play, television). Assess and record effectiveness.

EVALUATION FOR CHARTING

Describe any signs/symptoms of pain noted (such as those listed under **Characteristics**).

State ranges of vital signs.

Describe any successful measures used to reduce or eliminate pain.

Describe effectiveness of medications and any side effects noted.

RELATED NURSING DIAGNOSES

Actual Infection* *related to*
the invasion of the meninges by bacterial organisms

Compromised Family Coping *related to*
    a. seriousness of illness
    b. hospitalization
    c. potential for neurological or sensory sequelae

Injury: High Risk *related to*
    a. increased intracranial pressure
    b. infectious process
    c. seizure activity

Fluid Volume Deficit *related to*
    a. poor feeding
    b. vomiting
    c. fever

*Non-NANDA diagnosis.

5 MEDICAL DIAGNOSIS
Neural Tube Defects (Spina Bifida and Myelomeningocele)

PATHOPHYSIOLOGY Congenital malformations of the neural tube that occur during embryonic development are referred to as neural tube defects. Anencephaly (little or no development of brain tissue) or encephalocele (protrusion of part of the cranial contents through a midline defect in the skull) result if there is defective closure in the area of the developing embryonic head. Spina bifida results if the defective closure occurs lower in the spinal column.

Spina bifida occulta is the incomplete fusion of the vertebrae at a level in which the meninges or neural tissues are not exposed. An overlying dimple or tuft of hair may be the only indication of a spina bifida occulta. Neurologic or musculoskeletal disorders rarely accompany this condition. The lumbosacral area is the most common site for spina bifida occulta.

Spina bifida cystica is the incomplete fusion of one or more of the vertebral laminae, resulting in an external protrusion of the spinal tissue. When the sac contains meninges, spinal fluid, and neural tissue, the defect is called a myelomeningocele. Motor and sensory function below the sac are usually affected as the spinal nerve roots end in the sac. Myelomeningoceles most often occur in the lumbar or lumbosacral area of the spinal cord. Lesions at L3 or above result in total paraplegia, sensory loss, and bowel and bladder incontinence. The lower the myelomeningocele, the less severe the neurologic deficit. Abnormalities in brain development, including Chiari Type II deformity and hydrocephalus, often accompany myelomeningocele. Skeletal deformities, such as scoliosis, hip dislocation, and foot deformities, are also common.

A meningocele contains meninges and cerebrospinal fluid that have protruded through the unfused vertebral arches. Neurological complications are less severe than with myelomeningocele, as the spinal cord is not involved and the spinal nerve roots retain their function, even if displaced. Meningoceles also occur less commonly than myelomeningoceles.

Comprehensive care for the child with spina bifida is best provided by a multidisciplinary health care team. Surgical repair of these anomalies is usually performed soon after diagnosis to preserve neural tissue and to provide an anatomic barrier. When necessary, a ventriculoperitoneal shunt is placed to control progressive hydrocephalus. As the child grows, orthopedic care involving exercise, braces, casts, and surgery may be needed to promote mobility and prevent deformities. The goals of urological management are to promote urinary continence and to prevent infections, reflux, and renal damage. The child and family are often taught to perform clean intermittent catheterizations and to monitor for urinary tract infections. Bowel management often involves methods to help the child achieve continence. Dietary measures to alter stool consistency are also used.

NURSING DIAGNOSIS
Impaired Physical Mobility

DEFINITION   Limited ability of movement

POSSIBLY RELATED TO
Neuromuscular and sensory deficits secondary to neural tube defect

CHARACTERISTICS
Lower extremity motor weakness
Paraplegia
Flaccid paralysis of the lower extremities
Weakened abdominal and trunk musculature
Hip flexion
Knee extension
Scoliosis
Foot deformities
Dislocated joints
Small muscle bulk
Contractures
Fractures

EXPECTED OUTCOMES   Child will maximize ability of movement as evidenced by (state specific examples for each child).

POSSIBLE NURSING INTERVENTIONS
Assess and record child's activity level at least once/shift.

Assess and record any signs/symptoms of impaired physical mobility (such as those listed under **Characteristics**).

Ensure that child keeps scheduled appointments with occupational therapist and physical therapist as indicated.

Encourage child to participate as much as possible in self-care.

Make available activities within child's limitations (state specific examples for each child).

Allow adequate rest periods (state specific amount of rest needed for each child).

Perform scheduled active and passive range-of-motion exercises (at least every 4 hours).

Reposition child every 1 to 2 hours.

Ensure that child's body stays in proper alignment, whether in bed, chair, or wheelchair.

Assist child as necessary in using splints, braces, and other appliances.

When indicated, use Hoyer lift for totally dependent transfers. Use pivot or two-person transfer, as indicated.

Assess and record child's/family's knowledge of and participation in care regarding

identification of any signs/symptoms of impaired physical mobility (such as those listed under **Characteristics**).
monitoring of activity level and rest periods.
correct use of appliances.
correct handling and positioning techniques.
continuation of range-of-motion exercises, splinting, bracing, and occupational and/or physical therapy, as indicated.

Instruct child/family in any areas needing improvement. Record results.

EVALUATION FOR CHARTING
Describe child's level of mobility.

Describe any signs/symptoms of impaired physical mobility (such as those listed under **Characteristics**).

State child's ability to participate in self-care.

Describe any therapeutic measures used to improve physical mobility. State their effectiveness.

🏠 Describe child's/family's knowledge of and participation in care related to improving physical mobility. State any areas needing improvement and information provided. Describe child's family's responses.

NURSING DIAGNOSIS
Impaired Skin Integrity

DEFINITION   Interruption in integrity of the skin

POSSIBLY RELATED TO
Altered patterns of urinary and/or bowel elimination
Impaired mobility
Irritation from casts or braces

CHARACTERISTICS
Perineal skin breakdown or excoriation
Pressure sores
Reddened areas of skin
Incontinence (bladder and/or bowel)

EXPECTED OUTCOMES   Child will be free of signs/symptoms of impaired skin integrity as evidenced by

clean, intact skin.
natural skin color.
lack of

redness.
excoriation.
lesions.

POSSIBLE NURSING INTERVENTIONS
Assess and record skin condition every shift or PRN.

Handle child gently.

Bathe child daily (or as indicated) with water and a non-irritating soap.

Keep the perineal area clean and dry by

changing diapers/linens as soon as possible after
elimination or soiling.
using cloth diapers, when indicated.
using cotton underwear.
keeping area open to air when possible.

When indicated, allow the child to take sitz baths.

Apply topical medications on schedule. Assess and record effectiveness.

Use a barrier cream/ointment on schedule, as indicated.

Reposition child every 2 hours.

When indicated, use sheepskin surfaces, water beds, or egg-crate mattresses.

Use lotion to moisturize skin, when indicated.

Massage pressure points, as indicated.

Encourage compliance with bladder and/or bowel continence programs.

Assess and record child's/family's knowledge of and participation in care regarding

measures related to preventing or correcting impaired skin integrity.
medication administration.
compliance with bladder and/or bowel continence programs.

Instruct child/family in any areas needing improvement. Record results.

EVALUATION FOR CHARTING

Describe any potential or actual areas of skin breakdown.

Describe any therapeutic measures used to prevent or correct impaired skin integrity.

Describe child's/family's knowledge of and participation in care related to preventing or correcting impaired skin integrity. State any areas needing improvement and information provided. Describe child's/family's responses.

NURSING DIAGNOSIS
Impaired Home Maintenance Management

DEFINITION   Inability to provide and maintain a safe, optimal-growth-promoting home environment for the individual or family

POSSIBLY RELATED TO
Child's need for special equipment (e.g., wheelchair, crutches, braces, casts)

Child's need for assistance with hygiene, feeding, catheterizations, and/or mobility

Inadequate resources or use of resources, including lack of relief from caretaking, transportation problems, cleaning, and meals

Financial difficulties

Need to adapt or change home environment

Insufficient family organization and/or time management

Lack of knowledge

CHARACTERISTICS
Overtaxed caregiver

Child and/or family with poor hygiene

Report or verbalization of

  unclean and/or unsafe home environment
  offensive home environmental odors
  misuse or lack of use of special equipment

Offensive body odor of child/family

Unkempt child upon admission

Injured child upon admission

Misuse or lack of use of resources, special services, and supports

Verbalization of inability to manage care of the child and/or home

EXPECTED OUTCOMES   Child and/or primary caregiver will indicate that home maintenance management is improved as evidenced by

  identification of factors that make the child's home care difficult and possible ways to deal with these factors.

identification of factors that facilitate the child's home care.

demonstration of proper use of equipment and skills needed to care for the child at home (state specific examples for each child).

expression of satisfaction with the home situation.

lack of signs/symptoms of impaired home maintenance management (such as those listed under **Characteristics**).

demonstration of correct utilization of resources, special services, and supports.

POSSIBLE NURSING INTERVENTIONS

Assess and record any signs/symptoms of impaired home maintenance management (such as those listed under **Characteristics**) upon child's admission and PRN.

Assess and record causative or contributing factors of impaired home maintenance management.

Assist child/family in reducing or eliminating causative or contributing factors when possible (be specific).

When indicated, consult with social services for assistance in obtaining equipment, funds, respite care, transportation, and other supports.

When indicated, consult with service organizations and community agencies for assistance and support.

Encourage child and caregiver to verbalize concerns, problems, and feelings.

⌂ Assess and record child's/family's knowledge of and participation in care regarding

correct utilization of resources.
proper use of equipment.
proper skills in caring for child.

⌂ Instruct child/family in any areas needing improvement. Record results.

EVALUATION FOR CHARTING

Describe any signs/symptoms of impaired home maintenance management noted (such as those listed under **Characteristics**).

Describe any feelings, problems, and concerns expressed by the child/family.

Describe any therapeutic measures used to improve home maintenance management.

🔳 Describe child's/family's knowledge of and participation in care related to improving home maintenance management. State any areas needing improvement and information provided. Describe child's/family's responses.

RELATED NURSING DIAGNOSES

Body Image Disturbance *related to*
  a. bladder/bowel incontinence
  b. reduced muscle mass
  c. limited physical mobility secondary to neuromuscular deficit

Infection: High Risk *related to*
  a. chronic retention of urine
  b. repeated catheterizations
  c. ventriculoperitoneal shunt

Compromised Family Coping *related to*
  a. child's chronic illness
  b. demands of child's care
  c. lack of or inappropriate use of resources (financial, support)

Seizures

PATHOPHYSIOLOGY A seizure can be defined as a paroxysmal, uncontrolled episode of behavior that results from an alteration in brain function caused by abnormal electrical discharges from neuronal tissue. During a seizure, groups of neurons are activated all at once, disrupting normal brain function. This excessive discharge of electrical energy may remain localized in one part of the brain, may start in a focal area and spread to the rest of the brain, or may be generalized over the entire cortex without localized onset. Alterations of consciousness and/or motor, sensory, and autonomic function characterize seizure activity. The behavior exhibited reflects the type of abnormal electrical activity and the area of brain involvement. Seizure activity can occur as a single episode or recur intermittently.

Seizures can result from a number of conditions affecting the nervous system or from various systemic disorders. These conditions can include meningitis, encephalitis, brain tumors, head trauma, asphyxia, hypoglycemia, hypo- and hypernatremia, hypocalcemia, and degenerative neurological disorders. In many children the cause of recurrent seizures cannot be determined. This is referred to as idiopathic epilepsy.

Partial (focal) seizures involve abnormal firing of a group of neurons in one hemisphere of the brain, which may or may not spread to other areas. A simple partial seizure does not impair consciousness, but a complex one does. Localized motor (twitching of the face or an extremity or weakness of a muscle group) or sensory (tingling, numbness, or feeling of warmth) disturbances are characteristic of simple partial seizures. Complex partial seizures have widely varying manifestations that affect consciousness, behavior, thinking, and sensations (confusion, nonsensical speech, repetitive motor activity such as lip smacking, purposeless wandering, and/or altered visual or hearing sensations).

Generalized seizures affect the entire brain, and consciousness is always lost. These include generalized tonic-clonic seizures (formerly called grand mal seizures), absence seizures (formerly called petit mal seizures), myoclonic seizures, and atonic seizures (formerly called drop attacks). Generalized tonic-clonic seizures usually have five identifiable phases: flexion, extension or tonic (stiffening of the muscle groups), tremor, clonic (rapid succession of alternating involuntary muscle contraction and relaxation), and postictal. Absence seizures are characterized by a brief, sudden cessation of all motor activity, accompanied by a blank stare and loss of awareness, followed by a rapid return to consciousness and no memory of the seizure. Myoclonic seizures are characterized by one or more sudden jerks of muscle groups. Infantile spasms are a type of myoclonic seizures. Atonic seizures are characterized by a sudden decrease in muscle tone and a loss of consciousness.

Febrile seizures are a common disorder of early childhood, characterized by generalized tonic-clonic seizures associated with fever but without evidence of any known central nervous system infection or disorder. Usually the seizure lasts less than 15 minutes. These children generally have no neurological sequelae and little risk for subsequent epilepsy. Treatment involves fever reduction and management of the illness causing the fever.

Epilepsy is characterized by recurrent seizures. Although chronic, it will not necessarily last the child's lifetime, as remissions of childhood epilepsy do occur. Epilepsy is not a single disease entity but exists when a child has any number of underlying brain disorders.

The treatment goal for seizures is to prevent recurrent episodes. This can be accomplished through management of the specific cause of the seizures and the use of anticonvulsants.

PRIMARY NURSING DIAGNOSIS
Altered Level of Consciousness*

DEFINITION   Reduced or impaired state of awareness, ranging from mild to complete impairment (coma)

POSSIBLY RELATED TO
   Metabolic disorders
   Head trauma
   Central nervous system infections
   Asphyxia

---

*Non-NANDA diagnosis.

Degenerative neurological disorder
Drug intoxication
Neoplasms
Genetic disorders
Fever
Unknown etiology

CHARACTERISTICS
Change in level of consciousness and/or responsiveness
Fever
Tonic-clonic movements
Jerking
Twitching
Pupillary changes
Apnea
Grunting
Increased salivation
Eye rolling
Eye or head deviation to one side
Staring into space
Confusion
Cyanosis
Flushed appearance
Incontinence of urine/stool
Auras: unusual sensations (smells, flashing lights, buzzing
    sounds), abdominal pain, fear, and/or changes in behavior
Lip smacking
Plucking at clothes
Agitation
Wandering
Drowsiness and/or lethargy
Frothing from the mouth

EXPECTED OUTCOMES   Child will be free of seizure activity.

POSSIBLE NURSING INTERVENTIONS
Maintain seizure precautions per institutional policy, which
may include any or all of the following:

    keeping oxygen, suction, and airway equipment at bedside
    padding sides of bed or crib
    monitoring axillary temperatures
    supervising ambulation
    supervising mealtimes

using chest restraint when child is in a chair
having child wear protective helmet
keeping child away from sharp toys and furniture

Assess and record all seizure activity, including

precipitating event.
occurrence of an aura.
beginning and progression sequence.
duration.
type of movements.
eye movements.
tongue or lip biting.
apnea or color changes.
incontinence.
level of consciousness.
falls.
frequency.

If seizure does occur,

stay with child.
protect child from injury.
keep side rails padded and up if child is in a bed or crib.
place child on soft, flat surface.
move sharp objects away from child.
loosen any restrictive clothing.
position child to prevent upper airway obstruction and to
    facilitate drainage of secretions.
administer oxygen, as indicated.

Assess and record postictal state. Reorient child.

Maintain child's body temperature between 36.5°C and
37.2°C.

Administer anticonvulsants and antipyretics on schedule.
Assess and record effectiveness and any side effects (e.g.,
gingival hyperplasia, rash, sedation). When indicated, check
and record serum drug levels. Report any abnormalities to
the physician.

 Assess and record child's/family's knowledge of and
participation in care regarding

identification of signs/symptoms of altered level of

consciousness or seizure activity (such as those listed under **Characteristics**).

seizure precautions.

medication administration.

Instruct child/family in any areas needing improvement. Record results.

EVALUATION FOR CHARTING

State range of temperatures.

Describe any signs/symptoms of altered level of consciousness (such as those listed under **Characteristics**).

Describe any therapeutic measures used to restore appropriate level of consciousness. State their effectiveness.

State whether medications were administered on schedule and describe any side effects noted.

State current serum drug levels.

Describe child's/family's knowledge of and participation in care related to restoring an appropriate level of consciousness. State any areas needing improvement and information provided. Describe child's/family's responses.

NURSING DIAGNOSIS
Injury: High Risk

DEFINITION   Situation in which the child is at risk for sustaining damage or harm

POSSIBLY RELATED TO
Seizure activity

CHARACTERISTICS
Pain
Hemorrhage
Edema
Open wounds

EXPECTED OUTCOMES   Child will be free of injury during seizure activity.

POSSIBLE NURSING INTERVENTIONS

Maintain seizure precautions per institutional policy, which may include any or all of the following:

keeping oxygen, suction, and airway equipment at bedside
padding sides of bed or crib
monitoring axillary temperatures
supervising ambulation
supervising mealtimes
using chest restraint when child is in a chair
having child wear protective helmet
keeping child away from sharp toys and furniture

During seizure activity,

do not attempt to restrain child or use force.
do not attempt to put anything in child's mouth.
stay with child.
protect child's head from injury.
loosen any restrictive clothing.
ease child onto a soft, flat surface.

🏠 Assess and record child's/family's knowledge of and participation in care regarding

identification of signs/symptoms of injury (such as those listed under **Characteristics**).
seizure precautions.
any special home, swimming, or driving safety measures to be taken by child or adolescent.

🏠 Instruct child/family in any areas needing improvement. Record results.

EVALUATION FOR CHARTING

Describe any interventions implemented to prevent injury. State their effectiveness.

Describe any signs/symptoms of injury noted after seizure activity (such as those listed under **Characteristics**).

🏠 Describe child's/family's knowledge of and participation in care related to restoring an appropriate level of consciousness. State any areas needing improvement and information provided. Describe child's/family's responses.

RELATED NURSING DIAGNOSES

Ineffective Breathing Pattern *related to*
airway obstruction secondary to seizure activity

Knowledge Deficit: Child/Family *related to*
a. disease state
b. medications
c. seizure precautions

Compromised Family Coping *related to*
a. anxiety/fear secondary to unpredictable nature of seizures
b. fear of injury to child secondary to seizures
c. overprotection by family

Body Image Disturbance *related to*
a. unpredictable nature of seizures
b. safety/activity restrictions that may be placed on child
c. potential social stigmas

TEN

CARE OF CHILDREN WITH PULMONARY DYSFUNCTION

MEDICAL DIAGNOSIS

Apnea

PATHOPHYSIOLOGY   Apnea of infancy is defined as the cessation of breathing for 15 to 20 seconds, followed by a color change (visible pallor or cyanosis) and bradycardia. Analysis of arterial blood gases reveals the presence of acidosis. Apnea of infancy, also called infantile apnea (IA), may lead to brain damage and can be fatal. Although IA has been implicated as a possible cause of sudden infant death syndrome, there is no proven relationship between the two conditions.

The exact etiology of IA cannot always be determined. Extensive testing needs to be done to rule out specific and treatable causes such as airway obstruction, cardiac anomalies, seizures, infection, and electrolyte imbalance.

PRIMARY NURSING DIAGNOSIS
Ineffective Breathing Pattern

DEFINITION   Breathing pattern that results in inadequate oxygen consumption (failure to meet the cellular requirements of the body)

POSSIBLY RELATED TO
Specific condition such as

airway obstruction secondary to pulmonary pathology
central nervous system alteration
infection
dehydration
cardiac anomaly
electrolyte imbalance

Unknown cause

CHARACTERISTICS
Cessation of breathing for at least 15 to 20 seconds
Bradycardia

Pallor
Cyanosis
Hypotonia

EXPECTED OUTCOMES Infant will have an effective
breathing pattern as evidenced by

respiratory rate within acceptable range (state highest and
lowest rates for each infant).
clear and equal breath sounds bilaterally.
heart rate within acceptable range (state highest and lowest
rates for each infant).
absence of

pallor.
cyanosis.
hypotonia.

POSSIBLE NURSING INTERVENTIONS
Assess and record the following every 2 to 4 hours and PRN:

respiratory and heart rates
breath sounds
infant's color
infant's muscle tone

Ensure that sleeping infant remains on apnea monitor with
alarms appropriately set. Record frequency and duration of
any apneic episodes. Record type and duration of stimulation
needed.

Assist with pneumogram, cardiopneumogram, or
polysomnogram, as needed.

Administer medications (e.g., theophylline) on schedule.
Assess and record effectiveness and any side effects (e.g.,
tachycardia, irritability, vomiting).

Assess and record family's knowledge of and participation in
care regarding

setup and connection of apnea monitor.
response to apnea monitor alarm.
appropriate stimulation of infant, when indicated.
recording of apneic episodes and stimulation needed.
infant CPR.
medication administration.

identification of any signs/symptoms of ineffective
breathing pattern (such as those listed under
Characteristics).

 Instruct family in any areas needing improvement.
Record results.

EVALUATION FOR CHARTING

State highest and lowest respiratory and heart rates.

Describe breath sounds.

Describe infant's color and muscle tone.

Describe any apneic episodes and type and effectiveness of
stimulation.

State whether medications were administered on schedule.
Describe effectiveness and any side effects noted.

State results of any tests performed (pneumogram,
cardiopneumogram, or polysomnogram), when indicated.

 Describe family's knowledge of and participation in care
related to maintaining an effective breathing pattern. State
any areas needing improvement and information provided.
Describe family's response.

NURSING DIAGNOSIS
Compromised Family Coping

DEFINITION   Decreased ability of family members to manage
problems and concerns effectively

POSSIBLY RELATED TO

Unknown cause of illness
Hospitalization of infant
Fear secondary to responsibility for infant's survival when
infant is discharged from the hospital
Stress, anxiety, and fatigue from having to respond to apnea
monitor alarms

CHARACTERISTICS

Inability to leave infant's bedside
Inappropriate anger toward members of the health care team
Inability to meet own basic needs such as eating and resting
Inability to ask for and accept outside help

Failure to understand repeated explanations regarding illness, treatments, and procedures

EXPECTED OUTCOMES   Family will be able to cope effectively as evidenced by

ability to leave infant's bedside for short periods, especially to care for own basic needs such as eating meals and getting rest.

appropriate expression of anger toward staff or others.

ability to express fears and concerns to members of the health care team.

ability to accept outside help, when appropriate.

verbalized understanding of explanations regarding the illness, treatments, and procedures.

participation in infant's care.

POSSIBLE NURSING INTERVENTIONS

Assess and record family's stress level and ability to cope.

Communicate with family concerning infant's condition at least once/shift and PRN. This may require telephoning the family when members are not able to come to the hospital.

Encourage family to express feelings, fears, and concerns.

Encourage family members to meet own basic needs, such as eating and resting appropriately, and assist.

🏠 Identify and record any past or usually successful coping strategies used by family.

🏠 Provide family with outside help or assist members in seeking outside help (e.g., a visiting nurse agency, the electric company, a medical supply company, financial resources), when indicated.

🏠 Explain the course of the illness, treatments, and procedures to the family. Include reasons for treatments and procedures.

🏠 Support and encourage family's participation in infant's care.

Record results.

EVALUATION FOR CHARTING

Describe family's stress level.

State whether family members were able to leave infant's bedside long enough to meet their own basic needs.

Describe any feelings, fears, and concerns expressed by the family.

☗ State whether family is willing to accept outside help, as indicated.

☗ State whether family was able to understand information given about infant's illness.

☗ State whether family was able to understand the necessity and rationale for treatments and procedures.

☗ State any successful measures used to help family cope.

☗ Describe family's participation in infant's care.

RELATED NURSING DIAGNOSES

Altered Level of Consciousness* *related to*
hypoxia secondary to apneic episodes

Decreased Cardiac Output *related to*
bradycardia

Fear: Parental *related to*
a. breathing pattern of infant
b. responsibility for infant's survival when infant is discharged

Anticipatory Grieving: Family *related to*
the possibility of infant's death

---

*Non-NANDA diagnosis.

MEDICAL DIAGNOSIS
Asthma/Reactive Airway Disease

PATHOPHYSIOLOGY Asthma, or reactive airway disease (RAD), is the most common chronic respiratory disease of childhood, responsible for the majority of school absenteeism, physical disability, and hospitalization of children. Asthma is a complex disorder in which clinical pattern, severity, and natural history of the disease vary considerably. Many factors—including biochemical, immunological, infectious, metabolic, and psychological—can be involved. The impact of these factors varies from individual to individual.

Asthma, an episodic disorder that leads to airway obstruction, is characterized by recurrent reversible bronchospasms (smooth muscle contractions), edema, and inflammation of the mucous membranes lining the airways, leading to accumulation of tenacious secretions. Theoretically, this process is caused by damage to the airway epithelium from inflammatory processes, sensitizing the airway receptors and leading to exaggerated reflex responses. The sympathetic nervous system does not respond as it normally does to dilate the airways because there is only sparse nerve innervation secondary to the airway damage. Airway obstruction results and produces increased airway resistance. There is an increase in the work of breathing and in the elastic properties of the lungs. A ventilation-perfusion mismatch and changes in the arterial blood gases follows. Nonventilated portions of the lungs are still being perfused, leading to hypoxemia. Arterial PCO_2 may be decreased at first due to hyperventilation but tends to rise as the obstructive process worsens. Blood pH falls, leading to respiratory acidosis.

PRIMARY NURSING DIAGNOSIS
Impaired Gas Exchange
DEFINITION Alteration in the exchange of oxygen and carbon dioxide in the lungs and/or at the cellular level

POSSIBLY RELATED TO

Spasms of the smooth muscles of the bronchi and
bronchioles
Accumulation of tenacious secretions
Edema of the mucous membranes of the airways
Allergies
Respiratory infection

CHARACTERISTICS

Wheezing (inspiratory and/or expiratory)
Decreased breath sounds
Tachypnea
Retractions
Use of accessory muscles
Nasal flaring
Dyspnea
Prolonged expiratory time
Cough
Crackles, rhonchi
Tight feeling in the chest
Inability to take a deep breath
Anxiety
Fatigue
Hypoxia
Hypercarbia
Acidosis
Cyanosis
Hyperinflation of the lungs revealed on chest x-ray
Restlessness
Irritability
Lethargy

EXPECTED OUTCOMES   Child will have adequate gas
exchange as evidenced by

clear and equal breath sounds bilaterally.
respiratory rate within acceptable range (state specific highest
and lowest rates for each child).
absence of

retractions.
use of accessory muscles.
nasal flaring.
cough.

> tightness in chest.
> inability to take a deep breath.
> extreme anxiety.
> extreme fatigue.
> extreme restlessness.
> extreme irritability.
> extreme lethargy.
> cyanosis.

clear chest x-ray with appropriate A-P diameter.
oxygen saturation (via pulse oximeter) from 85% to 100%.
arterial pH of 7.35 to 7.45.
$PaCO_2$ from 35 to 45 mmHg.
PaO_2 from 75 to 100 mmHg.
arterial bicarbonate level of 22 to 28 mEq/L.

POSSIBLE NURSING INTERVENTIONS

Assess and record the following every 2 to 4 hours and PRN:

> breath sounds
> respiratory rate
> signs/symptoms of impaired gas exchange (such as those
>   listed under **Characteristics**

When using a pulse oximeter, record reading every 2 to 4 hours and PRN.

Assess and record arterial blood gas values, when indicated. Report any abnormalities to the physician.

Assess and record serum drug (such as theophylline) levels, when indicated. Report any abnormalities to the physician.

Check and record results of chest x-ray, when indicated.

Administer oxygen in the correct amount and route. Record percent of oxygen and route of delivery. Assess and record effectiveness of therapy.

Ensure that chest physiotherapy is performed on schedule. Record effectiveness of treatments and amount and characteristics of secretions.

Keep head of bed elevated at 30° to 45° angle.

Administer bronchodilators and steroids on schedule. Assess and record effectiveness and any side effects (e.g., tachycardia, GI disturbances).

⌂ Assess and record child's/family's knowledge of and participation in care regarding

> chest physiotherapy.
> medication administration.
> effective coughing in order to expectorate mucus.
> remaining calm while child is experiencing breathing difficulty; ways to regain control in crisis situation (e.g., assist child by positioning, breathe with child to calm child).
> use of games (e.g., blowing bubbles through a straw) to practice breathing exercise.
> identification of any signs/symptoms of impaired gas exchange (such as those listed under **Characteristics**).

⌂ Instruct family in any areas needing improvement. Record results.

EVALUATION FOR CHARTING

Describe breath sounds.

State highest and lowest respiratory rates.

Describe any signs/symptoms of impaired gas exchange noted (such as those listed under **Characteristics**).

State range of oxygen saturation.

State highest and lowest arterial blood gas values and state the ongoing physiological process (e.g. respiratory acidosis).

State results of any serum drug level and any therapeutic changes made.

State amount and route of oxygen delivery. Describe effectiveness.

Indicate whether chest physiotherapy was performed on schedule. Describe child's tolerance of procedure and its effectiveness. Describe characteristics of any secretions.

State whether head of bed was kept elevated.

State whether medications were administered on schedule. Describe effectiveness and any side effects noted.

⌂ Describe child's/family's knowledge of and participation in care related to improving gas exchange. State any areas

needing improvement and information provided. Describe child's/family's responses.

Knowledge Deficit: Child/Family

DEFINITION   Lack of information concerning the child's disease and care

POSSIBLY RELATED TO
Unfamiliarity with child's disease
Limited understanding of home management
Immediate and continuing management of breathing
    difficulty

CHARACTERISTICS
Verbalization by child/family indicating a lack of knowledge
    regarding asthma and the care needed
Relating incorrect information to members of the health
    care team
Inability to correctly repeat information previously explained
Inability to correctly demonstrate skills previously taught
    (e.g, medication administration, chest physiotherapy,
    breathing exercises)

EXPECTED OUTCOMES   Child/family will have an adequate knowledge base concerning the child's illness and care as evidenced by

ability to correctly state information previously taught
    regarding asthma and child's care (e.g., how to allergy-
    proof the home and correctly use hand-operated inhalers,
    appropriate exercise activities like swimming).
ability to correctly demonstrate skills previously taught (e.g.,
    medication administration, chest physiotherapy).
ability to relate appropriate information to the health
    care team.

POSSIBLE NURSING INTERVENTIONS
Listen to child's/family's concerns and fears.

🏠 Assess and record child's/family's knowledge of and
    understanding of child's illness.

⛨ Assess and record child's/family's knowledge of and participation in care regarding

> chest physiotherapy.
> breathing exercises.
> medication administration.
> identification of precipitating factors (e.g., stress, allergens, exercise).
> ways to allergy-proof the home.
> overdependence of child and/or overprotectiveness of parents.
> support organizations (such as American Lung Association).
> identification of any signs/symptoms of impaired gas exchange (such as those listed under **Characteristics**).

⛨ Instruct child/family in any areas needing improvement. Record results.

EVALUATION FOR CHARTING

⛨ State whether child/family verbalized a knowledge deficit.

⛨ State whether child/family were able to repeat information correctly and perform skills adequately. Describe ability.

⛨ Describe any measures used to facilitate child/family teaching.

RELATED NURSING DIAGNOSES

Fear: Child *related to*
  a. respiratory distress
  b. treatments and procedures
  c. unfamiliar surroundings
  d. hospitalization

Fluid Volume Deficit *related to*
  a. respiratory distress
  b. increased insensible water loss from rapid respiratory rate

Activity Intolerance *related to*
  a. dyspnea
  b. fatigue

Compromised Family Coping *related to*
  a. repeated hospitalization of child
  b. respiratory distress of child

Bronchiolitis

PATHOPHYSIOLOGY Bronchiolitis is a widespread inflammation and obstruction of the bronchioles resulting from a viral infection of the lower airways. The respiratory syncytial virus (RSV) is the causative organism in approximately 90% of diagnosed cases. Other causative organisms include the parainfluenza virus, rhinovirus, and adenovirus. The disease usually occurs in infants between 2 and 12 months of age, with the peak incidence at approximately 6 months of age. It rarely occurs in children more than 2 years of age.

The viral organism colonizes the bronchiole mucosa, which leads to necrosis. Edema and mucus obstruct the small airways, resulting in atelectasis. The infant is able to get air into the lungs but has difficulty expelling it because of plugs of mucus, which causes hyperinflation of the airways distal to the plugs. This airway plugging can interfere with gas exchange, and the infant may develop hypoxemia. Although the infant may experience severe respiratory distress during the first 3 days of hospitalization, the prognosis is generally good. Studies have shown that infants in about 50% of cases can develop subsequent episodes of wheezing associated with allergies.

PRIMARY NURSING DIAGNOSIS
Ineffective Breathing Pattern

DEFINITION   A breathing pattern that results in inadequate oxygen consumption (failure to meet the cellular requirements of the body)

POSSIBLY RELATED TO
   Inflammation of the lower airways secondary to a viral
   invasion

CHARACTERISTICS
   Tachypnea
   Retractions at rest

Nasal flaring
Crackles
Dry, hacking cough
Wheezing
Decreased breath sounds
Barrel-shaped chest
Cyanosis
Evidence of air trapping revealed on chest x-ray
Low-grade fever

EXPECTED OUTCOMES   Infant will have an effective
breathing pattern as evidenced by

respiratory rate within acceptable range (state highest and
lowest rates for each infant).
clear and equal breath sounds bilaterally.
absence of

cough.
nasal flaring.
retractions.
cyanosis.

clear chest x-ray with acceptable A-P diameter.
temperature within acceptable range of 36.5°C to 37.2°C.

POSSIBLE NURSING INTERVENTIONS
Assess and record the following every 4 hours and PRN:

respiratory rate, heart rate, and temperature
breath sounds
signs/symptoms of ineffective breathing pattern (such as
those listed under **Characteristics**). Notify physician of
any abnormalities.

Administer humidified oxygen in correct amount and route
of delivery. Record percent of oxygen and route of delivery.
Assess and record effectiveness of therapy.

Ensure that chest physiotherapy is performed on schedule.
Record effectiveness and child's tolerance of treatments.

When indicated, ensure that ribavirin aerosol is administered
on schedule per institutional protocol. Assess and record
effectiveness and any side effects (e.g., worsening of
respiratory status, hypotension).

Elevate head of bed at 30° angle (may use infant seat if infant can support head in midline position).

Ensure that bronchodilators are administered on schedule. Assess and record effectiveness and any side effects (such as tachycardia and GI disturbance).

Administer antibiotics (that may be given for a secondary bacterial infection) on schedule. Assess and record effectiveness and any side effects (e.g., rash, diarrhea).

When indicated, ensure that respiratory isolation is maintained.

Suction infant PRN if infant is unable to clear airway. Record amount and characteristics of secretions.

Check and record results of chest x-ray, when indicated.

Assess and record family's knowledge of and participation in care regarding

chest physiotherapy.
medication administration.
identification of any signs/symptoms of ineffective
    breathing pattern (such as those listed under
    Characteristics).

Instruct family in any areas needing improvement. Record results.

EVALUATION FOR CHARTING

State highest and lowest respiratory rates, heart rates, and temperatures.

Describe breath sounds.

Describe any signs/symptoms of ineffective breathing pattern noted (such as those listed under **Characteristics**).

State whether oxygen was administered and give amount and route of delivery. Describe effectiveness.

Indicate whether chest physiotherapy was performed on schedule. Describe infant's tolerance of procedure. State its effectiveness.

Indicate whether medications were administered on schedule. Describe effectiveness and any side effects noted.

State whether suctioning was needed. If so, describe any problems encountered during suctioning, the characteristics of the secretions, and the infant's response.

Describe any therapeutic measures used to maintain an effective breathing pattern. State their effectiveness.

State results of chest x-ray, when indicated.

🏠 Describe family's knowledge of and participation in care related to maintaining an effective breathing pattern. State any areas needing improvement and information provided. Describe family's response.

NURSING DIAGNOSIS
Fluid Volume Deficit

DEFINITION   Decrease in the amount of circulating fluid volume

POSSIBLY RELATED TO
Respiratory distress
Decreased fluid intake
Increased insensible water loss from rapid respirations

CHARACTERISTICS
Inability to tolerate fluids by mouth
Decreased urine output
Dry mucous membranes
Poor skin turgor
Sunken fontanel

EXPECTED OUTCOMES   Infant will have an adequate fluid volume as evidenced by

adequate fluid intake, IV and/or oral (state specific amount of intake needed for each infant).
adequate urine output (state specific highest and lowest outputs for each infant, minimum 1 to 2 ml/kg/hr).
urine specific gravity from 1.008 to 1.020.
moist mucous membranes.
rapid skin recoil.

POSSIBLE NURSING INTERVENTIONS
Keep accurate record of intake and output. Weigh diapers for output.

Assess and record

> IV fluids and condition of IV site every hour.
> signs/symptoms of fluid volume deficit (such as those listed under **Characteristics**) every 4 hours and PRN.

Check and record urine specific gravity every 4 hours or as ordered.

Give mouth care every 4 hours and PRN.

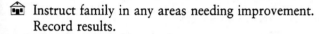 Assess and record family's knowledge of and participation in care regarding

> offering infant fluids, when indicated.
> monitoring of infant's intake and output.
> identification of any signs/symptoms of fluid volume deficit (such as those listed under **Characteristics**).

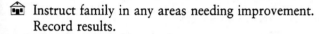 Instruct family in any areas needing improvement.
Record results.

EVALUATION FOR CHARTING

State intake and output.

Describe condition of IV site.

Describe status of mucous membranes, skin turgor, and fontanel.

State highest and lowest urine specific gravity values.

Describe any therapeutic measures used to improve fluid volume. State their effectiveness.

 Describe family's knowledge of and participation in care related to improving fluid volume. State any areas needing improvement and information provided. Describe family's response.

NURSING DIAGNOSIS
Sleep Pattern Disturbance

DEFINITION   Inability to achieve normal sleep pattern, causing interference with activities

POSSIBLY RELATED TO
Respiratory distress

Unfamiliar surroundings
Possible hypoxia

CHARACTERISTICS

Lethargy
Listlessness
Irritability
Constant crying
Fussy behavior

EXPECTED OUTCOMES   Infant will have an adequate sleep pattern as evidenced by

absence of listlessness and irritability.
alertness when awake.
ability to get the correct number of hours of sleep in 24 hours (state specific range for each infant).
absence of constant crying and fussy behavior.

POSSIBLE NURSING INTERVENTIONS

Assess and record the amount of sleep the infant gets in 24 hours.

Encourage family members to remain with infant when possible.

Allow infant to keep washable familiar objects in crib.

Assign same personnel to care for infant when possible.

Organize nursing care to allow infant uninterrupted rest periods.

Follow infant's normal naptime/bedtime routines as much as possible.

Assess and record any signs/symptoms of sleep pattern disturbance (such as those listed under **Characteristics**) every 8 hours and PRN.

EVALUATION FOR CHARTING

State how many hours of sleep infant gets in a 24-hour period. Determine if this is the appropriate amount for infant's age.

State whether family members were able to stay with infant and if this helped infant to sleep.

Describe any therapeutic measures used to improve sleep pattern. State their effectiveness.

Describe any signs/symptoms of sleep pattern disturbance noted (such as those listed under **Characteristics**).

RELATED NURSING DIAGNOSES

Altered Nutrition: Less than Body Requirements
related to
   a. respiratory distress
   b. refusal of solid foods
   c. lethargy

Fear: Parental *related to*
   a. hospitalization of small child
   b. knowledge deficit about disease state
   c. stress of seeing infant with respiratory distress

High Risk for Further Infection* *related to*
   a. increased respiratory secretions
   b. young age of child

---

*Non-NANDA diagnosis

MEDICAL DIAGNOSIS

Bronchopulmonary Dysplasia

PATHOPHYSIOLOGY Bronchopulmonary dysplasia (BPD) is believed to be caused by prolonged exposure to high oxygen concentrations and use of positive-pressure ventilation via endotracheal intubation. Prolonged use of these therapies results in thickening and necrosis of the alveolar wall and bronchiolar lining, which impairs the diffusion of oxygen from the alveoli to the capillaries. Use of an endotracheal tube for mechanical ventilation impairs ciliary action, preventing clearance of mucus and resulting in airway obstruction, atelectasis, and cystlike patterns that indicate developing emphysema. The thickening of the alveolar walls leads to respiratory acidosis and results in pulmonary hypertension, which can lead to right heart failure.

It is not always possible to prevent BPD. Oxygen should be administered in the lowest concentrations possible while adequate arterial oxygen tension is maintained. High-frequency ventilators, which require lower pressures, are sometimes used to help decrease lung damage. Most of the infants diagnosed with BPD were born prematurely with hyaline membrane disease present at birth. Babies who have mild BPD can usually be weaned from oxygen in a few weeks. infants with more severe disease may need oxygen therapy for many months.

Prognosis depends on the degree of lung damage sustained. If only the alveolar ducts and the alveoli are damaged, the prognosis is better since new growth of healthy alveoli is possible through early adolescence. Because of their minimal respiratory reserve, some infants with BPD have repeated hospitalizations for respiratory tract infections. Many have normal cardiopulmonary function by the age of 5 or 6 years.

PRIMARY NURSING DIAGNOSIS

Impaired Gas Exchange

DEFINITION Alteration in the exchange of oxygen and carbon dioxide in the lungs and/or at the cellular level

POSSIBLY RELATED TO
Long-term ventilator therapy
Barotrauma from mechanical ventilation
Prolonged high oxygen concentrations
Respiratory infection

CHARACTERISTICS
Tachypnea
Retractions
Rales
Diminished or unequal breath sounds
Wheezing
Barrel-chest appearance
Cyanosis
Resolving diffuse opacifications, atelectasis, and air cysts
    revealed on x-ray and indicating developing emphysema,
    flattened diaphragms, and hyperexpansion

EXPECTED OUTCOMES   Infant will maintain adequate gas
exchange as evidenced by

respiratory rate within acceptable range (state specific highest
    and lowest rates for each infant).
clear and equal breath sounds bilaterally.
absence of

retractions.
cyanosis.

oxygen saturation (via pulse oximeter) from 85% to 100%.

POSSIBLE NURSING INTERVENTIONS
Assess and record the following every 4 hours and PRN:

respiratory rate
breath sounds
signs/symptoms of impaired gas exchange (such as those
    listed under **Characteristics**). Notify physician of any
    abnormalities

Administer humidified oxygen in correct amount and route
of delivery. Record percent of oxygen and route of delivery.
Assess and record effectiveness of therapy.

Ensure that chest physiotherapy treatments and aerosol
bronchodilators are administered on schedule. Record
effectiveness of treatments. Assess and record effectiveness of

bronchodilators and any side effects (e.g., tachycardia, GI disturbance).

When using a pulse oximeter, record reading every 2 to 4 hours and PRN.

Suction PRN if infant is unable to clear airway. Record amount and characteristics of secretions.

Administer systemic bronchodilators (such as theophylline) on schedule. Assess and record their effectiveness and any side effects (e.g., tachycardia, irritability, vomiting).

Check and record results of chest x-ray, when indicated.

🏠 Assess and record family's knowledge of and participation in care regarding

> chest physiotherapy.
> medication administration.
> setup, connection, and maintenance of oxygen therapy.
> suctioning of infant.
> infant CPR.
> identification of any signs/symptoms of impaired gas exchange (such as those listed under **Characteristics**).

🏠 Instruct family in any areas needing improvement. Record results.

EVALUATION FOR CHARTING

State highest and lowest respiratory rates.

Describe breath sounds.

Describe any signs/symptoms of impaired gas exchange noted (such as those listed under **Characteristics**).

State whether oxygen was administered and give amount and route of delivery. Describe effectiveness.

Indicate whether chest physiotherapy was performed on schedule. Describe infant's tolerance of procedure. State its effectiveness.

State range of oxygen saturation.

State frequency of suctioning. Describe amount and characteristics of secretions. Describe infant's tolerance of procedure.

Indicate whether medications were administered on schedule. Describe effectiveness and any side effects noted.

State results of chest x-ray, when indicated.

Describe any therapeutic measures used to improve gas exchange. State their effectiveness.

⌂ Describe family's knowledge of and participation in care related to improving gas exchange. State any areas needing improvement and information provided. Describe family's response.

NURSING DIAGNOSIS
Fluid Volume Excess

DEFINITION   Increase in the amount of circulating fluid volume (which can eventually lead to interstitial or intracellular fluid overload)

POSSIBLY RELATED TO
Increased pulmonary vascular resistance
Right heart failure

CHARACTERISTICS
Sudden weight gain
Edema
Tachypnea
Crackles
Decreased urine output
Increased urine specific gravity (greater than 1.020)
Hepatosplenomegaly

EXPECTED OUTCOMES   Infant will resume fluid balance as evidenced by

lack of

sudden weight gain.
edema.
hepatosplenomegaly.

respiratory rate within acceptable range (state specific highest and lowest rates for each infant).
clear and equal breath sounds bilaterally.

adequate urine output (state specific highest and lowest
outputs for each infant, minimum 1 to 2 ml/kg/hr).
urine specific gravity from 1.008 to 1.020.

POSSIBLE NURSING INTERVENTIONS

Keep accurate record of intake and output. Be sure infant
does not exceed maximal intake ordered.

Assess and record

signs/symptoms of fluid volume excess (such as those
listed under **Characteristics**) every 4 hours and PRN.
amount and location of edema at least once/shift.
respiratory rate and breath sounds every 4 hours and
PRN.
urine specific gravity every 4 hours and PRN.

Weigh infant on same scale at same time each day.

Administer diuretics on schedule. Assess and record
effectiveness and any side effects (e.g., dehydration,
electrolyte imbalance).

Assess and record family's knowledge of and participation in
care regarding

medication administration.
monitoring of infant's intake and output.
identification of any signs/symptoms of fluid volume
excess (such as those listed under **Characteristics**).

Instruct family in any areas needing improvement.
Record results.

EVALUATION FOR CHARTING

State intake and output.

Describe any signs/symptoms of fluid volume excess noted
(such as those listed under **Characteristics**).

State highest and lowest respiratory rates.

Describe breath sounds.

Describe amount and location of edema.

State infant's weight and determine whether it has increased
or decreased since the previous weighing.

State whether medications were administered on schedule. Describe effectiveness and any side effects noted.

Describe family's knowledge of and participation in care related to resuming fluid balance. State any areas needing improvement and information provided. Describe family's response.

RELATED NURSING DIAGNOSES

Decreased Cardiac Output *related to*
a. pulmonary hypertension
b. right heart failure

Altered Nutrition: Less than Body Requirements *related to*
a. maximal respiratory effort requiring increased caloric consumption secondary to respiratory distress
b. difficulty sucking and breathing simultaneously
c. fatigue

Compromised Family Coping *related to*
a. need for repeated hospitalizations
b. difficulty in obtaining competent baby-sitters
c. financial burden
d. delayed infant growth and development
e. guilt (unfounded) when infant becomes ill and has to be admitted to the hospital

Infection: High risk *related to*
increased pulmonary secretions

Cystic Fibrosis

PATHOPHYSIOLOGY   Cystic fibrosis (CF) is the most common lethal genetic disease among Caucasians in North America. It is an autosomal recessive disease, meaning that both parents must be carriers and contribute one defective gene for a child to be born with CF. Each child born in these families has a 25% chance of having the disease, a 50% chance of being a carrier, and a 25% chance of neither having the disease nor being a carrier. The carrier rate is approximately one in every twenty white individuals. The incidence of the disease is one in every eighteen hundred live white births. Although it is rare, CF does also occur in the black and Asian populations. Prenatal diagnosis is now possible, but it is usually done only for families who already have a child diagnosed with CF. It is now possible to detect carriers by checking an individual's genes for the defect.

The child with CF has an inborn error of metabolism, which causes a generalized dysfunction of the exocrine (mucous-secreting) glands as well as of many other tissues and organs. The child may exhibit any or all of the major manifestations, which include chronic obstructive pulmonary disease; pancreatic insufficiency, which leads to malabsorption; and increased sweat electrolyte concentrations. The hepatic and reproductive systems are also affected. The basic biomedical defect is unknown; however, the specific gene has recently been identified. With the exception of the sweat and parotid glands, pathological changes are caused by abnormal secretions obstructing the various organ passageways (ducts). The progression and severity of the clinical manifestations in children with CF vary greatly.

Pulmonary manifestations develop in almost all patients and determine the prognosis of the individual. The major problems are an increased predisposition to infections and the presence of abnormal bronchial mucus, resulting in the production of viscid, purulent sputum. A vicious cycle ensues in which the thick mucus leads to obstruction of small airways and stasis of mucus, increasing the likelihood of infections. Infections in turn increase mucus production, resulting in obstruction and production of sputum. This obstructive cycle causes a decrease in gas exchange, leading to hypoxemia and hypercapnia. Hypoxemia and hypercapnia lead to pulmonary vasoconstriction and eventually to pulmonary hypertension. Cor pulmonale (right ventricular hypertrophy secondary to pulmonary hypertension) is a common complication. Other complications include hemoptysis due to pulmonary vascular changes and sinusitis caused by secretions filling the paranasal sinuses. Pulmonary symptoms include a productive cough, tachypnea, crackles, rhonchi, use of accessory muscles for breathing, and barrel-chest deformity. Digital clubbing is frequently seen.

Gastrointestinal symptoms result when abnormal secretions obstruct pancreatic ducts, leading to absence of pancreatic enzymes, which results in malabsorption of fats and proteins. Steatorrhea (fatty stools) and azotorrhea (nitrogen loss in the stool) are common. Some patients may present in the newborn period with meconium ileus.

Cystic fibrosis is diagnosed by family history, history of chronic pulmonary disease, history of malabsorption, and results of a sweat chloride test. A chloride concentration of 60 mEq/L or greater is considered diagnostic. The sweat of individuals with CF has abnormally high sodium and chloride concentrations; parents frequently complain of their infants tasting "salty" when kissed. The average life expectancy for a child with CF is approximately 27 years of age.

PRIMARY NURSING DIAGNOSIS
Ineffective Airway Clearance

DEFINITION Condition in which secretions cannot adequately be cleared from the airways

POSSIBLY RELATED TO
    Excessive mucus
    Bacterial infection

CHARACTERISTICS
    Decreased breath sounds
    Cough
    Tachypnea
    Dyspnea
    Wheezes, diffuse crackles, and rhonchi

Use of accessory muscles for breathing
Frequent respiratory infections
Barrel-chest deformity
Cyanosis
Digital clubbing

EXPECTED OUTCOMES   Child will have adequate airway clearance as evidenced by

clear and equal breath sounds bilaterally.
respiratory rate within acceptable range (state specific highest and lowest rates for each child).
lack of cyanosis and dyspnea.
absence of respiratory infection.
oxygen saturation (via pulse oximeter) from 85% to 100%.

POSSIBLE NURSING INTERVENTIONS

Assess and record the following every 4 hours and PRN:

breath sounds and any signs/symptoms of ineffective airway clearance (such as those listed under **Characteristics**). Notify physician of any abnormalities.
amount and characteristics of secretions

Ensure that chest physiotherapy treatments and administration of aerosol bronchodilators are done on schedule. Encourage child to cough during and after treatments. Record effectiveness of treatments. Assess and record for effectiveness of bronchodilators and any side effects (e.g., tachycardia, GI disturbance).

When using a pulse oximeter, record reading every 2 to 4 hours and PRN.

When indicated, administer oxygen in the correct amount and route. Record percent of oxygen and route of delivery. Assess and record effectiveness of therapy.

Instruct child to spit out secretions in a tissue and dispose of tissue in waste container.

Administer antibiotics on schedule. Assess and record effectiveness and any side effects (e.g., rash, diarrhea).

Encourage fluid intake in order to help liquify secretions.

Check and record results of chest x-ray and complete blood count (CBC), when indicated.

🏠 Assess and record child's/family's knowledge of and participation in care regarding

chest physiotherapy.
medication administration.
identification of any signs/symptoms of ineffective airway clearance (such as those listed under **Characteristics**).

🏠 Instruct child/family in any areas needing improvement. Record results.

EVALUATION FOR CHARTING

Describe breath sounds.

State highest and lowest respiratory rates.

Describe amount and characteristics of secretions.

Describe any signs/symptoms of ineffective airway clearance noted (such as those listed under **Characteristics**).

Indicate whether chest physiotherapy was performed on schedule. Describe child's tolerance of the procedure. State its effectiveness.

Indicate whether medications were administered on schedule. Describe effectiveness and any side effects noted.

State range of oxygen saturation.

State whether oxygen was administered and give amount and route of delivery. Describe effectiveness.

Describe any therapeutic measures used to improve airway clearance. State their effectiveness.

State results of chest x-ray and CBC when indicated.

🏠 Describe child's/family's knowledge of and participation in care related to improving airway clearance. State any areas needing improvement and information provided. Describe child's/family's responses.

NURSING DIAGNOSIS
Altered Nutrition: Less than Body Requirements

DEFINITION Insufficient nutrients to meet body requirements

POSSIBLY RELATED TO

Malabsorption secondary to absence of pancreatic enzymes
Infection

CHARACTERISTICS

Failure to gain weight
Voracious appetite (together with a failure to gain weight
    due to malabsorption)
Malabsorption of fat-soluble vitamins
Frequent, foul-smelling stools
Steatorrhea (fatty stools)
Azotorrhea (nitrogen loss in the stool)

EXPECTED OUTCOMES   Child will be adequately nourished
as evidenced by

absorption of adequate amount of calories, parenterally and/
    or orally (state specific amount for each child, usually 1½
    to 2 times the RDA for age for children with CF).
steady weight gain or lack of weight loss.

NURSING INTERVENTIONS

Keep accurate record of intake and output.

Assess and record every 8 hours and PRN for any
signs/symptoms of altered nutrition (such as those listed
under **Characteristics**).

Weigh child on same scale at same time each day.
Record results.

Maintain and record daily caloric count, as indicated.

Encourage child to eat by assessing likes/dislikes and, when
possible, providing foods that child likes to eat.

Offer between-meal snacks.

Organize care to conserve energy.

Administer medications (oral pancreatic enzymes and
vitamins) on schedule. It may be necessary to disguise the
taste of the enzymes in foods such as applesauce. Assess and
record effectiveness and any side effects.

 Initiate consultation with dietician, when indicated.

EVALUATION FOR CHARTING

State intake and output.

Describe any signs/symptoms of altered nutrition noted (such as those listed under **Characteristics**).

State current weight and determine whether it has increased or decreased since previous weighing.

State caloric intake when indicated.

Describe any therapeutic measures used to maintain adequate nutrition. State their effectiveness.

State whether medications were administered on schedule. Describe effectiveness and any side effects noted.

NURSING DIAGNOSIS
Compromised Family Coping

DEFINITION Decreased ability of family members to manage problems and concerns effectively

POSSIBLY RELATED TO
Child's long-term illness
Fatal disease
Financial considerations
Guilt secondary to the genetic nature of the disease

CHARACTERISTICS
Inability to leave child
Inappropriate anger toward other family members
Inability to meet own basic needs such as eating and resting
Inability to ask for and accept outside help
Failure to understand repeated explanations regarding the
    illness, treatments, and procedures

EXPECTED OUTCOMES Family will be able to cope effectively as evidenced by

ability to leave the child for short periods, especially to care
    for own basic needs such as eating meals and getting rest.
ability to express anger appropriately toward staff or others.
ability to express fears and concerns to members of the
    health care team.
ability to realize when it is appropriate to accept outside
    help.
verbalization of understanding explanations regarding the
    illness, treatments, and procedures.
participation in child's care.

POSSIBLE NURSING INTERVENTIONS

Communicate with family concerning child's condition at least once/shift and PRN. This may require telephoning the family when family members are not able to come to the hospital.

Encourage family members to express feelings, fears, and concerns.

Assist and encourage family members to meet own basic needs, such as eating and resting appropriately.

🏠 Identify and record any past or usually successful coping strategies used by the family.

🏠 Provide the family with outside help or assist members in seeking outside help, when indicated.

🏠 Explain the course of the illness, the treatments, and procedures to the family. Include reasons for treatments and procedures.

🏠 Encourage family involvement with CF support groups or a CF foundation.

🏠 Support family's participation in child's care. Record results.

EVALUATION FOR CHARTING

State whether family members were able to leave the child long enough to meet their own basic needs.

Describe any feelings, fears, and concerns expressed by the family.

🏠 State whether the family is willing to accept outside help as indicated.

🏠 State whether family members were able to understand information given to them about the child's illness.

🏠 State whether the family was able to understand the necessity and rationale for treatments and procedures.

🏠 State any successful measures used to help the family cope.

🏠 Describe family's participation in child's care.

RELATED NURSING DIAGNOSES

Knowledge Deficit: Child/Family *related to*
a. disease state and prognosis
b. treatments and procedures
c. home care maintenance

Body Image Disturbance *related to*
a. child's chronic long-term illness
b. delayed development of secondary sex characteristics
c. copious amounts of viscid, purulent sputum
d. inability to maintain average weight

Infection: High Risk *related to*
invasion of the respiratory tract by bacterial organisms

MEDICAL DIAGNOSIS

Foreign Body Aspiration

PATHOPHYSIOLOGY   A child could potentially aspirate any object put into the mouth. Children 6 months to 3 years are most generally affected. Food items such as nuts, popcorn, uncut hot dogs, and grapes are common hazards. Nonfood items such as buttons, coins, and small toy parts like eyes on stuffed animals are also commonly aspirated.

Any section of the airway, from the larynx to the bronchi, may be the site of a foreign body aspiration (FBA). Normally the airways expand on inspiration and contract on expiration. This helps explain the different degrees of obstruction possible. If a particle is very small, air could flow in and out around the object. Usually a wheeze is audible in this situation. When an aspirated object is a little larger, it may allow air to enter the airways, but the air distal to the obstruction is trapped during expiration due to narrowing of the airways on expiration. Some aspirated objects can be large enough to obstruct air flow in and out of the airways. The air distal to the obstruction is absorbed, and atelectasis results. The right main stem bronchus is the most common site because it is shorter and wider than the left main stem bronchus and comes off the trachea in a straighter angle.

The clinical manifestations and degree of severity of FBA depend on what has been aspirated and on its location. Whenever a child is afebrile and has a sudden onset of respiratory distress, FBA should be considered.

PRIMARY NURSING DIAGNOSIS
Ineffective Airway Clearance

DEFINITION   Condition in which secretions cannot adequately be cleared from the airways

POSSIBLY RELATED TO
    Airway obstruction by a small object (specify if object can
      be identified)

CHARACTERISTICS

INITIAL CHARACTERISTICS

Choking
Rhonchi
Wheezing
Gagging
Sudden, periodic coughing
Periods during which child is asymptomatic for days or
    weeks after initial onset of symptoms

SECONDARY CHARACTERISTICS

Fever
Dyspnea
Asymmetrical chest expansion
Decreased breath sounds over affected area
Recurrent pneumonia
Diaphragm low and fixed on the obstructed side as revealed
    on expiration chest x-ray (sometimes)

LOCATIONAL CHARACTERISTICS

Larynx:

hoarseness
croupy cough
inspiratory stridor
inability to vocalize

Trachea:

cough
dyspnea
hoarseness
cyanosis

Bronchus:

cough
blood-tinged sputum
dyspnea

EXPECTED OUTCOMES   Child will have adequate airway
clearance as evidenced by

clear and equal breath sounds bilaterally.
symmetrical chest expansion.

thin, clear secretions.

absence of any signs/symptoms of ineffective airway clearance (such as those listed under **Characteristics**).

ability to vocalize.

temperature within acceptable range of 36.5°C to 37.2°C.

POSSIBLE NURSING INTERVENTIONS

Assess and record the following every 4 hours and PRN:

breath sounds and temperature

signs/symptoms of ineffective airway clearance (such as those listed under **Characteristics**)

Assess and record amount and characteristics of any pulmonary secretions.

Ensure that chest physiotherapy is performed effectively and on schedule. Record effectiveness of treatments.

Ensure that aerosol bronchodilators are administered on schedule. Assess and record effectiveness and any side effects (e.g., tachycardia, nausea/vomiting).

Administer antibiotics on schedule. Assess and record effectiveness and any side effects (e.g., rash, diarrhea).

If indicated, administer antipyretics on schedule. Record effectiveness.

Explain to child/family any indicated procedure and its rationale.

Prepare child for surgical treatments such as bronchoscopy. Ensure that a high-humidity atmosphere is maintained following procedure.

Keep child NPO following bronchoscopy until gag reflex has fully returned.

Check and record results of chest x-ray, when indicated.

Assess and record child's/family's knowledge of and participation in care regarding

abdominal thrust to loosen or expel aspirated items (Heimlich maneuver).

hazards of aspiration in relation to developmental age of child.

chest physiotherapy.

medication administration.

identification of any signs/symptoms of ineffective airway clearance (such as those listed under **Characteristics**).

🏠 Instruct child/family in any areas needing improvement. Record results.

EVALUATION FOR CHARTING

Describe breath sounds.

State highest and lowest temperatures.

Describe any signs/symptoms of ineffective airway clearance noted (such as those listed under **Characteristics**).

State frequency of suctioning needed. Describe amount and characteristics of secretions.

Indicate whether chest physiotherapy was performed on schedule. Describe child's tolerance of procedure. State its effectiveness.

Indicate whether medications were administered on schedule. Describe effectiveness and any side effects noted.

Describe child's level of tolerance for any procedures that might have been done, such as bronchoscopy.

If bronchoscopy was done, indicate whether high-humidity mist was maintained and whether child's gag reflex has returned.

State results of chest x-ray, when indicated.

🏠 Describe child's/family's knowledge of and participation in care related to maintaining adequate airway clearance. State any areas needing improvement and information provided. Describe child's/family's responses.

NURSING DIAGNOSIS
Fear: Child

DEFINITION   Feeling of apprehension resulting from a known cause

POSSIBLY RELATED TO
Respiratory distress
Unfamiliar surroundings

Forced contact with strangers
Treatments and procedures
Hospitalization

CHARACTERISTICS

Uncooperativeness
Regressed behavior
Restlessness
Constant crying
Tachypnea
Tachycardia
Diaphoresis

EXPECTED OUTCOMES   Child will exhibit only a minimal amount of fear as evidenced by

ability to relate appropriately to family members.
ability to rest and sleep between treatments and procedures.
lack of constant crying.
respiratory rate within acceptable range (state specific highest and lowest rates for each child).
heart rate within acceptable range (state specific highest and lowest rates for each child).
lack of diaphoresis.

POSSIBLE NURSING INTERVENTIONS

Decrease child's fear when possible by

encouraging family members to stay with child.
encouraging family members to participate in care of child.
assigning same staff members to provide care for the child.
talking to child and explaining procedures and treatments and why they are necessary.
spending extra time with the child when family members are unable to be present.
encouraging family members to bring in familiar articles and toys from home.

Initiate age-appropriate therapeutic play, when indicated.

Assess and record any physiological signs/symptoms of fear (e.g., increased respiratory rate, increased heart rate, diaphoresis) when taking vital signs.

EVALUATION FOR CHARTING

State whether child manifested fear and describe any successful measures used to help alleviate the fear.

State whether child's fear decreases if family members stay and participate in child's care.

State highest and lowest respiratory and heart rates.

State whether diaphoresis was present.

NURSING DIAGNOSIS
Guilt: Parental/Family*

DEFINITION   State or condition in which the individual accepts blame, either appropriately or inappropriately

POSSIBLY RELATED TO
Accidental nature of child's illness
Discomfort child is experiencing
Delay in seeking health care

CHARACTERISTICS
Verbalization of blame
Overprotectiveness of ill child
Anger
Irritability

EXPECTED OUTCOMES   Parents/family will be able to deal with guilt feelings appropriately, as evidenced by

expression of fears/concerns to members of the health
   care team.
participation in child's care when possible.
acceptance of help, when indicated.

POSSIBLE NURSING INTERVENTIONS
Encourage family to ventilate and express feelings of guilt; give positive reinforcement for doing so.

Praise any positive family/child interaction observed.

Encourage family to participate in child's care when possible.

---

*Non-NANDA diagnosis.

Encourage and assist family in seeking outside help and/or counseling when appropriate.

EVALUATION FOR CHARTING

Describe any concerns and/or fears expressed by family.

State whether family participated in child's care.

Describe any successful measures used to help decrease family's guilt feelings.

State whether family sought outside counseling.

RELATED NURSING DIAGNOSIS

Fluid Volume Deficit *related to*
a. dyspnea
b. choking

Infection: High Risk *related to*
a. aspiration
b. invasive procedures

Knowledge Deficit: Parental *related to*
care and safety of a young child

7

Laryngotracheobronchitis/ Viral Croup

PATHOPHYSIOLOGY Laryngotracheobronchitis (LTB), the most common form of croup, is a viral infection that affects the larynx, trachea, and bronchi, thus involving both the upper and lower airways. The viral organism invades the mucosa lining of the airways, resulting in inflammation and edema. The inflammation and edema narrow the airways, sometimes obstructing them. This obstruction is greatest in the subglottic area, usually the narrowest part of the airways. The hallmark sound of children with LTB is inspiratory stridor, a shrill, harsh, "crowing" respiratory sound. This sound is the result of increased velocity and turbulence of airflow through a narrowed (extrathoracic) airway. When air passes through the constricted airway, the negative pressure tends to further narrow the already comprised airway, producing the stridor sound. Other common characteristics of LTB are hoarseness and a "barky" cough.

Laryngotracheobronchitis is more common in boys than in girls and typically occurs in children between 3 months and 4 years of age, with the peak incidence at 18 months of age. The child usually presents with a history of upper airway congestion, low-grade or no fever, normal activity, and hoarseness. The symptoms usually become worse at night. The most common viral agents causing LTB are parainfluenza viruses, influenza viruses, rhinoviruses, and the respiratory syncytial virus.

PRIMARY NURSING DIAGNOSIS
Ineffective Breathing Pattern

DEFINITION Breathing pattern that results in inadequate oxygen consumption (failure to meet the cellular requirements of the body)

POSSIBLY RELATED TO
Viral infection of the larynx, trachea, and bronchi

CHARACTERISTICS

Tachypnea
Inspiratory stridor
Hoarseness
"Barky" cough
Dyspnea
Diminished breath sounds bilaterally
Crackles and rhonchi
Substernal and suprasternal retractions
Fever
Tachycardia
Irritability and restlessness
Cyanosis (late sign)

EXPECTED OUTCOMES   Child will have an effective
breathing pattern as evidenced by

clear and equal breath sounds bilaterally.
respiratory rate within acceptable range (state specific highest
  and lowest rates for each child).
temperature within acceptable range of 36.5°C to 37.2°C.
absence of the following:

hoarseness
"barky" cough
extreme irritability
retractions

absence of signs/symptoms of increasing respiratory
  obstruction:

inspiratory stridor at rest
tachypnea (rate above 60/min at rest)
tachycardia (rate above 140/min at rest)
circumoral or orbital cyanosis
restlessness

absence of signs/symptoms of respiratory failure:

listlessness
decrease in stridor and retractions without clinical
  improvement
diminished breath sounds

POSSIBLE NURSING INTERVENTIONS

Assess and record the following every 2 to 4 hours and PRN:

breath sounds with vital signs
signs/symptoms of ineffective breathing pattern and
   increasing airway obstruction (such as those listed
   under **Characteristics**)

Ensure that cool mist is administered by ordered route of delivery.

Ensure that nebulized bronchodilators (such as racemic epinephrine) are administered on schedule. Assess and record effectiveness and any side effects (e.g., tachycardia, GI disturbances).

If indicated, administer antipyretics on schedule. Record effectiveness.

If indicated, administer antibiotics (sometimes given for secondary infections). Assess and record effectiveness and side effects (e.g., rash, diarrhea).

If indicated, administer steroids (e.g., dexamethasone) on schedule. Their effectiveness remains controversial. Assess and record effectiveness and any side effects (such as sodium retention and potassium loss).

If indicated, administer oxygen in the correct amount and route. Record percent of oxygen and route of delivery. Assess and record effectiveness of therapy. Be aware that more than 40% oxygen may mask symptoms of increasing respiratory distress. Arterial blood gases may be indicated. If indicated, assess and record arterial blood gas values. Report any abnormalities to the physician.

Deep suction only if specifically ordered. Suctioning may induce further airway obstruction. Record amount and characteristics of secretions.

Provide rest and a quiet atmosphere.

Assess and record child's/family's knowledge of and participation in care regarding

delivery of cool mist via humidifier at home.
maintenance of home humidifier (cleaning unit).
mist provided by steaming up bathroom (constant and
   careful supervision will be needed).
medication administration.

identification of any signs/symptoms of ineffective
breathing pattern and increasing airway obstruction
(such as those listed under **Characteristics**).

🏠 Instruct child/family in any areas needing improvement.
Record results.

EVALUATION FOR CHARTING

Describe breath sounds.

State highest and lowest respiratory rates, heart rates, and
temperatures.

Describe any signs/symptoms of ineffective breathing pattern
or increasing airway obstruction noted (such as those listed
under **Characteristics**).

State whether cool mist was administered and the route of
delivery. Describe effectiveness.

State whether medications were administered on schedule.
Describe effectiveness and any side effects noted.

State whether oxygen was needed. If so, state amount and
route of delivery. Describe effectiveness.

State whether suctioning was needed. If so, describe any
problems encountered during suctioning, the amount and
characteristics of the secretions, and the child's response.

Describe effectiveness of rest and quiet atmosphere.

🏠 Describe child's/family's knowledge of and participation in
care related to maintaining an effective breathing pattern.
State any areas needing improvement and information
provided. Describe child's/family's responses.

NURSING DIAGNOSIS
Fluid Volume Deficit

DEFINITION   Decrease in the amount of circulating
fluid volume

POSSIBLY RELATED TO
Respiratory difficulty

Sore throat and resulting decrease in intake by mouth
Increased insensible water loss from rapid respirations
Fever

CHARACTERISTICS

Anorexia
Inability to tolerate fluids by mouth
Decreased urine output
Vomiting
Tachypnea
Malaise
Dry mucous membranes
Poor skin turgor

EXPECTED OUTCOMES   Child will have an adequate fluid volume as evidenced by

adequate fluid intake, IV or oral (state specific amount of intake needed for each child).
adequate urine output (state specific highest and lowest outputs for each child, minimum 1 to 2 ml/kg/hr).
urine specific gravity from 1.008 to 1.020.
moist mucous membranes.
rapid skin recoil.
respiratory rate within acceptable range (state specific highest and lowest rates for each child).
temperature within acceptable range of 36.5°C to 37.2°C.
absence of anorexia, vomiting, and malaise.

POSSIBLE NURSING INTERVENTIONS

Keep accurate record of intake and output.

Assess and record

IV fluids and condition of IV site every hour.
signs/symptoms of fluid volume deficit (such as those listed under **Characteristics**) every 4 hours and PRN.
respiratory rate and temperature every 2 to 4 hours and PRN.

Check and record urine specific gravity every void or as ordered.

Give mouth care every 4 hours and PRN.

🔲 Assess and record child's/family's knowledge of and participation in care regarding

> offering child fluids when indicated.
> monitoring of child's intake and output.
> identification of any signs/symptoms of fluid volume deficit (such as those listed under **Characteristics**).

🔲 Instruct child/family in any areas needing improvement. Record results.

EVALUATION FOR CHARTING

State intake and output.

Describe condition of IV site.

State highest and lowest respiratory rates and temperatures.

Describe status of mucous membranes and skin turgor.

State highest and lowest urine specific gravity values.

Describe any therapeutic measures used to improve fluid volume. State their effectiveness.

Describe any signs/symptoms of fluid volume deficit noted (such as those listed under **Characteristics**).

🔲 Describe child's/family's knowledge of and participation in care related to improving fluid volume. State any areas needing improvement and information provided. Describe child's/family's responses.

RELATED NURSING DIAGNOSES

Fear: Child *related to*
   a. respiratory distress
   b. unfamiliar surroundings
   c. forced contact with strangers
   d. treatments and procedures
   e. mist tent
   f. restraints (may be needed to keep child under mist tent)

Activity Intolerance *related to*
   a. respiratory difficulty
   b. fatigue
   c. confinement to mist area

Altered Comfort* *related to*
  sore throat

Compromised Family Coping *related to*
  a. respiratory distress of child
  b. hospitalization of child
  c. guilt secondary to delay in seeking health care
  d. knowledge deficit regarding home care

---

*Non-NANDA diagnosis.

8

MEDICAL DIAGNOSIS

Pertussis (Whooping Cough)

PATHOPHYSIOLOGY   Pertussis, or whooping cough, is an acute bacterial respiratory infection caused by *Bordetella pertussis*, a gram-negative bacillus. This organism multiplies only in association with the respiratory epithelial cells, causing necrosis and desquamation of the superficial epithelium. When this process occurs in the small bronchi, bronchopneumonia develops. The accumulation of mucus secretions can also result in bronchiolar obstruction and atelectasis.

Pertussis progresses through three stages. During the catarrhal stage, which lasts 1 to 2 weeks, the symptoms of a mild upper respiratory tract infection—such as runny nose, sneezing, and cough—are present. The paroxysmal stage, lasting 2 to 4 weeks, is characterized by a paroxysmal or spasmodic cough, accompanied by a characteristic inspiratory whoop. Coughing spasms are often followed by vomiting. During the convalescent stage, which usually lasts 1 to 2 weeks, the severity of the symptoms and frequency of the cough gradually decrease. Complications of pertussis include apneic episodes, pneumonia, seizures, encephalopathy, and death.

Although pertussis can occur at any age, it is most common in infants and young children, with children under age 5 being at highest risk. Immunization has reduced the incidence and mortality rate of pertussis, but it does not provide permanent or complete immunity.

Transmission occurs with exposure to the aerosol droplets from the respiratory tract of infected individuals or from direct contact with their nasopharyngeal secretions. The incubation period is usually 7 to 10 days. The treatment of pertussis is symptomatic; however, erythromycin is used to shorten the period of communicability.

PRIMARY NURSING DIAGNOSIS
Ineffective Airway Clearance

DEFINITION   Condition in which secretions cannot adequately be cleared from the airways

POSSIBLY RELATED TO
> Accumulation of mucus secretions, including mucus plugs
> Bacterial infection of the lungs
> Spasmodic coughing episodes

CHARACTERISTICS
> Severe paroxysms of cough with an inspiratory whoop, often followed by vomiting
> Possible facial redness, cyanosis, bulging eyes, protrusion of the tongue, tearing, salivation, and distension of neck veins accompanying coughing episodes
> Diminished breath sounds
> Diffuse rhonchi and crackles
> Perihilar infiltrates, atelectasis, or emphysema revealed on chest x-ray
> Lethargy

EXPECTED OUTCOMES   Child will have adequate airway clearance as evidenced by

> lack of spasmodic coughing episodes.
> clear and equal breath sounds bilaterally.
> lack of lethargy.
> oxygen saturation (via pulse oximeter) from 85% to 100%.

POSSIBLE NURSING INTERVENTIONS
Assess and record the following every 4 hours and PRN:

> breath sounds
> coughing episodes and any accompanying signs
> any signs/symptoms of ineffective airway clearance or respiratory distress (e.g., tachypnea, retractions, nasal flaring, apnea, dyspnea, cyanosis). Notify physician of any abnormalities.

When using a pulse oximeter, record reading every 2 to 4 hours and PRN.

 Assist child/family in identifying and avoiding triggers of the coughing episodes (e.g., physical exertion, lying flat in bed).

Ensure that antibiotics (erythromycin) are administered on schedule. Assess and record effectiveness and any side effects (e.g., GI discomfort, rash).

When indicated, administer oxygen in correct amount and route. Record percent of oxygen and route of delivery. Assess and record effectiveness of therapy.

Ensure that chest physiotherapy is performed on schedule. Record effectiveness of treatments.

Suction gently if infant or child is unable to clear airway. Record frequency of suctioning and amount and characteristics of secretions.

Encourage fluid intake in order to help liquify secretions.

Elevate head of bed at a 30° angle (may use infant seat if infant can support head in midline position).

Check and record results of chest x-ray, when indicated.

Ensure that respiratory isolation is maintained.

🏠 Assess and record family's knowledge of and participation in care regarding

identification of any signs/symptoms of ineffective airway clearance (such as those listed under **Characteristics**) or respiratory distress.
medication administration.
chest physiotherapy.

🏠 Instruct family in any areas needing improvement. Record results.

EVALUATION FOR CHARTING

Describe breath sounds.

State frequency of suctioning. Describe amount and characteristics of secretions.

Describe any signs/symptoms of ineffective airway clearance (such as those listed under **Characteristics**) or respiratory distress noted. Describe frequency and severity of paroxysms of cough.

Describe any therapeutic measures used to improve airway clearance. State their effectiveness.

Indicate whether chest physiotherapy was performed on schedule. Describe child's tolerance of the procedure. State its effectiveness.

Indicate whether medications were administered on schedule. Describe effectiveness and any side effects noted.

State range of oxygen saturation.

State whether oxygen was administered and give amount and route of delivery. Describe effectiveness.

State results of chest x-ray, when indicated.

Describe family's knowledge of and participation in care related to improving airway clearance. State any areas needing improvement and information provided. Describe child's/family's responses.

NURSING DIAGNOSIS
Fear: Parental

DEFINITION   Feeling of apprehension resulting from a known cause

POSSIBLY RELATED TO
Child's spasmodic coughing episodes
Child's acute illness
Hospitalization of infant or young child
Communicability of child's illness to siblings
Guilt if child has not been immunized
Feelings of dread regarding child's outcome
Apprehension surrounding child's coughing episodes

CHARACTERISTICS
Avoidance of child or inability to leave child's side
Decreased attention span
Decreased communication
Inability to participate in child's care
Reports of somatic discomfort

EXPECTED OUTCOMES   Parent will exhibit only a minimal amount of fear as evidenced by

decreased reports of somatic discomfort.
ability to leave child's bedside for short periods, especially to

care for own basic needs such as eating meals and getting rest.

ability to express fears to members of the health care team or supportive family and friends.

participation in child's care.

ability to verbalize/understanding of explanations regarding child's illness, treatments, and procedures.

POSSIBLE NURSING INTERVENTIONS

Assess and record parental perception of threatening stimuli.

Communicate with parent concerning child's condition at least once/shift and PRN. Keep explanations simple and repeat them as necessary. Record interactions with parents.

🏠 Encourage parent to express fears to health care team, family, and/or friends.

🏠 Listen as parent expresses fears. If possible, encourage mastery of the situation (e.g., identifying and avoiding triggers of child's cough, responding appropriately to a coughing episode).

🏠 Encourage parent to meet basic needs, such as eating and resting appropriately, and assist.

🏠 Support parental participation in child's care. Record results.

EVALUATION FOR CHARTING

Describe any fears expressed by parent and any attempts made to cope with these fears.

🏠 State whether parent was able to leave the child long enough to meet own basic needs.

🏠 State whether parent was able to understand information given about the child's illness.

Describe parent's participation in child's care.

Describe any measures used to help decrease parental fears.

RELATED NURSING DIAGNOSES

Ineffective Breathing Pattern *related to*

a. spasmodic coughing episodes
b. infection of the lungs

Fluid Volume Deficit *related to*

a. vomiting after spasmodic coughing episodes
b. decreased fluid intake
c. drinking triggering spasmodic cough
d. fever

Altered Nutrition: Less than Body Requirements
related to

a. vomiting after spasmodic coughing episodes
b. decreased food intake
c. eating triggering spasmodic cough
d. increased caloric need related to increased energy
   expenditure secondary to fever or work of breathing

Impaired Home Maintenance Management *related to*

a. communicable disease
b. lack of knowledge

MEDICAL DIAGNOSIS

Pneumonia

PATHOPHYSIOLOGY Pneumonia is an inflammation of the lungs characterized by consolidation due to exudate filling the alveoli and bronchioles. Blood is shunted around these nonfunctioning areas, resulting in hypoxemia. Pneumonia can occur as a primary disease or as the result of another illness. It can be localized to one specific area (lobular pneumonia) or disseminated throughout the lungs (bronchopneumonia). The causative organism can be either bacterial, viral, or mycoplasmal. Bacterial pneumonia is commonly caused by pneumococcus, streptococcus, or staphylococcus. The respiratory syncytial virus (RSV) is the causative organism in the majority of viral pneumonias. Other causative organisms include influenza viruses, adenoviruses, rhinovirus, rubeola, and varicella. Mycoplasmal pneumonia generally occurs in older children and young adults.

PRIMARY NURSING DIAGNOSIS
Ineffective Breathing Pattern

DEFINITION Breathing pattern that results in inadequate oxygen consumption (failure to meet the cellular requirements of the body)

POSSIBLY RELATED TO
>   Infection of the lungs (state whether bacterial, viral, or mycoplasmal)

CHARACTERISTICS
>   Cough, unproductive in early stages but later becoming productive
>   Nasal discharge
>   Dyspnea
>   Tachypnea
>   Diminished breath sounds
>   Grunting respirations

Retractions
Fever
Diaphoresis
Crackles
Cyanosis
Leukocytosis
Evidence of infiltration revealed on chest x-ray

EXPECTED OUTCOMES   Child will have an effective
breathing pattern as evidenced by

respiratory rate within acceptable range (state specific highest
and lowest rates for each child).
clear and equal breath sounds bilaterally.
temperature within acceptable range of 36.5°C to 37.2°C.
absence of

cough.
nasal discharge.
cyanosis.
retractions.
diaphoresis.

white blood cell count within acceptable range (state specific
highest and lowest counts for each child).
clear chest x-ray.
oxygen saturation (via pulse oximeter) from 85% to 100%.

POSSIBLE NURSING INTERVENTIONS
Assess and record the following every 4 hours and PRN:

respiratory rate and temperature
breath sounds
signs/symptoms of ineffective breathing pattern (such as
those listed under **Characteristics**). Notify physician of
any abnormalities.

Ensure that chest physiotherapy is done on schedule. Record
effectiveness of treatments.

When indicated, administer humidified oxygen in correct
amount and route of delivery. Record percent of oxygen and
route of delivery. Assess and record effectiveness of therapy.

When indicated, administer antibiotics and antipyretics on
schedule. Assess and record their effectiveness and any side
effects (e.g., rash, diarrhea).

Check and record results of chest x-ray and complete blood count (CBC), when indicated.

Suction child PRN if child is unable to clear airway. Record amount and characteristics of secretions.

When using a pulse oximeter, record reading every 2 to 4 hours and PRN.

 Assess and record child's/family's knowledge of and participation in care regarding

chest physiotherapy.
medication administration.
identification of any signs/symptoms of ineffective breathing pattern (such as those listed under **Characteristics**).

 Instruct child/family in any areas needing improvement. Record results.

EVALUATION FOR CHARTING

State highest and lowest respiratory rates and temperatures.

Describe breath sounds.

Describe any signs/symptom of ineffective breathing pattern noted (such as those listed under **Characteristics**).

State whether oxygen was administered and give amount and route of delivery. Describe effectiveness.

Indicate whether chest physiotherapy was performed on schedule. Describe child's tolerance of the procedure. State its effectiveness.

Indicate whether medications were administered on schedule. Describe their effectiveness and any side effects noted.

Describe any therapeutic measures used to maintain an effective breathing pattern. State their effectiveness.

State results of chest x-ray and CBC, when indicated.

Indicate whether child needed suctioning; if so, state frequency. Describe amount and characteristics of secretions.

State range of oxygen saturation.

 Describe child's/family's knowledge of and participation in

care related to maintaining an effective breathing pattern.
State any areas needing improvement and information
provided. Describe family's response.

NURSING DIAGNOSIS
Fluid Volume Deficit

DEFINITION   Decrease in the amount of circulating
fluid volume

POSSIBLY RELATED TO
Respiratory distress
Decreased fluid intake
Increased insensible water loss from rapid respirations
Fever

CHARACTERISTICS
Loss of desire for food or liquids
Listlessness
Lethargy
Fever
Vomiting
Diarrhea
Dry mucous membranes
Poor skin turgor
Decreased urine output

EXPECTED OUTCOMES   Child will have an adequate fluid
volume as evidenced by

adequate fluid intake, IV and/or oral (state specific amount
  of intake needed for each child).
absence of

  lethargy.
  listlessness.
  vomiting
  diarrhea.

temperature within acceptable range of 36.5°C to 37.2°C.
moist mucous membranes.
rapid skin recoil.
adequate urine output (state specific highest and lowest
  outputs for each infant, minimum 1 to 2 ml/kg/hr).
urine specific gravity from 1.008 to 1.020.

POSSIBLE NURSING INTERVENTIONS

Keep accurate record of intake and output. Weigh diapers for output.

Assess and record

temperature every 4 hours and PRN.
IV fluids and condition of IV site every hour.
signs/symptoms of fluid volume deficit (such as those listed under **Characteristics**) every 4 hours and PRN.

Check and record urine specific gravity every 4 hours or as ordered.

Give mouth care every 4 hours and PRN.

Assess and record child's/family's knowledge of and participation in care regarding

offering/accepting of fluids, when indicated.
monitoring of child's intake and output.
identification of any signs/symptoms of fluid volume deficit (such as those listed under **Characteristics**).

Instruct child/family in any areas needing improvement. Record results.

EVALUATION FOR CHARTING

State highest and lowest temperatures.

State intake and output.

State condition of IV site.

Describe any signs/symptoms of fluid volume deficit noted (such as those listed under **Characteristics**).

State highest and lowest urine specific gravity values.

Describe any therapeutic measures used to improve fluid volume. State their effectiveness.

Describe child's/family's knowledge of and participation in care related to improving fluid volume. State any areas needing improvement and information provided. Describe child's/family's responses.

RELATED NURSING DIAGNOSES

Altered Nutrition: Less than Body Requirements
related to
- a. respiratory distress
- b. anorexia
- c. vomiting
- d. increased caloric consumption secondary to infection

Altered Comfort* *related to*
- a. headache
- b. chest pain

Activity Intolerance *related to*
- a. respiratory distress
- b. lethargy
- c. listlessness
- d. decreased fluid and food intake
- e. fever

Anxiety: Child *related to*
- a. hospitalization
- b. respiratory distress

---

*Non-NANDA diagnosis.

MEDICAL DIAGNOSIS
Tuberculosis

PATHOPHYSIOLOGY   Tuberculosis is a bacterial infection caused by tubercle bacillus, a member of the Mycobacteriaceae family. In the United States, disease caused by *Mycobacterium tuberculosis* is most common. In parts of the world that do not control tuberculosis in cattle or pasteurize milk, disease caused by *M. bovis* also exists.

Infection with *M. tuberculosis* occurs when microdroplets contaminated with infectious tuberculosis are inhaled and reach the terminal bronchioles and alveoli. Therefore, most primary lesions are in the lungs. At the focal site, an inflammatory reaction occurs, followed by a localized acute bronchopneumonia. The typical tubercle forms when the proliferating epithelial cells surround and encapsulate the multiplying bacilli in an attempt to wall off the invading organisms. The disease can also spread via intracellular multiplication of tubercle bacilli or via the blood stream from the focal site to the lymph system, the reticuloendothelial system, and other organ systems. The lymph nodes, meninges, and bone are frequently affected. The tuberculosis bacilli has the ability to remain dormant for many years. Reactivation of the disease may occur at a later date if the child's resistance decreases.

Children are usually infected with tuberculosis by adults with progressive cavitary lesions who discharge infected droplets into the air. Prolonged contact (such as through repeated exposure to coughing, kissing, and environmental dust) is necessary before a child will develop the active disease.

Children with tuberculosis may be asymptomatic or develop a broad range of symptoms. The infection often resolves spontaneously without progressing to a clinical disease. Hospitalization is usually needed only for children with the more serious forms of the disease, or to perform diagnostic tests. Isolation is rarely needed as most children with active primary pulmonary tuberculosis are noninfectious. Children are often considered noninfectious as their lesions are limited, output of bacilli is small, and cough is minimal or nonexistent.

Several factors increase the communicability of tuberculosis. Poverty and overcrowding can foster poor hygiene, and malnutrition and fatigue can lower one's resistance to the disease. Currently, the highest rates of infection are among minority groups (e.g., Hispanics, blacks, first-generation immigrants from high-risk countries such as Mexico or Vietnam). Patients with AIDS also have an increased incidence of tuberculosis.

PRIMARY NURSING DIAGNOSIS
Ineffective Airway Clearance

DEFINITION   Condition in which secretions cannot adequately be cleared from the airways

POSSIBLY RELATED TO
Bacterial infection of the lungs

CHARACTERISTICS
Persistent cough (slowly progressing over weeks to months)
Aching pain and tightness in the chest
Fever
Diminished breath sounds
Crackles
Rhonchi
Tachypnea
Wheezing
Stridor
Lobar infiltration, segmental atelectasis, lobar emphysema, or pleural effusion revealed on chest x-ray

EXPECTED OUTCOMES   Child will have adequate airway clearance as evidenced by

respiratory rate within acceptable range (state specific highest and lowest rates for each child).
clear and equal breath sounds bilaterally.
absence of

persistent cough.
aching pain or tightness in the chest.
stridor.

temperature within acceptable range of 36.5°C to 37.2°C.
improved chest x-ray, with absence of atelectasis and pleural
   effusion.

POSSIBLE NURSING INTERVENTIONS

Assess and record the following every 4 hours and PRN:

> respiratory rate and temperature
> breath sounds
> any signs/symptoms of ineffective airway clearance (such
>   as those listed under **Characteristics**)

Administer bacteriocidal antituberculosis agents (e.g.,
isoniazid, rifampin, streptomycin) on schedule. Assess and
record effectiveness and any side effects (e.g., GI discomfort,
hypersensitivity reactions, neurologic complications). If
indicated, administer antipyretics on schedule. Record
effectiveness.

When indicated, administer oxygen in correct amount and
route. Record percent of oxygen and route of delivery. Assess
and record effectiveness.

Ensure that chest physiotherapy is performed on schedule.
Record effectiveness.

Suction gently if infant or child is unable to clear airway.

Encourage fluid intake in order to help liquify secretions.

Elevate head of bed at 30° angle (may use infant seat if
infant can support head in midline position).

Check and record results of chest x-ray, when indicated.

When using a pulse oximeter, record reading every 2 to 4
hours and PRN.

If child produces sputum, instruct child to spit out secretions
in a tissue and dispose of tissue in waste container. Adhere
to Center for Disease Control (CDC) guidelines and/or
institutional policy for precaution/isolation techniques.

Assess and record child's/family's knowledge of and
participation in care regarding

> identification of any signs/symptoms of ineffective airway
>   clearance (such as those listed under **Characteristics**).

medication administration.
disposal of child's tissues.

🏠 Instruct family in any areas needing improvement.
Record results.

EVALUATION FOR CHARTING

Describe breath sounds.

State highest and lowest respiratory rates.

Describe any signs/symptoms of ineffective airway clearance noted (such as those listed under **Characteristics**).

Describe any therapeutic measures used to improve airway clearance. State their effectiveness.

Indicate whether chest physiotherapy was performed on schedule. Describe child's tolerance of the procedure. State its effectiveness.

Indicate whether medications were administered on schedule. Describe effectiveness and any side effects noted.

State whether oxygen was administered and amount and route of delivery. Describe effectiveness.

State results of chest x-ray, when indicated.

State range of oxygen saturation.

🏠 Describe child's/family's knowledge of and participation in care related to improving airway clearance. State any areas needing improvement and information provided. Describe child's/family's responses.

NURSING DIAGNOSIS

Knowledge Deficit: Parental

DEFINITION   Lack of information concerning the child's disease and care

POSSIBLY RELATED TO

Unfamiliarity with child's disease and its communicability
Cognitive or cultural-language limitations
Guilt secondary to child's acquiring disease

CHARACTERISTICS

Verbalization by parent indicating a lack of knowledge regarding tuberculosis and child's care

Relation of incorrect information to members of the health care team

Inability to correctly repeat information previously explained

Inability to correctly demonstrate skills previously taught (e.g., medication administration)

EXPECTED OUTCOMES   Parent will have an adequate knowledge base concerning the child's illness and care as evidenced by

ability to correctly state information previously taught regarding tuberculosis and the child's care (e.g., communicability, need to identify the person from whom the child contracted the illness, testing for other family members, home care, medication administration, compliance with treatment, future testing of child).

ability to correctly demonstrate skills previously taught (e.g., medication administration, hygiene).

ability to relate appropriate information to the health care team.

POSSIBLE NURSING INTERVENTIONS

Listen to parent's concerns and fears.

Assess and record parent's knowledge and understanding of child's illness.

Assess and record parent's knowledge of and participation in care regarding

hygiene.
nutrition.
activity level.
medication administration.
isolation from others who are susceptible.

Instruct parent in any areas needing improvement. Record results.

Assist and observe parent in performing skills previously taught regarding care of child. Record results.

Assign a primary nurse as usual spokesperson to parent.

When indicated, obtain an interpreter.

Dispel any incorrect information.

EVALUATION FOR CHARTING
State whether parent verbalized a knowledge deficit.

🏠 State whether parent was able to repeat information correctly.

🏠 State whether parent was able to adequately perform skills. Describe ability.

Describe any measures used to facilitate parent teaching.

RELATED NURSING DIAGNOSES

Activity Intolerance *related to*
a. fever
b. anorexia
c. increased respiratory effort

Altered Nutrition: Less than Body Requirements
related to
a. increased metabolic state
b. decreased food intake

Noncompliance *related to*
a. long duration of treatment
b. cognitive or cultural-language limitations

Impaired Home Maintenance Management *related to*
a. communicable disease
b. lack of knowledge
c. lack of resources and support systems

ELEVEN

CARE OF CHILDREN WITH UROGENITAL DYSFUNCTION

MEDICAL DIAGNOSIS

Acute Glomerulonephritis

PATHOPHYSIOLOGY Inflammation of the glomeruli is known as glomerulonephritis. Poststreptococcal glomerulonephritis is the most common type in children. Viruses, pharmacological and toxic agents, and autoimmune diseases may also be underlying causes of glomerulonephritis.

The specific pathophysiology of glomerulonephritis remains uncertain. Current theory suggests that glomerulonephritis results from immune-mediated injuries to the glomerulus. One type of injury is caused by antigen-antibody complexes that affix themselves in Bowman's capsule of the kidney, resulting in a proliferative and exudative process (immune complex disease). The antigen-antibody complexes become entrapped in the glomerular membrane, causing obstruction, inflammation, and edema in the kidney. The affected area of the kidney is infiltrated by white blood cells, and the glomerular endothelial and epithelial cells proliferate, become edematous, and occlude the glomeruli. Renal capillary permeability increases, and there is renal vascular spasm. These processes lead to decreased glomerular filtration. Water and sodium are retained, causing increased intravascular and interstitial fluid volume (edema). The edema is usually confined to the face, except in cases of severe disease when it may be more generalized. Proteinuria occurs when the nonoccluded glomeruli malfunction and allow large amounts of protein to leak into the glomerular filtrate. If the membranes rupture, red cells may pass into the urine (hematuria) as well. A child with glomerulonephritis also experiences oliguria and hypertension.

Injury to the glomerulus can also occur when antibodies are directed against antigens on the glomerular basement membrane (antiglomerular basement membrane disease). In this process, the complement system is activated, attracting the white blood cells to the glomerular basement membrane. These white blood cells, as in immune complex disease, initiate the damage to the glomerular basement membrane.

Primary Nursing Diagnosis
Fluid Volume Excess

DEFINITION   Increase in the amount of circulating fluid volume (which can eventually lead to interstitial or intracellular fluid overload)

POSSIBLY RELATED TO
Poststreptococcal infection
Antigen-antibody reaction
Pathological changes in the glomeruli

CHARACTERISTICS
Oliguria
Microscopic or gross hematuria (coke- or tea-colored urine)
Proteinuria
Increased specific gravity (>1.030)
Edema (usually facial, especially periorbital)
Hypertension
Headache
Sudden weight gain
Increased blood urea nitrogen (BUN)

EXPECTED OUTCOMES   Child will resume fluid balance as evidenced by

adequate urine output (state specific highest and lowest outputs for each child, minimum 1 to 2 ml/kg/hr).
clear, pale yellow urine.
blood pressure within acceptable range (state specific highest and lowest pressures for each child).
lack of

proteinuria.
hematuria.
edema.
headache.
sudden weight gain.

urine specific gravity from 1.008 to 1.020.
BUN from 5 to 18 mg/dL.

POSSIBLE NURSING INTERVENTIONS
Keep accurate record of intake and output. Be sure that child does not exceed maximum intake ordered. Record

characteristics of urine output, including presence of proteinuria and hematuria.

Check and record urine specific gravity every void or as indicated.

Assess and record

> signs/symptoms of fluid volume excess (such as those listed under **Characteristics**) every 4 hours and PRN.
> amount and location of edema at least once/shift.
> blood pressure every 4 hours and PRN.
> laboratory values, as indicated. Report abnormalities to the physician.
> condition of IV site every hour.

Weigh child on same scale at same time each day. Determine if weight has increased or decreased since previous weighing.

Administer diuretics (e.g., furosemide) and antihypertensive medications (e.g., hydralazine) on schedule. Assess and record effectiveness and any side effects (e.g., headache, nausea/vomiting, diarrhea, tachycardia).

When indicated, restrict dietary sodium and/or potassium.

⌂ Assess and record child's/family's knowledge of and participation in care regarding

> monitoring of intake and output.
> fluid restriction.
> identification of signs/symptoms of excess fluid volume (such as those listed under **Characteristics**).
> medication administration.
> diet restrictions, when indicated.

⌂ Instruct child and family in any areas needing improvement. Record results.

EVALUATION FOR CHARTING

State intake and output. Describe characteristics of urine output.

Describe any signs/symptoms of fluid volume excess (such as those listed under **Characteristics**).

State highest and lowest blood pressures.

State child's weight and determine whether it has increased or decreased since the previous weighing.

State highest and lowest urine specific gravity values.

State current laboratory values.

Describe condition of IV site.

State whether medications were administered on schedule. Describe effectiveness and any side effects noted.

Describe any therapeutic measures used to improve fluid balance. State their effectiveness.

🏠 Describe child's/family's knowledge of and participation in care related to improving fluid balance. State any areas needing improvement and information provided. Describe responses.

NURSING DIAGNOSIS
Body Image Disturbance

DEFINITION Condition in which the child has a negative self-view

POSSIBLY RELATED TO
Facial/periorbital edema
Sudden weight gain

CHARACTERISTICS
Verbalization of displeasure in body
Refusal to look in mirror
Refusal to participate in care or play and social activities
Decreased interest in appearance

EXPECTED OUTCOMES Child will indicate acceptance of body image as evidenced by

ability to verbally describe self positively.
ability to look in the mirror.
willingness to participate in care.
willingness to participate in play and social activities.
developmentally appropriate interest in appearance.

POSSIBLE NURSING INTERVENTIONS

Assess and record any signs/symptoms of body image disturbance (such as those listed under **Characteristics**).

Assess and record child's/family's ability to accept altered body image.

Encourage child to express feelings, fears, or concerns regarding appearance.

Clarify any misconceptions child may express regarding illness and change in appearance.

Provide child with opportunities for age-appropriate therapeutic play.

Encourage child/family to participate in care when possible.

Encourage child to maintain usual state of grooming and appearance.

Encourage child/family to focus on nonphysical qualities.

📷 Assess and record child's/family's knowledge of and participation in care regarding promoting a positive self-image.

📷 Instruct child/family in any areas needing improvement. Record results.

EVALUATION FOR CHARTING

Describe child's/family's ability to accept altered body image.

Describe any methods successful in helping child/family cope with child's altered body image.

State whether child/family participated in care.

State whether child showed appropriate interest in his or her appearance.

📷 Describe child's/family's knowledge of and participation in care related to promoting a positive self-image. State any areas needing improvement and information provided. Describe child's/family's responses.

RELATED NURSING DIAGNOSES

Activity Intolerance *related to*
fatigue

Impaired Skin Integrity *related to*
   a. immobility
   b. edema

Knowledge Deficit: Child/Parental *related to*
   home care secondary to diet restrictions and medication
   administration

Altered Nutrition: Less than Body Requirements
related to
   anorexia

MEDICAL DIAGNOSIS
Chronic Renal Failure

PATHOPHYSIOLOGY   In chronic renal failure (CRF), kidney function deteriorates over time as the nephrons suffer irreversible damage. The causes of CRF vary, with congenital abnormalities and infections of the kidneys and urinary tract being the most common. Other causes include glomerulonephritis, acute tubular necrosis, diabetes mellitus, immune system disorders, metabolic disorders, and obstructions.

Insult to the kidneys results in tissue scarring and structural and functional damage to the nephrons, especially to the glomeruli. Initially undamaged nephrons compensate, but eventually nephron function deterioration becomes secondary to injury from hyperfiltration (the increased filtration load) and renal insufficiency. The glomerular filtration rate (GFR) continues to decrease, impairing the body's ability to excrete nitrogenous wastes, causing metabolic, biochemical, and clinical disturbances.

There are three stages of CRF. In Stage I, the child has decreased renal reserve but is asymptomatic and has normal blood urea nitrogen (BUN) and serum creatinine levels. In Stage II, the child suffers renal insufficiency. More than 75% of the nephrons are destroyed, reducing the GFR to 25% of normal, and BUN and serum creatinine levels are rising. In end stage renal disease (ESRD), Stage III, 90% of the nephrons have been destroyed, the GFR is 10% of normal, and BUN and serum creatinine levels rise sharply.

Azotemia and/or uremia, an elevation in BUN and creatinine levels, occurs as renal function decreases and nitrogenous wastes are retained. Metabolic acidosis occurs for several reasons: the blood levels of acids increase because of their decreased excretion, the kidney is unable to excrete hydrogen ions, the distal tubules' ability to produce ammonia is decreased, and urinary bicarbonate wasting related to impaired tubular function occurs. Decreased GFR and abnormal reabsorptive function in damaged tubules result in fluid alterations and electrolyte imbalances as well.

Sodium and fluid excretion may initially increase as the undamaged nephrons try to compensate by filtering an increased solute load, causing diuresis with possible dehydration. As renal failure progresses, the very low GFR and the continued alterations in the kidneys' dilutional ability cause sodium and fluid retention. An activated renin-angiotensin system leads to hyperaldosteronism, further compounding sodium and water retention. Hypoproteinemia, caused by the excessive loss of serum proteins through the damaged glomeruli, can compound the already existing edema.

As long as fluid and acid-base balance are maintained, hyperkalemia is not a problem in children with CRF. Hyperkalemia can occur, though, from the ingestion of a large potassium load, from hemolysis, as metabolic acidosis ensues, or from a catabolic state associated with fever.

Impaired renal absorption of calcium and decreased tubular excretion of phosphorus result in hypocalcemia and hyperphosphatemia, which in turn cause a rebound effect of increased parathyroid hormone production. Calcium absorption from the gastrointestinal tract is reduced as the increased phosphorus level impairs the kidney's ability to produce usable vitamin D. Hypocalcemia causes bone resorption and bone abnormalities collectively known as renal osteodystrophy.

Impaired red cell production and a shortened red blood cell life span due to uremia result in anemia. Impaired release of stored iron, inadequate iron intake, and the detrimental effects of nitrogenous wastes on platelet function lead to bleeding tendencies and also contribute to the anemia. The severity of the anemia is proportional to the decline in renal function.

The child with CRF can develop growth retardation, affected by such factors as the etiology of the primary disease, the age of onset, acidosis, and the presence of renal osteodystrophy.

The onset of CRF is insidious, with the symptoms often presenting only after severe kidney damage has occurred. The child with CRF may present with edema, symptomatic hypertension, gross hematuria, or a urinary tract infection. Most children with chronic renal failure are treated conservatively with pharmacologic, dietetic, and supportive therapy. Dialysis or kidney transplantation are considered when conservative measures no longer allow the child to function normally or when uremia is no longer preventable.

PRIMARY NURSING DIAGNOSIS
Altered Metabolic Function*

DEFINITION   Imbalance or altered utilization of specific body biochemicals

POSSIBLY RELATED TO
Accumulation of nitrogenous waste products, decreased ammonia excretion, decreased acid excretion, and fluid and electrolyte imbalances secondary to irreversibly damaged nephrons

CHARACTERISTICS
Elevated BUN (>20 mg/dL)
Elevated serum creatinine level (>1.5 mg/dL)
Decreased serum bicarbonate (<20 mEq/L)
Skin dryness
Pruritis (uremic frost)
Uremic breath
Nausea
Vomiting
Anorexia
Uremic neuropathy (muscle cramps, tetany, weakness, muscle wasting)
Uremic encephalopathy (irritability, lethargy, seizures)

EXPECTED OUTCOMES   Child will have improved metabolic function as evidenced by

BUN from 5 to 18 mg/dL.
serum creatinine from 0.3 to 1.0 mg/dL.
serum bicarbonate >20 mEq/L.
lack of signs/symptoms of altered metabolic balance (such as those listed under **Characteristics**).

POSSIBLE NURSING INTERVENTIONS
Assess and record

signs/symptoms of altered metabolic function (such as those listed under **Characteristics**) every 4 hours and PRN.

---
*Non-NANDA diagnosis.

laboratory values, as indicated. Report any abnormalities to the physician.

When indicated, ensure that peritoneal dialysis is done according to institutional policy, including

maintaining a closed sterile system.
using aseptic technique whenever the system is opened.
warming the dialysate.
obtaining daily cultures (e.g. site, fluid).
changing the tubing and catheter site dressing using sterile technique.

When indicated, ensure that child keeps scheduled hemodialysis appointments. Assess and record condition of access site.

When indicated, restrict dietary protein intake (approximately 1.5 g/kg/24 hr).

Administer sodium bicarbonate tablets on schedule. Assess and record effectiveness.

Initiate and maintain consultation with dietician.

⌂ Initiate and maintain consultation with visiting nurses and/or other home care providers.

⌂ Consult social services to assist the family in identifying and using available resources (e.g., financial, transportation).

⌂ Assess and record child's/family's knowledge of and participation in care regarding

identification of signs/symptoms of altered metabolic function (such as those listed under **Characteristics**).
dietary protein restrictions.
compliance with dialysis schedule and techniques.
appropriate use of services of health care professionals and other available resources.

⌂ Instruct child/family in any areas needing improvement. Record results.

EVALUATION FOR CHARTING
State current laboratory values.

Describe any signs/symptoms of altered metabolic function (such as those listed under **Characteristics**).

State whether medications were administered on schedule. Describe effectiveness and any side effects noted.

State whether dialysis was used. Describe procedure and child's response.

Describe any therapeutic measures used to improve metabolic function. State their effectiveness.

🏠 Describe child's/family's knowledge of and participation in care regarding improving metabolic function. State any areas needing improvement and information provided. Describe responses.

NURSING DIAGNOSIS

Fluid Volume Imbalance: Deficit (Intravascular) and/or Excess (Extravascular or Intravascular)

DEFINITION   Decrease in the amount of circulating fluid volume *and/or* interstitial fluid overload *or* increased intravascular volume (which can eventually lead to interstitial or intracellular fluid overload)

POSSIBLY RELATED TO
Reduced renal function due to irreversible nephron damage secondary to

> glomerular diseases
> congenital abnormalities of the kidneys or urinary tract (e.g., renal hypoplasia, severe bilateral vesicoureteral reflux)
> pyelonephritis with reflux
> hereditary renal diseases
> miscellaneous disorders

CHARACTERISTICS
Initial polydipsia
Diuresis
Nocturia or polyuria (in renal insufficiency where more than 75% of the nephrons are destroyed and GFR is 25% of normal)
Oliguria
Edema

Hypertension
Either dehydration or circulatory overload with tachycardia,
  tachypnea, and crackles
Unconcentrated urine

EXPECTED OUTCOMES   Child will have improved fluid
balance as evidenced by

adequate urine output (state specific highest and lowest
  outputs for each child, minimum 1 to 2 ml/kg/hr).
lack of

  edema.
  dehydration.
  circulatory overload, accompanied by tachycardia,
    tachypnea, and/or crackles.
  polydipsia.

blood pressure within acceptable range (state specific highest
  and lowest pressures for each child).

POSSIBLE NURSING INTERVENTIONS
Keep accurate record of intake and output. If Foley catheter
is in place, note hourly output. Maintain aseptic technique
when emptying urine and caring for catheter.

Restrict or replace fluids, as indicated. Assess and record
child's response.

Assess and record

  signs/symptoms of fluid imbalance (such as those listed
    under **Characteristics**) every 4 hours and PRN.
  blood pressure every 4 hours and PRN.
  IV fluids and condition of IV site every hour.

Weigh child on same scale at same time each day.

When indicated, administer diuretics and antihypertensives
on schedule (ensure that dose has been adjusted to avoid
toxicity from inadequate renal clearance). Assess and record
effectiveness and any side effects (e.g., headache, nausea/
vomiting, diarrhea, tachycardia).

When indicated, restrict dietary sodium intake.

When indicated, ensure that peritoneal dialysis is done
according to institutional policy, including

maintaining a closed sterile system.

using aseptic technique whenever the system is opened.

warming the dialysate.

obtaining daily cultures (e.g. site, fluid).

changing the tubing and catheter site dressing using sterile technique.

When indicated, ensure that child keeps scheduled hemodialysis appointments. Assess and record condition of access site.

Record child's response to dialysis.

Initiate and maintain consultation with dietician.

Initiate and maintain consultation with visiting nurses and/or other home care providers.

Consult social services to assist family in identifying and using available resources (e.g., financial, transportation).

Assess and record child's/family's knowledge of and participation in care regarding

monitoring of intake and output.

medication administration.

dietary changes.

identification of any signs/symptoms of fluid imbalance (such as those listed under **Characteristics**).

compliance with dialysis schedule and techniques.

appropriate use of services of health care professionals and other available resources.

Instruct child/family in any areas needing improvement. Record results.

EVALUATION FOR CHARTING

State intake and output.

Describe condition of IV site.

State highest and lowest blood pressures.

Describe any signs/symptoms of fluid imbalance noted (such as those listed under **Characteristics**).

State child's weight and determine whether it has increased or decreased since previous weighing.

State whether medications were administered on schedule. Describe effectiveness and any side effects noted.

State whether dialysis was used. Describe procedure and child's response.

⌂ Describe child's/family's knowledge of and participation in care regarding improving fluid balance. State any areas needing improvement and information provided. Describe responses.

RELATED NURSING DIAGNOSES

Electrolyte Imbalance: Sodium Excess, Potassium Excess, Calcium Losses, Phosphate Losses* *related to* irreversibly damaged nephrons

Altered Nutrition: Less than Body Requirements *related to*
   a. anorexia
   b. nausea
   c. vomiting
   d. inadequate intake
   e. catabolic state

Altered Growth and Development *related to*
   a. frequent biochemical and metabolic disturbances secondary to irreversible dysfunction
   b. noncompliance with treatment plan

Body Image Disturbance *related to*
   a. altered growth and development
   b. dependency upon a dialysis machine
   c. edema

---

*Non-NANDA diagnosis.

MEDICAL DIAGNOSIS
Nephrotic Syndrome

PATHOPHYSIOLOGY Nephrotic syndrome, a condition that results in alteration of renal function, is characterized by hypoproteinemia, edema, hyperlipidemia, proteinuria, ascites, and decreased urinary output. It usually affects preschool children and can be classified as congenital, idiopathic, or secondary to another disease. Congenital nephrotic syndrome is rare and responds poorly to the usual therapy. Infants generally succumb to this form of the disease in the first or second year of life. The secondary form of the disease develops during the course of other illnesses, such as acute or chronic glomerulonephritis, systemic lupus erythematosus, or diabetes mellitus, or it may occur as the result of drug toxicity. Idiopathic nephrotic syndrome, also called minimal change nephrotic syndrome (MCNS), is the most common form of the disease (approximately 90%). The cause of MCNS is unknown.

The pathogenesis of nephrotic syndrome is not clearly understood. A disturbance in the basement membrane of the glomeruli leads to increased permeability, which allows protein (especially albumin) to leak into the urine (proteinuria). This shift of protein out of the vascular system causes fluid from the plasma to seep into the interstitial spaces. Edema and hypovolemia result. The reduced vascular volume stimulates the renin-angiotensin system, which in turn leads to the secretion of aldosterone and antidiuretic hormone (ADH). Aldosterone increases the distal tubular reabsorption of sodium and water, adding to the edema already present. The hyperlipidemia is thought to occur because the lipoproteins are of higher molecular weight than albumin and therefore are not lost in the urine.

PRIMARY NURSING DIAGNOSIS

Fluid Volume Imbalance: Deficit (Intravascular)/Excess (Extravascular)*

DEFINITION   Disturbance in the amount of circulating fluid volume with a decrease in intravascular fluid volume and an interstitial fluid overload

POSSIBLY RELATED TO
Protein loss in the urine secondary to increased permeability of the glomeruli

Increased water and sodium reabsorption from renal tubules secondary to increased secretion of aldosterone

CHARACTERISTICS
Marked generalized edema

Ascites

Possible diarrhea secondary to edema of the intestinal mucosa

Dramatic weight gain

Hypoproteinemia

Hyperlipidemia

Proteinuria

Decreased urine output

Frothy, dark-colored urine

Blood pressure within acceptable limits or slightly decreased (usually)

EXPECTED OUTCOMES   Child will have an adequate intracellular and extracellular fluid volume as evidenced by

lack of

edema.
ascites.
hypoproteinemia.
hyperlipidemia.
proteinuria.
diarrhea.

return to usual weight.

---

*Non-NANDA diagnosis.

adequate urine output (state specific highest and lowest outputs for each child, minimum 1 to 2 ml/kg/hr).

clear, pale yellow urine.

blood pressure within acceptable range (state specific highest and lowest pressures for each child).

POSSIBLE NURSING INTERVENTIONS

Keep accurate record of intake and output. Record characteristics of urine output.

Assess and record every 4 hours and PRN:

blood pressure
abdominal girth
signs/symptoms of fluid imbalance (such as those listed under **Characteristics**)
strip-test on urine for presence of protein
laboratory values, as indicated. Report any abnormalities to the physician

Weigh child on same scale at same time each day without clothes.

Handle edematous areas gently. Males may need to wear a scrotal support if scrotal edema is present.

Administer steroids (prednisone) on schedule. Assess and record effectiveness and any side effects (e.g., sodium retention, potassium loss).

If indicated, administer diuretics (to combat edema) and antacids (to help prevent complication of GI bleeding from steroid therapy) on schedule. Assess and record effectiveness and any side effects (e.g., hypokalemia, dehydration).

Assess and record child's/family's knowledge of and participation in care regarding

monitoring of intake and output.
test for protein in urine.
medication administration.
recognition of subtle signs/symptoms of infection; side effects of steroids may mask signs of infection.
identification of any signs/symptoms of fluid imbalance (such as those listed under **Characteristics**).

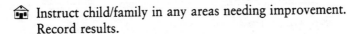 Instruct child/family in any areas needing improvement. Record results.

EVALUATION FOR CHARTING

State intake and output. Describe characteristics of urine output.

State highest and lowest blood pressures.

State current abdominal girth and indicate whether it has increased or decreased since previous measurement.

State range of urine protein testing.

Describe any signs/symptoms of fluid imbalance noted (such as those listed under **Characteristics**).

State current weight and indicate whether it has increased or decreased since previous weighing.

State whether medications were administered on schedule. Describe effectiveness and any side effects noted.

Describe any therapeutic measures used to maintain adequate fluid balance. State their effectiveness.

 Describe child's/family's knowledge of and participation in care related to maintaining adequate fluid volume. State any areas needing improvement and information provided. Describe child's/family's responses.

NURSING DIAGNOSIS

Altered Nutrition: Less than Body Requirements

DEFINITION   Insufficient nutrients to meet body requirements

POSSIBLY RELATED TO

Malnutrition secondary to protein loss and poor appetite
Poor intestinal absorption secondary to edema of the
intestinal mucosa

CHARACTERISTICS

Anorexia
Lethargy

Hypoproteinemia
Diarrhea

EXPECTED OUTCOMES Child will be adequately nourished as evidenced by

absorption of adequate amount of calories (state specific amount for each child).
return of appetite.
lack of hypoproteinemia.

POSSIBLE NURSING INTERVENTIONS

Keep accurate record of intake and output.

Assess and record any signs/symptoms of altered nutrition (such as those listed under **Characteristics**) every 4 hours and PRN.

Ensure that child gets prescribed diet (usually high in protein with no added table salt).

Encourage child to eat by assessing likes/dislikes and, when possible, providing foods that child likes to eat.

Organize care to conserve energy.

Assess and record child's/family's knowledge of and participation in care regarding

diet high in protein with no added table salt.
organization of care and activity of child in order to conserve energy.
identification of any signs/symptoms of altered nutrition (such as those listed under **Characteristics**).

Instruct child/family in any areas needing improvement. Record results.

EVALUATION FOR CHARTING

State intake and output.

Describe any signs/symptoms of altered nutrition (such as those listed under **Characteristics**).

Describe any therapeutic measures used to maintain adequate nutrition. State their effectiveness.

Describe child's/family's knowledge of and participation in care related to improving nutritional status. State any areas

needing improvement and information provided. Describe child's/family's responses.

RELATED NURSING DIAGNOSES

Infection: High Risk *related to*
    a. edema fluid being excellent culture medium
    b. thin and stretched skin secondary to edema
    c. lowered resistance secondary to steroid therapy

Knowledge Deficit: Child/Family *related to*
    disease state and home care

Impaired Skin Integrity *related to*
    edema

Body Image Disturbance *related to*
    edema

MEDICAL DIAGNOSIS
Vesicoureteral Reflux

PATHOPHYSIOLOGY   Vesicoureteral reflux (VUR) is the abnormal backflow of urine from the bladder into the ureters and possibly into the kidneys. Normally urine flows downward from the kidneys through the ureters into the bladder. The ureters are positioned at the posterior, lower aspect of the bladder at an oblique angle and tunnel through the bladder mucosa for a short distance before opening into the bladder. When the bladder becomes full of urine and voiding begins, the pressure in the bladder is increased and the bladder musculature contracts, compressing the tunneled portion of the ureters (similar to a valve) and preventing backflow of urine into the ureters. When voiding is complete, the bladder relaxes and the ureteral openings may drain once again.

Reflux occurs when the mechanism for compressing the tunneled portion of the ureters malfunctions. Primary reflux occurs with a congenital malformation in which the ureters enter the bladder at an abnormal acute angle and the tunneling of the ureters in the bladder mucosa is shortened, resulting in decreased compression. When pressure builds in the bladder, urine refluxes up into the ureters. If pressure is high enough, the urine can reflux into the kidneys and eventually cause hydronephrosis and renal damage. When voiding is complete, the bladder wall relaxes and the urine that was refluxed into the ureters returns to the bladder. Secondary reflux occurs as a result of chronic infection or from increased pressure secondary to bladder outlet obstruction. When infection is present, the resulting edema renders the valvular mechanism of constricting the tunneled portion of the ureters incompetent. Vesicoureteral reflux ranges from mild to severe, with grading system from I to V used to describe the degree. In Grade I, urine is refluxed into the lower ureters only; Grade V indicates gross reflux and dilatation of the ureters, renal pelvis, and calyces.

Most cases of VUR can be treated with conservative (nonsurgical) medical management, which includes continuous low-dose antibacterial therapy with frequent urine cultures. The goal of therapy is to prevent urinary tract infections. If reflux is mild, it usually resolves spontaneously. Surgical correction is employed when (1) there is a significant anatomic abnormality, (2) the reflux is severe enough to cause ureteral dilatation and upper urinary tract dysfunction, and (3) there is noncompliance with medical therapy or intolerance to antibiotics. When surgery is indicated, the ureters are reimplanted into the bladder at an oblique angle and the tunneled portion of the ureters in the submucosal wall is lengthened to correct the angle at which the ureters enter the bladder.

POSTOPERATIVE NURSING CARE PLAN FOR URETERAL IMPLANTATION

PRIMARY NURSING DIAGNOSIS
Infection: High Risk

DEFINITION   Condition in which the body is at risk for being invaded by microorganisms

POSSIBLY RELATED TO
>Surgical procedure
>Invasive urinary devices (urinary stents, suprapubic catheter)

CHARACTERISTICS
>Fever
>Redness
>Swelling
>Purulent wound drainage
>Foul-smelling urine
>Cloudy, hazy, or thick urine
>Lower abdominal pain
>Lethargy
>Anorexia
>Chills
>Leukocytosis

EXPECTED OUTCOMES   Child will be free of infection as evidenced by

>body temperature between 36.5°C and 37.2°C.
>clear, pale yellow urine.
>return of appetite.

white blood cell count(WBC) within acceptable range (state specific highest and lowest counts for each child).

lack of signs/symptoms of infection (such as those listed under **Characteristics**).

POSSIBLE NURSING INTERVENTIONS

Assess and record

temperature every 4 hours and PRN.

IV fluids and condition of IV site every hour.

signs/symptoms of infection (such as those listed under **Characteristics**) every 4 hours and PRN.

Maintain good handwashing technique.

Keep accurate record of intake and output. Use aseptic technique when emptying urine collection bags. Keep all measurements from stents (ureteral catheters used to maintain patency and divert urine while healing occurs) and catheter separate. Check and record urine output every hour for the first 24 hours and then at least every 4 hours. Decreased output from a stent could indicated obstruction. Record characteristics of urine.

Secure tubing attached to stents and catheter with tape in order to prevent displacement. Include a stress loop for additional protection.

Use aseptic technique when dressing changes are indicated.

Unattended children may need wrist restraints to prevent dislodgement of tubes.

Administer antibiotics on schedule. Assess and record effectiveness and any side effects (e.g., rash, diarrhea).

Administer antipyretics as directed. Assess and record effectiveness.

Check and record results of WBC. Notify physician if WBC results are out of the stated range.

Ensure that proper collection of urine specimens for culture are obtained as indicated. Make sure that specimens are sent to the laboratory immediately after collection. Record results when available.

 Assess and record child's/family's knowledge of and participation in care regarding

handwashing technique.

home care and prevention of recurrent urinary tract
    infections, including

- recognition of signs/symptoms.
- administration of antibiotics when indicated.
- need for reminding child to empty bladder
  frequently.
- proper collection of urine specimens, when
  indicated.
- need for reminding child to wear clean cotton
  underwear.
- good hygienic habits. Teach females to wipe the
  perineal area from front to back.
- avoidance of harsh detergents and bubble baths.
- reminding child to drink liquids frequently.
  (Cranberry juice can help keep urine acidic.)
- avoidance of tight-fitting clothing.
- reminding sexually active adolescent to urinate as
  soon as possible after intercourse.

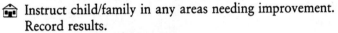 Instruct child/family in any areas needing improvement.
Record results.

EVALUATION FOR CHARTING

State highest and lowest temperatures.

Describe condition of IV site.

Describe any signs/symptoms of infection (such as those
listed under **Characteristics**).

State intake and output. Describe characteristics of urine.

State whether antibiotics were administered on schedule.
Describe effectiveness and any side effects noted.

State whether antipyretics were administered as directed.
Describe their effectiveness in reducing fever and increasing
child's level of comfort.

State results of WBC and urine cultures, if available.

Describe any therapeutic measures used to treat or help
prevent infection. State their effectiveness.

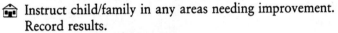 Describe child's/family's knowledge of and participation in
care regarding treatment of future infections. State any areas
needing improvement and information provided. Describe
child's/family's responses.

NURSING DIAGNOSIS
Pain

DEFINITION   Condition in which an individual experiences severe discomfort

POSSIBLY RELATED TO
Surgical incisions
Bladder spasms

CHARACTERISTICS
Verbal communication of pain
Crying unrelieved by usual comfort measures
Decreased activity, self-imposed
Physical signs/symptoms:

tachycardia
tachypnea/bradypnea
increased blood pressure
diaphoresis

EXPECTED OUTCOMES   Child will be free of extreme pain as evidenced by

verbal communication of decreased pain.
lack of constant crying.
increase in activity.
heart rate, respiratory rate, and blood pressure within
acceptable ranges (state specific parameters for each child).
decrease in or lack of diaphoresis.

POSSIBLE NURSING INTERVENTIONS
Assess and record any signs/symptoms of pain (such as those listed under **Characteristics**) every 2 hours and PRN.

Handle child gently.

Encourage family members to stay and comfort child when possible.

Administer analgesics and/or antispasmodics (for relief of bladder and ureter spasms) on schedule. Assess and record effectiveness and any side effects (e.g., GI disturbance, vertigo).

When indicated, institute additional pain relief measures, such as relaxation and music. Assess and record effectiveness.

Use diversional activities and distraction measures (e.g., toys, play activities, television) when appropriate.

EVALUATION FOR CHARTING

Describe any signs/symptoms of pain noted (such as those listed under **Characteristics**).

State range of vital signs.

State whether analgesics and/or antispasmodics were administered. Describe effectiveness and any side effects noted.

Describe any therapeutic measures used to decrease pain. State their effectiveness.

RELATED NURSING DIAGNOSES

Knowledge Deficit: Child/Family *related to*
  a. postoperative care of child
  b. prevention of further urinary tract infections

Compromised Family Coping *related to*
  a. hospitalization of child
  b. guilt (if parents/family were noncompliant with medical management in past)

Fear: Child *related to*
  a. hospitalization
  b. forced contact with strangers
  c. treatments and procedures

Activity Intolerance *related to*
  a. immobilization secondary to protection of tubes
  b. postoperative state

Urinary Tract Infection/ Pyelonephritis

PATHOPHYSIOLOGY   Urinary tract infections (UTI) are caused by bacterial invasion of a normally sterile area in the urinary tract. Cystitis occurs when the infection is limited to the bladder or lower urinary tract; involvement of the upper urinary tract or kidneys is called pyelonephritis. Organisms can enter the system through the blood stream (blood-borne), but more often they enter through the genital area, ascending through the urethra into the bladder. Facilitating entry of bacteria into the urinary system are structural factors (e.g., the short urethra and its close proximity to the anus in females), anatomical anomalies (e.g., obstruction, which may lead to reflux of urine from the bladder through the ureters to the kidneys because of the high voiding pressure needed to overcome the obstruction), urinary stasis (e.g., inadequate bladder innervation or neurogenic bladder), and introduction of urinary catheters. The bacterial organisms usually responsible are *Escherichia coli* (75% to 90% of the time), *Klebsiella,* enteric *Streptococci,* and *Staphylococcus epidermidis.*

The inflammation resulting from the bacterial invasion causes irritability and spasms of the bladder wall. The inflammation may also lead to hematuria. Changes in the bladder wall can occur after repeated infections, which may damage the vesicoureteral valves (where ureters enter the bladder) and result in reflux of urine into the ureters, especially during voiding. The ureters can become dilated and allow access of urine and bacteria into the upper urinary tract. Bacteria that reach the kidneys can cause inflammation, edema, necrosis of the renal cortex, scarring, and loss of renal tissue. The normal concentrating and filtering mechanisms of the kidneys may also be impaired.

Clinical manifestations vary with age and the area involved along the urinary tract. Urinary tract infections are more frequent in females except during the newborn period. The higher incidence of UTIs in males during that period is thought to be due to the increased incidence of anatomic abnormalities.

PRIMARY NURSING DIAGNOSIS
Actual Infection*

DEFINITION   Condition in which microorganisms have invaded the body

POSSIBLY RELATED TO
Bacterial invasion of urinary tract secondary to

    entry of organisms through blood or perineal area
    anatomic anomaly
    inadequate bladder innervation (neurogenic bladder)

CHARACTERISTICS

INFANTS: CYSTITIS OR PYELONEPHRITIS

    Vomiting
    Diarrhea
    Irritability
    Lethargy
    Poor feeding
    Slow weight gain
    Unexplained jaundice
    Fever or hypothermia
    Abdominal distention
    Weak urine stream
    Frequency or infrequent voiding
    Strong-smelling urine
    Persistent diaper rash

CHILDREN: CYSTITIS

    Dysuria
    Frequency
    Urgency
    Lower abdominal pain
    Foul-smelling urine
    Hematuria
    Incontinence
    Enuresis

---

*Non-NANDA diagnosis.

CHILDREN: PYELONEPHRITIS

Fever
Chills
Nausea
Anorexia
Vomiting
Malaise
Lower back pain over costovertebral angle
Cloudy, hazy, or thick urine
Leukocytosis

EXPECTED OUTCOMES   Child will be free of infection as evidenced by

body temperature between 36.5°C and 37.2°C.
clear, pale yellow urine.
return of appetite.
urine specific gravity from 1.008 to 1.020.
white blood cell count (WBC) within acceptable range (state specific highest and lowest counts for each child).
lack of signs/symptoms of infection (such as those listed under **Characteristics**).

POSSIBLE NURSING INTERVENTIONS

Assess and record

temperature every 4 hours and PRN.
IV fluids and condition of IV site every hour.
signs/symptoms of infection (such as those listed under **Characteristics**) every 4 hours and PRN.

Keep accurate record of intake and output. Record characteristics of urine.

Maintain good handwashing technique.

Administer antibiotics on schedule. Assess and record effectiveness and any side effects (e.g. rash, diarrhea).

Administer antipyretics/analgesics as directed. Assess and record effectiveness.

Check and record urine specific gravity every void or as directed.

Check and record results of WBC. Notify physician if WBC results are out of the stated range.

Ensure that urine specimens for culture are obtained as indicated. Make sure that the specimens are sent to the laboratory immediately after collection. Record results when available.

Assess and record child's/family's knowledge of and participation in care regarding

> handwashing technique.
> urine specimen collection.
> identification of any signs/symptoms of infection (such as those listed under **Characteristics**).

Instruct child/family in any areas needing improvement. Record results.

EVALUATION FOR CHARTING

State highest and lowest temperatures.

Describe condition of IV site.

Describe any signs/symptoms of infection (such as those listed under **Characteristics**).

State intake and output. Describe characteristics of urine.

State whether antibiotics were administered on schedule. Describe effectiveness and any side effects noted.

State whether antipyretics/analgesics were administered as directed. Describe effectiveness in reducing fever and increasing child's level of comfort.

State results of WBC and urine cultures, if available.

Describe any therapeutic measures used to treat the infection. State their effectiveness.

Describe child's/family's knowledge of and participation in care regarding treatment of infection. State any areas needing improvement and information provided. Describe child's/family's responses.

NURSING DIAGNOSIS
Knowledge Deficit: Child/Family

DEFINITION Lack of information concerning the child's disease and care

POSSIBLY RELATED TO
Disease state
Cause of infection
Recognition of signs/symptoms
Prevention of recurrent infections
Sensory overload
Cognitive or cultural-language limitations

CHARACTERISTICS
Verbalization by child/family indicating lack of knowledge
Relation of incorrect information to members of the health
care team
Request for information

EXPECTED OUTCOMES   Child/family will have an adequate
knowledge base concerning the child's disease state and care as
evidenced by

ability to correctly state information previously taught
regarding home care, including prevention of recurrent
infections.
ability to relate appropriate information to the health
care team.

POSSIBLE NURSING INTERVENTIONS
Listen to child's/family's concerns and fears.

Assess and record child's/family's knowledge concerning the
disease state and care of the child.

Prepare child/family for any tests (e.g., IV pyelogram, voiding
cystourethrogram) by explaining the procedure and the
rationale for doing the procedure.

🏠 Provide child/family with information about the disease state,
including

definition and etiology.
treatments and prognosis.
home care and prevention of recurrence by
• recognition of signs/symptoms.
• administration of antibiotics for entire prescribed
course (even though child usually gets better before
antibiotic therapy is completed).
• reminding child to empty bladder frequently.
• proper collection of urine specimens when indicated.

- reminding child to wear clean cotton underwear.
- good hygienic habits. Teach females to wipe the perineal area from front to back.
- avoidance of harsh detergents and bubble baths.
- reminding child to drink liquids frequently. (Cranberry juice can help keep urine acidic.)
- avoidance of tight-fitting clothing.
- reminding sexually active adolescent to urinate as soon as possible after intercourse.

EVALUATION FOR CHARTING

State whether child/family verbalized a knowledge deficit.

State whether child/family were able to repeat information correctly.

State whether parents were able to perform skills previously taught (e.g., proper urine specimen collection). Describe ability.

Describe any measures used to facilitate child/family teaching.

RELATED NURSING DIAGNOSES

Fluid Volume Deficit *related to*
a. vomiting
b. diarrhea
c. fever

Pain *related to*
spasms of bladder wall secondary to inflammation

Fear: Child *related to*
a. pain
b. hospitalization
c. treatments and procedures

Compromised Family Coping *related to*
a. hospitalization of child
b. pain experienced by child

Twelve

CARE OF CHILDREN WITH FAILURE TO THRIVE

MEDICAL DIAGNOSIS

Failure to Thrive

DESCRIPTION Failure to thrive (FTT) is when infants and children fail to grow and gain weight at a normal rate. The weight, and sometimes the height, fall below the third percentile on standard growth curves. Failure to thrive is classified as either organic or inorganic in origin. Organic FTT is the result of physical factors such as congenital heart defects, gastrointestinal disorders, central nervous system abnormalities, chronic infections, endocrine disorders, metabolic disorders, and genetic abnormalities. Inorganic FTT is the result of an environmental or social cause; there are no physical findings. Inorganic FTT occurs more often than organic FTT and is caused by a disturbance in the relationship between the child and the primary caregiver. The reasons for the disturbed relationship vary; the parent may be inexperienced and lack information concerning infant development and nutritional requirements, or the child may be the result of an unwanted, unplanned pregnancy. Children with inorganic FTT who suffer from emotional deprivation can experience delays in emotional, social, motor, language, and intellectual development.

PRIMARY NURSING DIAGNOSIS
Altered Nutrition: Less than Body Requirements

DEFINITION Insufficient nutrients to meet body requirements

POSSIBLY RELATED TO
    Disturbance in child/primary caregiver relationship
    Neglect
    Emotional deprivation
    Parental knowledge deficit
    Congenital anomaly or other physical condition
    Malabsorption

Loose stools
Decreased food intake

CHARACTERISTICS
Vomiting
Diarrhea
Rumination
Anorexia or voracious appetite
Apathy
Lethargy
Dehydration
Weight below the third percentile
Sudden or rapid decline in growth rate

EXPECTED OUTCOMES   Child will be adequately nourished
as evidenced by

lack of

vomiting.
diarrhea.
rumination.
anorexia.
apathy.
lethargy.
dehydration.

steady weight gain (state how much would be reasonable for
each child).
adequate caloric intake (state range of calories needed for
each child).

Possible Nursing Interventions

Keep accurate record of intake and output, including calorie
count of intake.

Weigh child on same scale at same time each day without
clothes. Record results and compare to previous weight.

Assess and record any signs/symptoms of altered nutrition
(such as those listed under **Characteristics**) every 4 hours
and PRN.

Feed child on schedule. Record amount accurately and
record infant's response to feedings.

Assist, observe, and record child/parental interaction during feedings. Note parental feeding technique, when appropriate. In some instances, the child may need to be fed exclusively by the nurse.

Provide role modeling and education to parents for feeding skills, infant care, and nurturing in a nonthreatening and nonjudgmental manner. Provide positive feedback for appropriate behaviors.

📠 Assess and record family's knowledge of and participation in care regarding

> observation of nurse's feeding techniques.
> feeding techniques.
> monitoring of child's weight gain and caloric consumption.
> ability to nurture child.
> identification of signs/symptoms of altered nutrition (such as those listed under **Characteristics**).

📠 Instruct family in any areas needing improvement. Record results.

EVALUATION FOR CHARTING

State intake, output, and calorie count.

State current weight and determine whether it has increased or decreased since previous weighing.

Describe any signs/symptoms of altered nutrition noted (such as those listed under **Characteristics**).

State whether child was fed on schedule. Describe child's tolerance of feedings, including effectiveness of any feeding techniques used. Describe child/parent interaction during feedings and parental feeding techniques when appropriate.

📠 Describe family's knowledge of and participation in care related to improving nutritional status. State any areas needing improvement and information provided. Describe family's response.

NURSING DIAGNOSIS
Altered Growth and Development

DEFINITION Failure to gain weight at an acceptable rate for age group and failure to progress in expected tasks and skills according to chronologic age

POSSIBLY RELATED TO
Disturbance in child/primary caregiver relationship
Neglect
Emotional deprivation
Environmental problems (e.g., lack of stimulation)
Parental knowledge deficit
Congenital anomaly or other physical condition
Nutritional deficit

CHARACTERISTICS
Weight below the third percentile
Sudden or rapid decline in growth rate
Apathy
Withdrawn behavior
No fear of strangers (at an age when fear of strangers would
   be a normal finding)
Avoidance of eye-to-eye contact
Minimal smiling
Passivity
Indifference to caregivers
Intense watchfulness
Delayed and/or minimal vocalization
Repetitive behaviors (e.g., head banging, rocking.)
Other characteristics varying with age and state of
   development for infant. At all ages, normal growth and
   development will be delayed; for example, a 4-month-old
   may not be able to attain behaviors such as

   grasping toys and bringing them to mouth.
   using both hands when attempting to pick up objects.
   pulling to sitting position with little head lag.
   recognizing familiar faces.
   laughing out loud.

EXPECTED OUTCOMES   Child will demonstrate adequate
growth and developmental progression as evidenced by

   steady weight gain (state how much would be reasonable for
      each child).
   adequate caloric intake (state range of calories needed for
      each child).
   lack of continued regressed behavior (such as those listed
      under **Characteristics**).
   beginning to attain developmental milestones according
      to age.

POSSIBLE NURSING INTERVENTIONS

Keep accurate record of intake and output, including calorie count of intake.

Weigh child on same scale at same time each day without clothes. Record results and compare to previous weight.

Assess and record developmental progression of child.

Assess and record any signs/symptoms of altered growth and development (such as those listed under **Characteristics**) every 4 hours and PRN.

Feed child on schedule. Record amount accurately and record infant's response to feedings.

Assist, observe, and record child/parental interaction during feedings. Note parental feeding technique when appropriate. In some instances, the child may need to be fed exclusively by the nurse.

Provide role modeling and education to parents for feeding skills, infant care, and nurturing in a nonthreatening and nonjudgmental manner. Provide positive feedback for appropriate behaviors.

Provide adequate stimulation for child. Place bright and colorful objects, such as mobiles, within reach.

Talk to child with direct eye contact during interactions.

Touch and stroke child during contact. Hold and cuddle child at intervals.

🏠 Assess and record family's knowledge of and participation in care regarding

observation of nurse's feeding techniques.
feeding techniques.
monitoring of child's weight gain and caloric consumption.
assistance with developmental progression of child by adequate stimulation.
ability to nurture child.
identification of signs/symptoms of altered growth and development (such as those listed under **Characteristics**).

Instruct family in any areas needing improvement.
Record results.

EVALUATION FOR CHARTING
State intake, output, and calorie count.

State current weight and determine whether it has increased or decreased since previous weighing.

State whether child was fed on schedule. Describe child's tolerance of feedings, including effectiveness of any feeding techniques used. Describe child/parent interaction during feedings and parental feeding techniques when appropriate.

Describe child's level of developmental task/skill attainment.

Describe any successful measures used to help child attain developmental milestones.

Describe any signs/symptoms of altered growth and development noted (such as those listed under **Characteristics**).

 Describe family's knowledge of and participation in care related to improving optimal growth and development. State any areas needing improvement and information provided. Describe family's response.

NURSING DIAGNOSIS
Altered Parenting

DEFINITION   Inability of the child's primary caregiver to provide a nurturing environment

POSSIBLY RELATED TO
Disturbance in child/primary caregiver relationship
Parental knowledge deficit
Low self-esteem
Multiple stressors and unmet needs
Abuse or neglect of caregiver as child
Congenital anomaly or other physical condition of child
Physical and mental health problem (e.g., retardation, depression, chemical dependency, immaturity, adolescent parent)

CHARACTERISTICS

Ambivalent feelings about child
Unwanted pregnancy and child
Lack of expression
Indifference when caring for child
Failure to plan for future or care of child
Handling of child only when necessary
Annoyance and revulsion at diaper changes
Lack of timely response to child's needs
Negative statements about motherhood and parenting

EXPECTED OUTCOMES Parent will demonstrate appropriate parenting behaviors as evidenced by

increased attachment behaviors (e.g., holding child in the
face position during feedings, seeking eye contact with
child, smiling and talking to child, and holding child
close).
participation in child's care.
provision of age-appropriate stimulation for child.
verbalization of positive feeling regarding child and child's
appearance.
willingness to seek help and information about child's care.

POSSIBLE NURSING INTERVENTIONS

Assess and record parent's interactions with child each shift
and PRN.

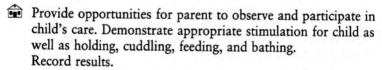 Provide opportunities for parent to observe and participate in
child's care. Demonstrate appropriate stimulation for child as
well as holding, cuddling, feeding, and bathing.
Record results.

Encourage parent to incorporate infant's care into daily
routine.

Allow parent to express feelings regarding infant's defect (if
one is present) and any feeding difficulties.

Initiate social services consultation to help parent identify
available supports and resources.

Encourage and provide positive verbal feedback when parent
demonstrates healthy behaviors in interacting with child.
Record results.

Assess and record parent's knowledge of and participation in care regarding

> positive bonding or caring behaviors.
> feeding techniques.
> acceptance of help from appropriate community agencies/ social services.
> attendance at parenting support groups.
> identification of signs/symptoms of altered parenting (such as those listed under **Characteristics**).

 Instruct parent in any areas needing improvement. Record results.

EVALUATION FOR CHARTING

Describe any signs/symptoms of altered parenting noted (such as those listed under **Characteristics**).

Describe any therapeutic measures used to promote appropriate parenting. State their effectiveness.

 Describe parent's knowledge of and participation in care related to improving parenting role. State any areas needing improvement and information provided. Describe parent's response.

RELATED NURSING DIAGNOSES

Knowledge Deficit: Parental *related to*
a. parenting role
b. nurturing behaviors
c. feeding techniques

Anxiety: Parental *related to*
a. knowledge deficit
b. failure to appropriately nurture child

Compromised Family Coping *related to*
a. knowledge deficit
b. inadequate support systems
c. maturational crises
d. unmet expectations

THIRTEEN

CARE OF CHILDREN WHO HAVE BEEN MALTREATED

MEDICAL DIAGNOSIS
Child Maltreatment

DESCRIPTION Child maltreatment is a term applied to physical abuse or neglect, emotional abuse or neglect, or sexual abuse, usually by adult caregivers. Maltreatment occurs in children of all ages, all socioeconomic classes, and all races, religions, ethnic groups, and nationalities.

Child neglect is the form of child maltreatment most often reported. It can be further classified into physical or emotional neglect. Physical neglect can be defined as deprivation of necessities such as food, clothing, shelter, supervision, protection, medical care, and education. Emotional neglect occurs when the child is denied affection, attention, love, and emotional nurturance. Children who are neglected can present with failure to thrive, malnutrition, poor hygiene, inappropriate dress (e.g., without a coat in winter), untreated infections, frequent colds and injuries, and lack of immunizations. The child may be inactive and passive. Older children who are victims of neglect can become drug or alcohol addicted, may resort to vandalism or shoplifting, and may frequently be absent from school. Clinical manifestations of emotionally neglected children include enuresis, feeding disorders (such as rumination), and sleep disorders.

Physical abuse is the nonaccidental injury (NAI) of a child, usually by a parent or adult caregiver. This condition is also sometimes called battered child syndrome (BCS) or Kempe's syndrome. The etiology of physical abuse is not known, but certain characteristics seem to predispose children to it. Abusing parents may have had poor nurturing during their own childhood, have negative feelings toward the pregnancy or unwanted pregnancy, have been neglected or abused as a child, have unrealistic expectations for the child, have inadequate knowledge of normal child development, have mismatched temperament with the child, experience poverty and/or unemployment, be emotionally immature, lack patience, be preoccupied with themselves, be involved in an unstable marriage, be unable to identify resources, and/or have difficulty controlling aggressive impulses. Other environmental factors that may contribute are prematurity of the infant, illegitimacy of the infant, brain damage or disability of an infant, alcoholism, and drug addiction. Behaviors of the physically abused child include wariness of physical contact with adults, apparent fear of parents, failure to cry during painful procedures, apprehensiveness at the sound of other children crying, indiscriminate display of affection, aggressiveness, and withdrawal behavior.

Evidence of physical abuse can include bruises or welts on ears, eyes, mouth, torso, buttocks, genital areas, and calves; immersion, pattern, friction, or scald burns; fractures of the skull, face, nose, orbit, long bones, and ribs; multiple or spiral fractures caused by twisting motion; head trauma such as subdural hematoma; areas of baldness and swelling from hair being pulled out; intracranial trauma due to violent shaking; injury that does not fit the description; and fractures in various stages of healing.

A perplexing form of physical abuse that is sometimes hard to detect is the Münchausen syndrome by proxy (MSP). This type of abuse occurs when one person fabricates or induces illness in another person—generally the mother fabricating an illness in the child in order to gain attention. The mother may add her blood to the child's urine in order to simulate hematuria or may present a false history. In more severe forms of MSP, the mother may suffocate the child to cause apnea or seizures.

Emotional abuse can occur when parents instill attitudes of worthlessness, inferiority, or self-rejection in a child by constant negative criticism and verbal assault. This type of abuse is extremely difficult to identify. Physical signs may include eating disorders (vomiting), sleep disorders, enuresis, speech disorders (stuttering), and developmental delay. Behavioral signs may include hyperactivity, aggressiveness or passivity, depression, complacency, substance abuse, runaway behavior, and suicidal behavior.

Sexual abuse is the use of a child for the sexual gratification of an adult. Most common is intrafamilial involving the father-daughter or the stepfather-daughter relationship. The many forms of sexual abuse include lewd conversation, genital viewing, fondling of the genitals and breasts, oral sex, vaginal intercourse, anal penetration, child pornography, and child prostitution. Behavioral indicators of the abusing adult can include rigid role perception within the family, a need to dominate the family, lack of social and emotional contacts outside the family, and rationalization of the behavior as being educational and pleasurable to the child.

Behavioral signs of the sexually abused child include advanced knowledge of adult sexual behavior, excessive bathing, unusual interest in the genital area, poor peer relations, depression, extreme shyness, and increased aggressive or hostile behavior. Physical indicators in the child can include difficulty in walking or sitting; bruises, bleeding, or lacerations of external genital, vaginal, or anal areas; torn, stained, or bloody clothing; pain on urination; recurrent urinary tract infections; vaginal/penile discharge; and/or pregnancy.

Treatment of children abused or neglected in any way requires a team approached by physicians, nurses, and social workers. Treatment includes a diagnostic interview, physical assessment and treatment of injuries, laboratory tests, reports to a child welfare agency, psychosocial interviews with the child and family, careful record keeping, and family therapy.

NURSING CARE PLAN FOR CHILD VICTIMS OF PHYSICAL ABUSE

PRIMARY NURSING DIAGNOSIS

Actual Injury*

DEFINITION   Situation in which the child has sustained damage or harm

POSSIBLY RELATED TO
>   Bruises and welts on face, lips, mouth, back, buttocks, thighs, or torso; pattern descriptive of object used (e.g., hand, belt buckle)
>   Burns on soles of feet, palms of hands, back, or buttocks; pattern descriptive of object used (e.g., cigar, cigarette); absence of "splash" marks
>   Fractures and dislocations of skull, nose, or facial structures; spiral fracture from twisting
>   Head trauma, including subdural hematomas from blows to the head or from being dropped; intracranial trauma from violent shaking; areas of baldness and swelling from hair being pulled out
>   Multiple new or old fractures in various stages of healing

---

*Non-NANDA diagnosis.

Lacerations and abrasions on mouth, lips, gums, eyes,
 genitals; descriptive marks such as from human bites
Incompatibility between the history and the injury

CHARACTERISTICS
Suggestive physical findings (see **Possibly Related To**)

CHILD BEHAVIORS

Wariness of physical contact with adults
Fear of parents
Extreme aggressiveness or withdrawal
Apprehension when other children cry
Indiscriminate affection shown toward anyone
Vacant stare or frozen watchfulness; no eye contact
Failure to cry from pain

PARENTAL BEHAVIORS

Explanation that does not fit the injury
Lengthy time interval between occurrence of the injury and
 seeking of medical attention
Conflicting stories about the "accident" or injury
Lack of awareness of normal developmental stages of
 children
Description of own childhood as unhappy or abusive
Difficulty controlling aggressive impulses
Reluctance to look at or handle child
Inability to comfort child during painful or invasive
 procedures
Blame placed on child for the injury
Infrequent visits to see the hospitalized child

EXPECTED OUTCOMES Child will be free of further injury.

POSSIBLE NURSING INTERVENTIONS
Assess and record any signs/symptoms of injury (such as
those listed under **Characteristics**) every 4 hours and PRN.
See specific nursing care plan related to child's physical
injury (e.g., burns, fractures).

Handle child gently.

Accurately record behaviors of child and parents (do not
interpret behaviors). Record child/parent interaction. ·

Assign same nurses to care for child when possible.

Demonstrate acceptance and affection for child even when child does not return it.

Use behavior modification, including praise, to foster positive behavior from the child.

Demonstrate and role model for parents alternative ways to interact with and discipline child in a nurturing, nonthreatening, nonjudgmental manner.

Allow parents to ventilate and discuss feelings about being parents.

Refer parents to self-help groups such as Parents Anonymous, when indicated.

🏠 Educate parents about useful resources such as

telephone hotlines for parents who feel they are about to lose control.
sources of funds for necessities such as food.
information on low-cost health care.
day-care programs.
before- and after-school child-care programs.

🏠 Assess and record family's knowledge of and participation in care regarding

understanding normal developmental stages of children.
use of available resources.
keeping appointments with agencies and health care facilities.
demonstration of appropriate interaction with child.
cooperation with authorities.

🏠 Instruct child/family in any areas needing improvement. Record results.

EVALUATION FOR CHARTING

Describe any signs/symptoms of injury noted (such as those listed under Characteristics).

Describe any interventions and their effectiveness in preventing further injury.

🏠 Describe family's knowledge of and participation in care related to preventing further injury. State any areas needing improvement and information provided. Describe responses.

NURSING DIAGNOSIS
Knowledge Deficit: Parental

DEFINITION   Lack of information concerning the child's disease and care

POSSIBLY RELATED TO
>   Lack of knowledge concerning normal developmental stages of children
>   Lack of knowledge concerning appropriate interaction with child

CHARACTERISTICS
>   Verbalization by parents indicating lack of knowledge
>   Relation of incorrect information to members of the health care team
>   Requests for information

EXPECTED OUTCOMES   Parents will have an adequate knowledge base concerning child care as evidenced by

>   ability to correctly state information previously taught.
>   ability to relate appropriate information to the health care team.

POSSIBLE NURSING INTERVENTIONS
>   Listen to parent's concerns and fears.
>
>   Assess and record parent's knowledge concerning normal childhood growth and development and appropriate parent/child interaction.
>
>   Provide parents with any available literature or booklets on normal childhood growth and development.
>
>   Accurately record behaviors of child/parents. (Do not interpret behaviors.) Record child/parent interaction.
>
>   Assign same nurses to care for child when possible.
>
>   Demonstrate acceptance and affection for child even when child does not return it.
>
>   Use behavior modification, including praise, to foster positive behavior from the child.
>
>   Demonstrate and role model for parents alternative ways to interact with and discipline the child in a nurturing, nonthreatening, nonjudgmental manner.

Allow parents to ventilate and discuss feelings about being parents.

Refer parents to self-help groups such as Parents Anonymous, when indicated.

🏠 Educate parents about useful resources such as

telephone hotlines for parents who feel they are about to lose control.
sources of funds for necessities such as food.
information on low-cost health care.
day-care programs.
before- and after-school child-care programs.

🏠 Assess and record family's knowledge of and participation in care regarding

normal developmental stages of children.
use of available resources.
keeping appointments with agencies and health care facilities.
demonstration of appropriate interaction with child.
cooperation with authorities.

🏠 Instruct child/family in any areas needing improvement. Record results.

EVALUATION FOR CHARTING

State whether parents verbalized a knowledge deficit.

Describe any measures used to facilitate parent teaching.

🏠 State whether parents were able to demonstrate behaviors previously taught.

RELATED NURSING DIAGNOSES

Fear: Child *related to*
a. repeated maltreatment
b. powerlessness
c. possible separation from parents
d. forced contact with strangers

Pain *related to*
injury

Altered Parenting *related to*
   a. poor role model
   b. unrealistic expectations of child
   c. knowledge deficit of normal developmental stages of children

Anxiety: Child *related to*
   a. hospitalization
   b. possible separation from parents

Fourteen

Care of Children
Post-Suicide
Gesture/Attempt

Status Post-Suicide Gesture/Attempt

PATHOPHYSIOLOGY Suicide is the third leading cause of death in the 15- to 24-year-old category, following accidents and homicides. In children under the age of 15, the incidence of suicide is low but rising. The actual number of suicides may be higher than documented since many deaths in which suicide is not clearly evident are attributed to accidents or natural causes.

Suicidal methods vary with sex and age. Girls are more likely to use passive methods, such as ingestion of pills, whereas boys use quicker methods, such as hanging or shooting. Preadolescents most commonly jump from heights, but they may also ingest a poison or medication, hang or stab themselves, or run into traffic. The incidence of poison or medication ingestion as a suicidal gesture or attempt increases with age.

Girls are two to three times more likely to attempt suicide than boys, but boys are more likely to succeed. A suicide gesture is really a cry for help without a true desire to die; often these gestures go unnoticed. The child or adolescent who makes a suicide attempt truly wants to die. It is often difficult to distinguish between a suicidal gesture and an attempt at the time of the incident. All suicidal behavior should be taken seriously. In determining the intent and lethality of the suicidal behavior, factors to consider include whether or not the child or adolescent had a plan or acted on impulse, the accessibility of the plan, and the possibility and probability of the child's being rescued as foreseen by the child or adolescent.

After a suicidal gesture or attempt, the child or adolescent may be admitted to a general pediatric unit for several days so that the patient's frame of mind, home environment, and family situation may be adequately assessed. After a thorough evaluation, a decision is made as to whether the child or adolescent will require inpatient or outpatient psychiatric care. The nursing staff on the general pediatric unit should provide a safe environment while the child is being evaluated. In-depth therapy is not expected of the pediatric nursing staff.

PRIMARY NURSING DIAGNOSIS

Self-Harm and High Risk for Additional Self-Harm*

DEFINITION   Situation in which the child sustains and is at risk of sustaining harm

POSSIBLY RELATED TO

Depressed mood
Feelings of worthlessness
Overwhelming feelings of hopelessness
Powerlessness
Family conflicts
School problems or failures
Inability to meet increased demands or expectations
Irrational feelings of guilt
Loss of a loved one
Prolonged grief
Despair
Loneliness
Low self-esteem
Thought disorders
Deteriorating home environment
Abuse
Chronic illness
Misinterpretation of reality
Anger turned inward

CHARACTERISTICS

Self-destructive behavior (e.g., ingesting poison or medication, slitting wrists, jumping from heights, hanging, running into traffic, stabbing)
History of a suicidal plan
Behaviors toward getting affairs in order, including giving away belongings
Statements indicating a desire to kill self, suicidal ideation

---

*Non-NANDA diagnosis.

Statements of hopelessness or worthlessness
Preoccupation with death and dying
Withdrawal from family and peers
Eating or sleep disturbances

EXPECTED OUTCOMES   Child will not harm self as evidenced by

lack of further suicide attempts.
verbalization of a decrease in suicidal ideation.
verbalization of feelings of hope.
verbalization of feelings of increased self-esteem.
age-appropriate behavior (e.g., reinvolvement with family and peers).
willingness to contract, in writing, not to harm self.
lack of signs/symptoms of self-harm (such as those listed under **Characteristics**).

POSSIBLE NURSING INTERVENTIONS

Ensure the child's safety by

placing the child on suicide (and possibly elopement) precautions with 1:1 staffing (sitter), when indicated. Assess the child every 15 minutes if a sitter is not indicated. Document child's status on flowsheet.
removing all potentially dangerous objects from the child's room and belongings (e.g., pins, glass, cans, belt, shoestrings, mirrors, razors).
explaining to child that he or she will be protected from any self-harm.
dressing child in hospital clothing (so he or she will be less likely to leave the hospital).

Child's room should be located near the nurses' station.

Initiate a psychiatric consultation upon admission. Refer child/family to appropriate community resources.

Provide child with a consistent caregiver (primary nurse).

Document any suicidal ideation or gestures.

Document child's mood, affect, behavior, and interactions each shift and PRN.

Minimize stimulation; may include limiting visitors.

Encourage child to recognize suicidal feelings and to alert the staff to these feelings. Use a written, no-suicide contract with the child, as indicated.

Encourage child to verbalize feelings.

Allow child to participate in the formulation of goals.

Assess and record any signs/symptoms of self-harm (such as those listed under **Characteristics**).

Assess and record child's/family's knowledge of and participation in care regarding

> identification of signs/symptoms of self-harm (such as those listed under **Characteristics**) or behaviors indicating increased risk for self-harm.
> need for therapy.
> identification and use of available community resources.
> health care team's recommendations for care.

Instruct child/family in any areas needing improvement. Record results.

EVALUATION FOR CHARTING

Describe any signs/symptoms of self-harm noted (such as those listed under **Characteristics**).

Describe child's suicide status.

Describe any therapeutic measures used to ensure child's safety. State their effectiveness.

Describe child's/family's knowledge of and participation in care related to the prevention of self-harm by the child. State any areas needing improvement and information provided. Describe child's/family's responses.

NURSING DIAGNOSIS
Altered Thought Processes

DEFINITION State in which the individual's thoughts create a disruption of the individual's mental status

POSSIBLY RELATED TO
Depression
Substance abuse

Loss
Thought disorders
Peer pressure
Conflict
Isolation
Rejection by others
Irrational guilt

CHARACTERISTICS

Misinterpretation of reality
Impaired ability to make decisions
Impaired ability to solve problems
Distractibility
Disorientation/confusion
Cognitive dissonance
Delusions
Hallucinations
Poor impulse control
Altered interpersonal interactions
Inappropriate reactions to stimuli

EXPECTED OUTCOMES   Child will have increased appropriate thought processes as evidenced by

orientation to person, place, and time.
ability to differentiate between fantasy and reality.
improved ability to make decisions.
improved ability to solve problems.
appropriate response to stimuli.
lack of

delusions.
hallucinations.
impulsivity.
signs/symptoms of altered thought processes (such as those listed under **Characteristics**).

POSSIBLE NURSING INTERVENTIONS

Assess and record any signs/symptoms of altered thought processes (such as those listed under **Characteristics**).

Provide reality testing every 4 hours and PRN.

Provide child with a consistent caregiver (primary nurse).

Minimize stimulation; may include limiting visitors.

📬 Encourage child to verbalize feelings.

Initiate a psychiatric consultation upon admission. Refer the child/family to appropriate community resources.

Allow child to participate in the formulation of goals.

📬 Support child's appropriate attempts to problem solve and make decisions.

📬 Assist child in identifying appropriate coping behaviors.

📬 Assist child in identifying appropriate supports.

📬 Assess and record child's/family's knowledge of and participation in care regarding

> identification of signs/symptoms of altered thought
> processes (such as those listed under **Characteristics**).
> need for therapy.
> identification and use of available community resources.
> appropriate actions.

📬 Instruct child/family in any areas needing improvement. Record results.

EVALUATION FOR CHARTING

Describe any signs/symptoms of altered thought processes noted (such as those listed under **Characteristics**).

Describe any therapeutic measures used. State their effectiveness.

📬 Describe child's/family's knowledge of and participation in care related to managing altered thought processes. State any areas needing improvement and information provided. Describe child's/family's responses.

NURSING DIAGNOSIS
Powerlessness

DEFINITION   State in which an individual perceives that he/she has had a loss of control

POSSIBLY RELATED TO
Depression
Substance abuse

Lack of knowledge
Peer pressure

CHARACTERISTICS

Verbalization of lack of control
Failure to participate in care
Apathy
Aggressive or violent behavior
Acting-out behavior
Depression
Inability to make decisions (age-appropriate)

EXPECTED OUTCOMES   Child/adolescent will demonstrate a decrease in powerlessness as evidenced by

verbalization of increased feelings of control.
increased decision-making ability.
increased participation in care.
lack of signs/symptoms of powerlessness (such as those listed under **Characteristics**).

POSSIBLE NURSING INTERVENTIONS

Assess and record any signs/symptoms of powerlessness (such as those listed under **Characteristics**) every 4 hours and PRN

Allow child to express feelings.

Explain procedures and rules to child.

Allow child to make choices or decisions (e.g., when to bathe, menu selection) whenever possible, but do not offer options if none exist.

Allow child to participate in the formulation of goals.

Provide child with appropriate knowledge (e.g., available resources).

Provide child with a consistent caregiver.

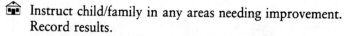 Assess and record child's/family's knowledge of and participation in care regarding

identification of any signs/symptoms of powerlessness (such as those listed under **Characteristics**).
appropriate actions.

Instruct child/family in any areas needing improvement. Record results.

EVALUATION FOR CHARTING

Describe any signs/symptoms of powerlessness noted (such as those listed under **Characteristics**).

Describe any therapeutic measures used. State their effectiveness.

🏠 Describe child's/family's knowledge of and participation in care related to decreasing powerlessness. State any areas needing improvement and information provided. Describe child's/family's responses.

RELATED NURSING DIAGNOSES

Knowledge Deficit: Child *related to*
a. lack of awareness of available supports and resources
b. under-utilization of supports and resources

Compromised Individual Coping *related to*
a. depression
b. poor self-esteem
c. helplessness

Compromised Family Coping *related to*

a. guilt
b. social isolation of family
c. child's behavior

REFERENCES

Allen, B. P. (1987). Youth suicide. *Adolescence, 86,* 271–290.

Axton, S.E. (1986). *Neonatal and pediatric care plans.* Baltimore: Williams & Wilkins.

Axton, S. E., & Fugate, T. (1989). *Neonatal and pediatric critical care plans.* Baltimore: Williams & Wilkins.

Bailey, D. J., Andres, J. M., Danek, G. D., & Pineiro-Carrero, U. M. (1987). Lack of efficacy of thickened feedings as a treatment for gastroesophogeal reflux. *Journal of Pediatrics, 110* (2), 187–189.

Barnett, D. J. (1988). The clinician's guide to pediatric AIDS. *Contemporary Pediatrics, 5,* 24–47.

Behrman, R. E., Vaughan, V. C., & Nelson, W. E., (Eds.). (1987). *Nelson textbook of pediatrics.* (13th ed.). Philadelphia: Saunders.

Blanchet, E. D. (Ed.). (1988). *AIDS: A health care management response.* Rockville, MD: Aspen.

Boland, M., & Gaskill, T. D. B. (1984). Managing AIDS in children. *The American Journal of Maternal/Child Nursing, 9,* 384–389.

Carpenito, L. J. (1987). *Handbook of Nursing Diagnosis* (2nd ed.). Philadelphia: Lippincott.

Carpenito, L. J. (1987). *Nursing Diagnosis: Application to clinical practice* (2nd ed.). Philadelphia: Lippincott.

Charache, S., Lubin, B., & Reid, C. D. (Eds.). (1989). *Management and therapy of sickle cell disease.* Washington, DC: U.S. Government Printing Office.

Chenevey, B. (1987). Overview of fluids and electrolytes. *Nursing Clinics of North America, 22,* (4), 749–756.

Cooke, S. S. (1986). Major thermal injury—The first 48 hours. *Critical Care Nurse, 6,* (1), 55–63.

Cowan, M. J., Hellman, D., Chudwin, D., Wara, D. W., Chang, R. S., & Ammann, A. J. (1984). Maternal transmission of acquired immune deficiency syndrome. *Pediatrics, 73* (3), 382–386.

Doenges, M. E., & Moorhouse, M. F. (1988). *Nurses' pocket guide: Nursing diagnoses with interventions* (2nd ed.). Philadelphia: F. A. Davis.

Durham, J. D., & Cohen, F. L. (Eds.). (1987). *The person with AIDS: Nursing perspectives.* New York: Springer.

Fink, B. W. (1975). *Congenital heart disease: A deductive approach to its diagnosis.* Chicago: Year Book Publishers.

Fischback, F. T. (1984). *A manual of laboratory tests* (2nd ed.). Philadelphia: Lippincott.

Fochtman, D., & Raffensperger, J. G. (1976). *Principles of nursing care for the pediatric surgery patient* (2nd ed.). Boston: Little, Brown.

Foster, R. L. R., Hunsberger, M. M., & Anderson, J. J. T., (Eds.). (1989). *Family-centered nursing care of children.* Philadelphia: Saunders.

Frumkin, L. R., & Leonard, J. M. (1987). *Questions and answers on AIDS.* Oradell, NJ: Medical Economic Books.

Govoni, L. E., & Hayes, J. E. (1988). *Drugs and nursing implications* (6th ed.). Norwalk, CT: Appleton & Lange.

Guenter, P., & Slocum, B. (1983). Hepatic disease: Nutritional implications. *Nursing Clinics of North America, 18* (1), 71–79.

Hazinski, M. F. (Ed.). (1984). *Nursing care of the critically ill child.* St. Louis: Mosby.

Heiss, R. (1987). Immunology of AIDS. *Pediatric Annals, 16* (6), 495–503.

Hockenberry, M. J., & Coody, D. K. (Eds.). (1986). *Pediatric oncology and hematology.* St. Louis: Mosby.

Keith, J. S. (1985). Hepatic failure: Etiologies, manifestations, and management. *Critical Care Nurse, 5* (1), 60–86.

Kirshner, B. S. (1988). Inflammatory bowel disease in children. *Pediatric Clinics of North America, 35* (1), 189–208.

Krane, E. J. (1987). Diabetic ketoacidosis: Biochemistry, physiology, treatment, and prevention. *Pediatric Clinics of North America, 34* (4), 935–957.

LeBoeuf, M. B., & Greco-Gallagher, M. (1987). Standardized care plan for the child with bacterial meningitis. *Critical Care Nurse, 7* (5), 66–76.

McNamara, J. G. (1989). Immunologic abnormalities in infants infected with human immunodeficiency virus. *Seminars in Perinatology, 13* (1), 35–43.

Malsteed, R. T. (1985). *Pharmacology: Drug therapy and nursing considerations* (2nd ed.). Philadelphia: Lippincott.

Marlow, D. R., & Redding, B. A. (1988). *Textbook of pediatric nursing* (6th ed.). Philadelphia: Saunders.

Metheny, N. M. (1987). *Fluid and electrolyte balance: Nursing considerations.* Philadelphia: Lippincott.

Moorhouse, M. F., & Doenges, M. E. (1990). *Nurse's clinical pocket manual: Nursing diagnoses, care planning, and documentation.* Philadelphia: F. A. Davis.

Moses, A. M. (1977, July). Diabetes insipidus and ADH regulation. *Hospital Practice, 12,* (7) 37–44.

Mott, S. R., James, S. R., & Sperhac, A. M. (1990). *Nursing care of children and families* (2nd ed.). Redwood City, CA: Addison-Wesley.

Murphy, C. M. (1984). *Quick reference to pediatric nursing.* Philadelphia: Lippincott.

Muscari, M. E. (1987). Adolescent suicide attempts by acetaminophen ingestion. *The American Journal of Maternal/Child Nursing, 12,* 32–35.

Naccarato, M. K., & Kresevic, D. M. (1989). Caring for adults who have cystic fibrosis. *American Journal of Nursing, 89* (11), 1462–1465.

Nelson, N. P., & Beckel, J. (Eds.). (1987). *Nursing care plans for the pediatric patient.* St. Louis: Mosby.

New nursing skillbook: Monitoring fluid and electrolytes precisely (2nd ed.). (1984). Nursing 84 Books, Springhouse, PA: Springhouse.

Novak, D. A., & Balistreri, W. F. (1985). Management of the child with chronic cholestasis. *Pediatric Annals, 14* (7), 488–492.

Osgood, P. F. (1989). Management of burn pain in children. *Pediatric Clinics of North America, 36* (4), 1001–1013.

Pahwa, S. (1988). Human immunodeficiency virus infection in children: Nature of immunodeficiency, clinical spectrum, and management. *Pediatric Infectious Disease Journal, 7* (5), S61–S71.

Pinney, M. (1981). Foreign body aspiration. *American Journal of Nursing, 81* (3), 521–522.

Pinney, M. (1981). Pneumonia. *American Journal of Nursing, 81* (3), 517–518.

Pizzo, P. A. (1989). Emerging concepts in the treatment of HIV infection in children. *JAMA, 262* (14), 1989–1992.

Robbins, S. L. (1984). *Pathologic basis of disease.* Philadelphia: Saunders.

Russman, B. S., & Gage, J. R. (1989). Cerebral palsy. In J. D. Lockhart (Ed.). *Current problems in pediatrics* (pp. 69–111). Chicago: Year Book Medical Publishers.

Schafer, P., Kelly, M. K., Lehr, K., & Saracco, J. (1988). *Nursing care plans for the child: A nursing diagnosis approach.* Norwalk, CT: Appleton and Lange.

Schwartz, S. I., Shires, G. T., Spencer, F. C., & Storer, E. H. (1979). *Principles of surgery.* New York: McGraw-Hill.

Simkins, R. (1981). Asthma: Reactive airways disease. *American Journal of Nursing, 81* (3), 522–524.

Simkins, R. (1981). The crises of bronchiolitis. *American Journal of Nursing, 81* (3), 515–516.

Simkins, R. (1981). Croup and epiglottitis. *American Journal of Nursing, 81* (3), 519–520.

Smith, M. J., Goodman, J. A., & Ramsey, N. L. (1987). *Child and family: Concepts of nursing practice* (2nd ed.). New York: McGraw-Hill.

Speer, K. M. (1990). *Pediatric care plans.* Springhouse, PA: Springhouse.

Sperling, M. A. (1987). Outpatient management of diabetes mellitus. *Pediatric Clinics of North America, 34* (4), 919–934.

Steele, S., Hughes, J., Beaty, N., Echols, K., & Lewis, D. (1987). *Special people with special needs.* Funded by a grant from the U.S. Department of Education, Office of Special Education and Rehabilitation Services.

Swearington, P. L., (Ed.). (1986). *Manual of nursing therapeutics: Applying nursing diagnoses to medical disorders*. Menlo Park, CA: Addison-Wesley.

Tamborlane, W. V., & Davis, P. B. (1986). Diabetes mellitus in children and adolescents. *Connecticut's Current Therapy*, 443–450.

Vanden Belt, R. J., Ronan, J. A., & Bedynek, J. L. (1979). *Cardiology: A clinical approach*. Chicago: Year Book Medical Publishers.

Voyles, J. B. (1981). Bronchopulmonary dysplasia. *American Journal of Nursing, 81* (3), 510–514.

Vulcan, B. M. (1987). Acute bacterial meningitis in infancy and childhood. *Critical Care Nurse, 7* (5), 53–65.

Ward-Wimmer, D. (1988). Nursing care of children with HIV infection. *Nursing Clinics of North America, 23* (4), 719–729.

Whaley, L. F., & Wong, D. L. (1987). *Nursing care of infants and children* (3rd ed.). St. Louis: Mosby.

Whaley, L. F., & Wong, D. L. (1991). *Nursing care of infants and children* (4th ed). St. Louis: Mosby.

Wong, D. L., & Whaley, L. F. (1986). *Clinical handbook of pediatric nursing* (2nd ed.). St. Louis: Mosby.

Index

I

IA (infantile apnea), 326. *See also* Apnea

IBD. *See* Inflammatory bowel disease

Idiopathic scoliosis, 267–268. *See also* Scoliosis

Idiopathic thrombocytopenia purpura (ITP)
family coping and, compromised, 193
fear and, child and family/parental, 192–193
fluid volume deficit and, 193
injury and, 190–191
knowledge deficit and, child and family/parental, 193
pathophysiology, 189–190
physical mobility and, impaired, 193

Immunoglobulins, intravenous, 190

Individual coping, compromised, 453

Infantile apnea (IA), 326. *See also* Apnea

Infection. *See also* Acquired immunodeficiency syndrome; Cellulitis
acquired immunodeficiency syndrome and, 227–229
appendicitis and, 92–96
bacterial meningitis and, 303, 308
bowel obstruction and, 103–105, 110
bronchiolitis and, 343
bronchopulmonary dysplasia and, 349
burns and, 81
cardiac catheterization and, 11
cellulitis and, 235–237
chronic liver failure and, 223
cleft lip/cleft palate and, 116, 118–120
congenital heart disease and, 21, 25
cystic fibrosis and, 357
esophageal atresia and, 127, 131
foreign body aspiration and, 364
fractures and, 254
gastroenteritis and, 135
gastroesophageal reflux and, 143
Hirschsprung disease and, 152–154
hydrocephalus and, 302
infective endocarditis and, 45
neoplasms and, 199–202
nephrotic syndrome and, 411
neural tube defects and, 316

Infection—cont'd
osteomyelitis and, 262–264
pyloric stenosis and, 171–173
septic arthritis and, 273–276
sickle cell disease and, 211–214
tracheoesophageal fistula and, 127, 131
urinary tract infection and, 419–421
vesicoureteral reflux and, 413–415

Infective endocarditis
activity intolerance and, 42–44
anxiety and, family/parental, 45
breathing pattern and, ineffective, 45
cardiac output and, decreased, 40–42
consciousness and, altered level of, 45
infection and, 45
pathophysiology, 39–40
Streptococci and, 39

Inflammatory bowel disease (IBD)
body image disturbance and, 163
Crohn's disease, 157, 158
family coping and, compromised, 163
fluid volume deficit and, 158–161
growth/development and, altered, 163
nutrition and, altered, 162
pain and, 161–162
pathophysiology, 157–158
ulcerative colitis, 157–158

Injury. *See also* Burns
acute rheumatic fever and, 51
bacterial meningitis and, 308
child maltreatment and, 438–440
hemophilia and, 183–186
idiopathic thrombocytopenia purpura and, 190–191
neoplasms and, 202–204
nonaccidental, 436
seizures and, 321–322

Interventions. *See* specific diagnoses

Intravascular fluid imbalance. *See* Fluid volume deficit

Intussusception, 100–101

ITP. *See* Idiopathic thrombocytopenia purpura

J

Joint inflammation, 46

JRA. *See* Juvenile Rheumatoid Arthritis